Major Problems in Obstetrics and Gynecology

A series of monographs designed to explore in depth specific problems in these related disciplines, and to offer reviews of the most complete and up-to-date information available on topics in the study of human reproduction and of the female reproductive system.

Other monographs in this Series:

Already published:

Cohen: *Laparoscopy, Culdoscopy and Gynecography: Technique and Atlas*

Plentl and Friedman: *Lymphatic System of the Female Genitalia*

Burrow: *The Thyroid Gland in Pregnancy*

Janovski and Paramanandhan: *Ovarian Tumors*

Burghardt: *Early Histological Diagnosis of Cervical Cancer*

Roland: *Response to Contraception*

Vollman: *The Menstrual Cycle*

Neuwirth: *Hysteroscopy*

Dexeus, Carrera and Coupez: *Colposcopy*

Cavanagh, Comas and Rao: *Septic Shock*

Charles: *Infections in Obstetrics and Gynecology*

Graff and Kuhn: *Coagulation Disorders in Obstetrics*

Goldstein and Berkowitz: *Gestational Trophoblastic Disease*

To be published:

Bieniarz: *Angiography and Placental Localization*

Knapp: *Radical Surgery of Pelvic Cancer*

Brown: *Ultrasonography in Obstetrics and Gynecology*

Perlmutter: *Human Sexuality*

Weinberger: *Hypertension in Pregnancy*

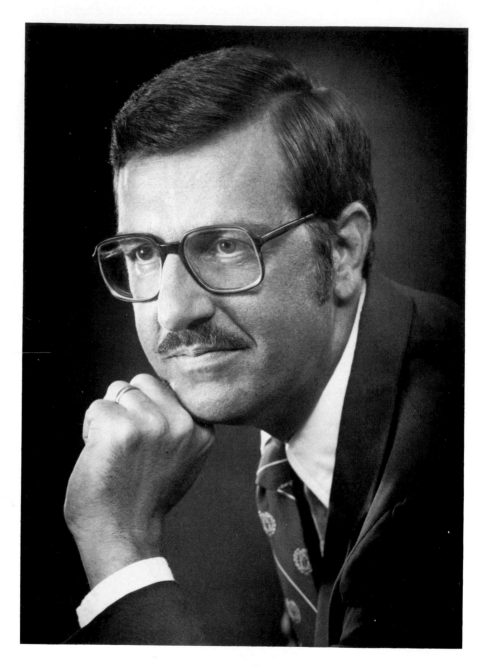

EDUARD G. FRIEDRICH, JR.
H.A.B., M.D., L.L.D.

VULVAR DISEASE

SECOND EDITION

EDUARD G. FRIEDRICH, JR.

H.A.B., M.D., L.L.D. (Hon.)

President and First Secretary General
International Society for the Study of Vulvar Disease
Professor and Chairman
Department of Obstetrics and Gynecology
University of Florida

VOLUME 9 IN THE SERIES

MAJOR PROBLEMS IN OBSTETRICS AND GYNECOLOGY

EMANUEL A. FRIEDMAN, M.D.

Consulting Editor

1983
W.B. SAUNDERS COMPANY
Philadelphia • London • Toronto • Mexico City • Rio de Janeiro • Sydney • Tokyo

W. B. Saunders Company: West Washington Square
Philadelphia, PA 19105

1 St. Anne's Road
Eastbourne, East Sussex BN21 3UN, England

1 Goldthorne Avenue
Toronto, Ontario M8Z 5T9, Canada

Apartado 26370—Cedro 512
Mexico 4, D.F., Mexico

Rua Coronel Cabrita, 8
Sao Cristovao Caixa Postal 21176
Rio de Janeiro, Brazil

9 Waltham Street
Artarmon, N.S.W. 2064, Australia

Ichibancho, Central Bldg., 22-1 Ichibancho
Chiyoda-Ku, Tokyo 102, Japan

Library of Congress Cataloging in Publication Data

Friedrich, Eduard G., 1937–
 Vulvar disease.

 (Major problems in obstetrics and gynecology; v. 9)
 Includes bibliographical references and index.
 1. Vulva—Diseases. I. Title. II. Series. [DNLM:
1. Vulvar diseases—Diagnosis. 2. Vulvar diseases—
Therapy. 3. Vulvar neoplasms—Diagnosis. 4. Vulvar
neoplasms—Therapy. W1 MA492C v. 9 / WP 200 F911v]
RG39.M25 vol. 9 1983 [RG261] 618s 82-24100
ISBN 0-7216-1096-X [618.1'6]

Vulvar Disease   ISBN 0-7216-1096-X

Last digit is the print number: 9   8   7   6   5   4   3   2   1

DEDICATION
again to God

*Whose reality alone gives meaning
to all the facets of our
existence—and in Whose
service it is a joyful
privilege to care
for others.*

> "One truly sees only that which one already knows."
>
> GOETHE

Foreword

What does the reader expect of a foreword? A knowledge of the author and his character; an accurate evaluation of his ability to discern the significant from the insignificant; a careful and critical survey of the material in the text and the accuracy of presentation? Yes, all of these and more!

Ed Friedrich's words in many conferences, publications, and discussions have spoken and now again *speak* for themselves. An unequalled thoroughness in the evaluation of data, a discerning and questioning mind, and a mastery of the language are the hallmarks of his presentations, written or spoken. His personal contributions to our knowledge of vulvovaginal disease have been documented in many incisive publications; his presentations at innumerable conferences are heralded by accolades; and his willingness to persist in answering his questioning audience all attest to his enthusiasm for and interest in his profession. His dedication to excellence and a basic professional and societal integrity have characterized our relationship, now extending over more than 20 years. To this must be added the current status of the International Society for the Study of Vulvar Disease. Without his persistent efforts to promote this unique but remarkably productive organization, it might have foundered on the rocks of immaturity and the current plethora of embryonic societies. Today his presidency of this now well-recognized entity attests to his continuing efforts to elucidate the intricacies of vulvovaginal disease.

In spite of these personal remarks, the author of the foreword must be objective and thorough in his evaluation of the production as well as have a knowledge of the field with an ability to discern the accuracy and completeness of the text. This second edition of *Vulvar Disease* complements and improves upon the first. The material is as up to date as tomorrow. The chapter on surgical procedures is a demonstration of the excellence and conciseness of this volume. Each operative technique is explained in sufficient detail to furnish the reader with a brief but realistic evaluation of the procedure and references to substantiate the indications and complications. To understand the basics of vulvovaginal disease; to be able to evaluate the clinicopathologic entities and the variations thereof; and to be able to look into the future of this complicated melange of socioscientific entities, this text must be a priority item for the gynecologist/obstetrician, pathologist, and generalist. His or her answers to the many practical, as well as the exotic, problems will be found herein.

J. DONALD WOODRUFF, M.D.
Johns Hopkins Hospital
Baltimore, Maryland

Preface

What endeavor is truly worthy of the time that can be allotted to it? For me, the effort spent preparing this second edition will be justified if the book becomes as useful as the first edition has been. I am grateful to the many physicians from various practice settings who have taken the time to let me know that they enjoyed the earlier work. I hope they will not be disappointed with the present effort. I have added a chapter on Vulvar Surgery to familiarize everyone who encounters vulvar problems with the surgical techniques available. Another chapter on Special Problems has been included to address those areas that are extremely important, but do not fit the simple recognition categories. Vulvar pain and vestibular papillae are discussed in this section for the first time. Short biographies have been scattered throughout the text to acquaint you with those great physicians who have made important contributions to this field over the years. The organization of the chapters illustrating the disease categories is essentially unchanged, but many have been expanded and new photographs have been added. A new paragraph accompanies each entity, listing other lesions to be considered in the differential diagnosis.

The pace of discovery waxes and wanes. But in the field of vulvar disease, that pace has been rapid during the last seven years. When this book was first published, I tried to include the latest articles on a given disease and only rarely was there a choice. Now almost all of the further reading suggestions have been replaced from an expanding library of literature.

This book is not my work alone. Once again, the W. B. Saunders Company, through Mr. Albert Meier, has cooperated fully and supported my efforts and ideas to bring you a unique book designed for practical clinical application. Dr. Edward J. Wilkinson, gynecologic pathologist and close colleague, has been a steady source of inspiration and personal guidance. Mr. Thomas M. Swiss, friend of a lifetime, has similarly encouraged my work and provided an invaluable perspective. Drs. Ross J. Baldessarini, Daniel R. Considine, Frederick J. Hofmeister, and Gerald A. Sieggreen, sound clinicians and good friends, have generously shared their experience, while my companions Dr. Charles S. Mahan and Dr. John W. C. Johnson have often relieved my administrative burdens. Drs. Dale Brown, C. P. Douglas, P. J. Krupp, and C. M. Ridley contributed valuable data and portraits for the biographies. Ruth Ann Klockowski and Joan Magyari labored intensively with the manuscript. I am grateful to them all, for it is they who, with my family, have enabled me, by the grace of God, to complete the work.

EDUARD G. FRIEDRICH, JR.

Contents

Chapter 1
INTRODUCTION 1

Chapter 2
VAGINITIS 9

Chapter 3
DIAGNOSIS AND THERAPY 35

Chapter 4
SURGICAL PROCEDURES 61

Chapter 5
MANAGEMENT OF NEOPLASIA 89

Chapter 6
RED LESIONS 108

Chapter 7
WHITE LESIONS 129

Chapter 8
DARK LESIONS 149

Chapter 9
ULCERS 166

Chapter 10
SMALL TUMORS 189

Chapter 11
LARGE TUMORS 216

Chapter 12
SPECIAL PROBLEMS 237

INDEX 249

INTRODUCTION

Through the centuries, in the arts and in the sciences, the vulva has been richly ignored. Cave paintings and ancient pottery identified the female by conical shapes representing breasts added to the basic form. Even as painting and sculpture developed, the vulva remained covered with innocent foliage or discreetly invisible; though it was hardly necessary, since in most positions of the human female form, the vulva is hidden. If there were vulvologists in ancient China, they had a difficult time; the diagnostic doctor's "dolls," used by the discreet patient to point out the location of her symptoms, did not show the vulva. And embryologically, it is a negative result—the phenotypic genitalia that develop in the absence of testosterone effect. It is really not surprising, then, that the vulva was accorded little attention by those who first began to apply science to medicine. Not until this century did things begin to change.

The sculptures of Rodin broke many traditions. He dared to raise the leg of "Iris—Messenger of the Gods" and so was obliged to sculpt the vulva. Modern artists like Judy Chicago now celebrate it in beautiful designs like the opening of flowers. And medicine is catching up.

Early texts of gynecology only mentioned the vulva and identified one or two common symptoms as if they were diseases, e.g., pruritus vulvae. It required a physician with the special zeal of Frederick Taussig, M.D., of St. Louis to collate what was known about the vulva into book form. He first published his work on *Diseases of the Vulva* in 1923, and it quickly became the nationwide standard for vulvar disease. He was alone in the field for almost twenty years, and his thoughts and ideas on vulvar disease became firmly established in this country.

Frederick J. Taussig was born in Brooklyn, New York, in 1872, received his basic education there, and obtained his A.B. degree from Harvard in 1893. He went to St. Louis and received his M.D. degree from Washington University in 1898. The equivalent of internship and residency was performed in St. Louis and also at the Imperial and Royal Elizabeth Hospital in Vienna, Austria.

On return to St. Louis, he entered private practice and became clinical professor of gynecology and professor of clinical obstetrics at the Washington University Medical School. It is significant that from 1911 on, he was attending gynecologist at the Barnard Free Skin and Cancer Hospital. He was certainly interested in oncology. It was probably cancer of the vulva

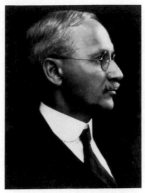

Frederick J. Taussig, M.D.

that first drew his attention to that organ, but the experience of practicing in a large dermatologic center may have also kindled an interest in the benign vulvar diseases.

That interest led to the writing of his book Diseases of the Vulva, *first published in a monograph series in 1923. In his preface, he notes that the vulva occupies a borderland between dermatology and gynecology, and laments its insufficient study. Both drawings and black-and-white photographs were used to illustrate the work, which influenced American medical thought on the subject over the next thirty years.*

Dr. Taussig was the recognized authority of his day on vulvar cancer and by extension on all of vulvar disease. He was an influential member of all the prestigious organizations in Obstetrics and Gynecology, and as a lecturer he was in great demand. His ideas were accepted with little question, and he commanded the respect of all when speaking within his field of special knowledge and when operating for vulvar carcinoma.

Elsewhere in the world, there was little interest in vulvar disease. The great medical centers of Europe were occupied with advances in obstetrics and gynecological surgery. Dermatology was a newborn specialty, concentrating on venereal diseases and vaccination. However, one dermatologist in Great Britain, Dr. Elizabeth Hunt, developed an interest in vulvar disease and became a pioneer among dermatologists after publication of her highly successful book on the subject. She, then, represented for England what Taussig represented for the United States.

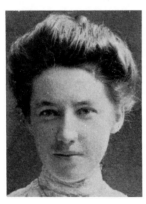

Elizabeth Hunt, M.D.

Elizabeth Hunt was born at Omagh in County Tyrone, Ireland, in 1876. She received a B.A. degree from the University of Ireland and subsequently married a surgeon, Dr. T. H. Hunt, who died in 1918. Elizabeth then entered the Liverpool Medical School, achieved her M.D. degree in 1924, and studied dermatology in Vienna, Paris, and London. She practiced as head of the dermatology department of the Royal Sussex County Hospital until her retirement in 1945.

She was honored by election as an Emeritus Member of the British Association of Dermatologists shortly before her death in 1977. Such recognition was long her due. In addition to her other accomplishments, she had a definite interest in vulvar disease and was a careful observer and clinician. She published her book Diseases Affecting the Vulva *in 1940. The book ran to four editions, and she established in England the tradition which Taussig had established in the United States. That tradition has now been extended by Dr. C. M. Ridley, a consultant dermatologist in London, whose scholarly monograph,* The Vulva, *has carried the work forward in the United Kingdom.*

In the United States, Taussig's ideas were essentially unchallenged until 1969, when Herman L. Gardner and Raymond H. Kaufman wrote their first edition on *Benign Diseases of the Vulva and Vagina*. Kaufman, the wise and gentle scholar from New York, joined with Gardner, the astute Texas clinician, and produced a true first in American gynecology, a book devoted to the vulva that did not deal primarily with cancer. A pathologist as well as an obstetrician-gynecologist, Kaufman emphasized the pathophysiology of vulvar diseases as well as their clinical aspects. He supported and explored new avenues of research and published extensively. His collaboration with Gardner marked a new era of activity and interest in vulvar disease that was not limited to the United States. At the same time, Janovski and Douglas first published their *Diseases of the Vulva* in German as *Erkrankungen der Vulva*. DiPaola and Balina in Argentina composed the message in Spanish and published *Enfermedades de le Vulva*, and the renowned French dermatologist Jean Hewitt assembled the information in *Pathologie de la Vulve*.

At the Sixth World Congress of the International Federation of Obstetricians and Gynecologists in New York City in 1970, a group of physicians interested in vulvar research came together at a round-table meeting. The meeting was extended to extra sessions when each discovered how much information there was to share, and within that *seminar impromptu* was born the idea of an International Society for the Study of Vulvar Disease. The group was to consist of gynecologists, dermatologists, and pathologists from around the world who concentrated their clinical or investigative efforts on diseases of the vulva. The suggestion first came from Herman L. Gardner, who agreed to serve as Organizing Vice President. Guillermo R. DiPaola from Buenos Aires became the first President; Eduard G. Friedrich, the founding Secretary and later Secretary-General; and Kane Zelle, the Treasurer. By-laws were established and kindred spirits were recruited to attend the first Congress of the Society in Spain in 1973. Since then, the group has expanded to over 100 fellows from 24 nations who meet every two years to share with enthusiasm their latest knowledge.

The symbol of the Society (Fig. 1) reflects the international cooperation necessary for building the arch of knowledge of vulvar disease on a global scale. As one of its initial tasks, the Society devised, debated, and in 1976, recommended the adoption of a new nomenclature for white lesions and intraepithelial neoplasia. These suggestions have largely been accepted by physicians in all three specialities and have been incorporated into current terminology. They achieved the desired abolition of the concept of "leukoplakia," a vague term

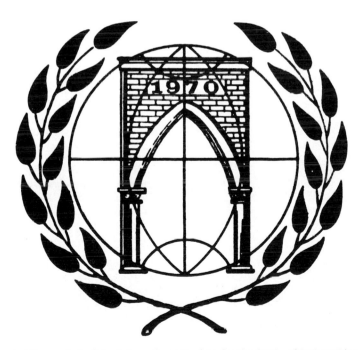

Figure 1. The symbol of the International Society for the Study of Vulvar Disease.

that had been used for decades to describe white lesions and that carried strong, if inaccurate, connotations of malignancy. They substituted the benign concept of *dystrophy,* a term that had no attached preconceptions. The need for education of other physicians in the field of vulvar disease was met by the Society's encouragement and support of annual postgraduate courses on the subject. As a small action group of committed investigators, the Society is dedicated to the ignition of interest in others and will continue to play a key role in the dissemination of new knowledge gained through the work of its fellows.

The development of the Society, the publication of the books, the fresh attitude toward investigation all represent a great total effort by many people over many years. This was beautifully stated by Kahlil Gibran in his book *Jesus, the Son of Man:*

> You shall not be yourself alone. You are in the deeds of other men, and they though unknowing are with you all your days.

Indeed, we all stand upon the shoulders of our predecessors and are dependent upon that heritage. That understanding is personified by J. Donald Woodruff, M.D. Always concerned about the acknowledgment of earlier authors, Woodruff himself contributed a steady stream of articles on all aspects of vulvar disease to the American medical literature. A tireless lecturer, he carried the message across the United States and to many other countries.

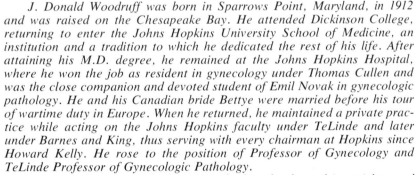

J. Donald Woodruff was born in Sparrows Point, Maryland, in 1912 and was raised on the Chesapeake Bay. He attended Dickinson College, returning to enter the Johns Hopkins University School of Medicine, an institution and a tradition to which he dedicated the rest of his life. After attaining his M.D. degree, he remained at the Johns Hopkins Hospital, where he won the job as resident in gynecology under Thomas Cullen and was the close companion and devoted student of Emil Novak in gynecologic pathology. He and his Canadian bride Bettye were married before his tour of wartime duty in Europe. When he returned, he maintained a private practice while acting on the Johns Hopkins faculty under TeLinde and later under Barnes and King, thus serving with every chairman at Hopkins since Howard Kelly. He rose to the position of Professor of Gynecology and TeLinde Professor of Gynecologic Pathology.

His contributions to the literature, both in books and in articles, and the frequent use of his abilities as an outstanding lecturer have shaped much of gynecologic thought. He has been honored with the responsibilities of high office in many societies, among them President of the American Association of Obstetricians and Gynecologists (now the American Gynecological and Obstetrical Society) and President of the Johns Hopkins Medical and Surgical Association. He served as the second President of the International Society for the Study of Vulvar Disease and wisely guided its early development.

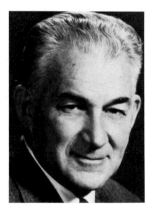

J. Donald Woodruff, M.D.

His interest in vulvar disease began when Emil Novak asked him to review a case of in situ neoplasia of the vulva, a case in fact of extramammary Paget's disease. With typical thoroughness, that review included a literature survey and a hunt for other cases, which culminated in 1955 in the landmark paper Paget's Disease of the Vulva. *That paper re-established the entity with authority and once again called attention to vulvar disease. Perhaps its greatest effect was on his own interest, for he then became concerned with all aspects of vulvar pathology. As a true clinician-investigator in the tradition of Sir James Paget and Emil Novak, he looked upon each entity as a challenge full of fresh correlations. It is simultaneously a privilege and an inspiration to be in his presence, and hundreds count him as their mentor. Among those stands the author, with gratitude and warm affection for the inspiration and support of a professional lifetime.*

Dr. Woodruff sought out and encouraged the interest of others. One such was Peter J. Lynch, M.D., a renowned dermatologist and a teacher of medicine, who recognized a kindred spirit in Dr. Woodruff and shared his interest in the cutaneous diseases of the vulva. Dr. Lynch in turn, along with other dermatologists, influenced members of that specialty, increasing their awareness of vulvar pathology and enlisting their participation in the work of the International Society for the Study of Vulvar Disease. The book *Dermatology for the House Officer,* written by Dr. Lynch, is a prime source for clinical reference, laden with pearls of dermatologic diagnosis and therapy.

Thus, the ripples spread across the surface of the pond involving more and more people in the ever-expanding waves of knowledge. And as a result of all this combined interest and energy, we now know a great deal more than before about the human vulva and the diseases that affect it.

A visit to the zoo is sufficient to impress anyone with the fact that in some animals—monkeys, baboons, and chimpanzees—the vulvar skin, the sexual skin, is something special. It looks different and undergoes obvious changes. Such display probably serves an important function for those species, and draws our attention to the fact that human sexual skin, vulvar skin, is similarly special. Yet we are only just beginning to understand the many ways in which this is true.

The envelope of skin that encloses the body serves as a front-line interface with the environment. It is a membrane that allows, favors, or discourages the passage of substances. Among the most important of these is water. Water is lost at identifiable rates from all body surfaces. We now know that the transepidermal water loss of the labia exceeds that of reference forearm skin by a large amount. The vulva is indeed "wetter" as part of its normal state. This basic fact in turn has many other implications.

The ability of skin to absorb compounds placed on its surface depends upon a number of factors including the hydration state of the stratum corneum. The inherent "wetness" of the vulva may explain the rapid uptake of various steroids and other chemicals by scrotal and vulvar skin. It may also explain the increased response to irritants noted on the vulva.

The phenomenon of contact irritation is familiar to anyone who has seen a case of poison ivy. Certainly the magnitude of the reaction depends on the potency of the irritant as well as the responsiveness of the epithelium. But holding the irritant constant and using the forearm skin for reference, the vulva shows a definite propensity to irritant reaction.

The hydration/permeability of the vulvar stratum corneum also determines, to some extent, the microenvironment of the skin surface. Some organisms do well on dry surfaces, while others require high moisture conditions. The quantitative microbiology of the vulva depends upon these factors. Diphtheroids, *Staphylococcus aureus,* and micrococci abound in numbers that exceed the rates known for other sites. Yeasts and gram-negative rods are also present in significant quantity. For these reasons, the vulva requires special hygienic attention, both for routine purposes and during episodes of disease, and should be kept as dry as possible. Obese women find this an almost impossible task. Stress urinary incontinence frequently accompanies obesity and further aggravates the situation, since the constant presence of irritating urine will inevitably result in the equivalent of a diaper rash. Simple rinsing with clear water after voiding, the use of talcum powder during the day, and the avoidance of tight-fitting lingerie at night can do much to avoid many of the simple skin irritations caused by lack of air circulation and constant moisture. When thorough drying is absolutely essential, the patient may lie down at home with her heels together and her knees drawn up and spread widely apart. A small fan, or portable hair dryer set on *COOL,* may then be directed toward the vulva. This will assure at least a brief period of dry air circulation and may be repeated at intervals throughout the day.

Nonabsorbent materials act to keep the vulva moist and the vaginal irritants in more or less continuous contact. Therefore, in the presence of any exudative vulvovaginal disorder, synthetic underwear should not be worn and cotton garments or those with a cotton crotch should be used instead. Because some dyes are themselves irritating, white is the preferred color. Many common detergents contain arsenicals; if these are incompletely rinsed from the underwear, they may act as topical irritants. Panties should therefore be rinsed well after separate washing in pure soap solution without the use of presoaks or enzymes.

Vaginal deodorants, perfumed soaps, and "hygiene" sprays serve absolutely no physiologic purpose. Such cosmetics, however, may be harmful insofar as they may produce sensitivity reactions. Therefore, since they are of no definite benefit and are sources of at least potential harm, the use of these products should be discouraged. When irritation has resulted from their use, plain mineral oil should be used as a vulvar cleanser for a time until the irritation subsides. Any objectionable odor in the normal vulvar area that persists after thorough bathing is coming from the vagina, and no amount of propellant or perfume applied topically will alleviate this problem.

We still know relatively little of the normal "basic science" of the vulva. Much needs to be done in the cellular biology, tissue chemistry, and organ physiology of the vulva. As this is accomplished, our understanding of disease processes and prevention will also increase. Until then, we remain dependent upon clinical observation and experience, and that is the purpose of this book: to share with each of you, my readers, those insights, tips, correlations, and ideas that have occurred in my practice.

This book was written to be read, not simply consulted. Its organization and illustrations are designed to enhance your reading pleasure. This is not a reference text. Instead, I have added a list of publications for further reading at the end of each chapter. There, I have indicated those articles I think you'll enjoy if you have further interest in the subject. I have chosen them because they represent landmarks in the progress of our understanding or because they are significant works of current knowledge and review. They, in turn, will lead you to more articles and may be sufficient to initiate an odyssey of personal study.

Rather than for reference or research, this book is for the clinician, the one who sees and does—the doctor in primary care, in ambulatory gynecology, in general office practice, in dermatology, or wherever the woman patient is seen.

And for all of you, it is meant to be a handbook for recognition. For this reason, the chapters that illustrate the disease entities do so according to the way they present in the office. Not as fungal disorders or primary dermatoses or benign neoplasms do they present, but rather more simply as red, white, or dark lesions, ulcers, little tumors, and big tumors. Within these groups may be recognized most vulvar diseases. The diagnosis can then be confirmed and treatment begun. Further research may then be accomplished based on the knowledge gained from patient experience.

I chose most of the photographs from my private collection to show you the typical and important varietal features of the disease discussed. I am grateful to those others who made their own collections available to me for use in this book. The format maintains wide margins for a purpose: Write in them. Use them to annotate the photographs with your own observations and to record your ideas and correlations.

It is my final hope that you will truly enjoy the process of reading and using this book in the everyday expansion of those ripples in the pond, as they touch you and your patients.

FURTHER READING

Aly, R., Britz, M.B., and Maibach, H.I.: Quantitative microbiology of human vulva. Brit. J. Dermatol. 101:445–448, 1979.
A basic investigation into the vulvar microenvironment.

Britz, M.B., and Maibach, H.I.: Human labia majora skin: transepidermal water loss in vivo. Acta Dermatovener. 59(s85):23–25, 1979.
Basic physiologic work establishing important characteristics of vulvar skin.

DiPaola, G.R., and Balina, L.M.: Enfermedades de la Vulva. Editoria Medica Panamericana S.A., Buenos Aires, 1970.
The Spanish language work that documented the insights and observations of an Argentinian gynecologist and dermatologist.

DiPaola, G.R., and Friedrich, E.G.: The International Society for the Study of Vulvar Disease. Int. J. Gynaecol. Obstet. 14:565–566, 1976.
A brief history of the society and physicians who contributed to its early development.

Gardner, H.L., and Kaufman, R.H.: Benign Disease of the Vulva and Vagina. 1st ed. The C.V. Mosby Company, St. Louis, 1969.
The first American text since Taussig's to deal with the problem in book length and to spark a new era of interest.

Huguier, J., and Hewitt, J.: Pathologie de la Vulve. Masson et Cie editeurs, Paris, 1970.
The French summation of a grand seminar called to discuss and present many aspects of the subject.

International Society for the Study of Vulvar Disease. New nomenclature for vulvar disease. Obstet. Gynecol. 47.122–124, 1976.
A landmark recommendation for change that popularized the concept of dystrophy.

Janovski, N.A., and Douglas, C.P.: Diseases of the Vulva. Harper & Row Publishers, Hagerstown, Md., 1972.
The English version of the work first published in German four years earlier.

Lynch, P.J.: Dermatology for the House Officer. The Williams & Wilkins Company, Baltimore, 1982.
A plain-talking, problem-oriented gem of a book for frequent clinical reference.

Ridley, C.M.: The Vulva. W. B. Saunders Company, Ltd., London, 1975.
The reference work for vulvar disease that lists all pertinent literature and discusses the problems from a dermatologist's viewpoint.

Woodruff, J.D.: Paget's disease of the vulva. Obstet. Gynecol. 5:175–185, 1955.
The landmark paper that marked the beginning of Woodruff's interest in vulvar disease generally and Paget's disease in particular—thereby influencing the host of pupils who studied under him and followed his lead.

2

VAGINITIS

The vaginal mucosa has only a few of the nerve endings needed for the sensations of pain and light touch. For this reason, many vaginal infections are asymptomatic until the discharge reaches the vulva, where such nerve endings are abundant. The problem is then perceived as a sensation of itching, burning, or pain. Thus, vaginitis often presents as a vulvar disease. Facility and expertise in the differential diagnosis and treatment of vaginitis is therefore a prerequisite for the successful management of vulvar problems. There is nothing particularly difficult about the treatment of vaginitis if one understands the ecology of the vagina and has the patience to employ a few simple diagnostic techniques. For the vagina is like a river with its own ecosystem of interdependent factors subject to imbalance and pollution. Like a good trout fisherman, the physician must know how to "read the stream" in order to assess those factors.

In addition to a microscope, the necessary equipment consists of a roll of nitrazine pH paper (range 4.5 to 7.5), small dropper bottles of fresh physiologic saline and 10 per cent KOH solution, along with microscopic slides and coverslips (Fig. 2). These items are readily obtainable and can be conveniently kept in the examining table drawer, where they will be available for immediate use. If they are kept in any other location, the time and trouble necessary to find them, when in the middle of an examination, leads to the strong temptation of "not to bother this time." The result may be an inaccurate diagnosis followed by inappropriate and ineffective therapy.

By taking a brief but careful history, delineating the patient's major symptom, noting the presence and character of the vaginal discharge, and combining this with an observation of the vaginal pH and wet smear morphology, almost every case can be classified into one of the major categories listed in Table 1.

Table 1. The Major Categories of Vaginitis

	CANDIDA	GARDNERELLA	TRICHOMONAS	ATROPHY
Complaint	Pruritus	Odor	Discharge	Bleeding
pH	4–5	5–6	5–7	6–7
Discharge	Thick—cheesy	Scant—creamy	Thin—copious	Scant—purulent
Wet smear	Hyphae	Clue cells	Motile protozoa	WBC—parabasals

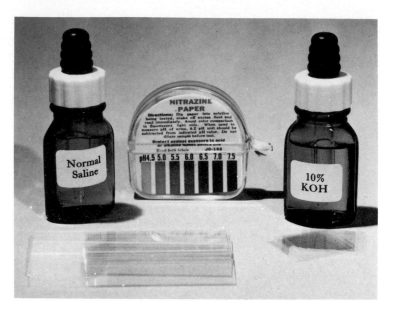

Figure 2. Basic materials required for the differential diagnosis of vaginitis.

Each case, whether recurrent or primary, whether you are the first physician to see the problem or the last in a long list of consultants, should be approached as a unique entity. This "fresh look" approach is essential and ought to be employed each and every time.

Tearing off a small piece of nitrazine paper and placing it in the anterior or lateral fornix gives an immediate pH reading and takes only a few seconds to perform. A small amount of representative discharge is mixed on a slide with a few drops of saline and a coverslip is gently placed on top of the preparation. A similar slide is made using 10 per cent KOH. These slides should be observed under both low and high dry magnification. Close down the iris diaphragm of the microscope to diminish the light intensity for sharper contrast. Assistants quickly learn to interpret these smears, but if the clinician performs the microscopic examination personally, the time spent is short and the information gained is crucial. Excellent therapeutic measures are available for vaginitis and will give good results if properly applied after an accurate diagnosis.

ECOLOGY

The vagina must be appreciated as a complex and sensitive ecosystem (Fig. 3). The squamous epithelium of the vagina is exquisitely responsive to the influence of the steroid hormones. Both in childhood and after menopause, in the absence of estrogen, the vaginal epithelium is thin and undifferentiated. Estrogen causes a thickening of the epithelium and a differentiation into the well-recognized layers (basal, intermediate, and superficial) characteristic of the reproductive years. The percentage of superficial cells present on a vaginal smear is an approximate indicator of the amount of estrogenic activity. Progesterone, on the other hand, produces a relative decrease in the number of superficial cells while promoting the number of intermediate cells.

A great deal of glycogen is present within the vaginal epithelial cells. As an organ, the vagina is second only to the liver in total amount of contained glycogen. The formation of glycogen and its deposition in an available form within the cells constitutes another of the estrogenic effects. Glycogen is abundant and most available within the superficial cell layers. Thus, estrogen is seen to be responsible for the development of a thick vaginal epithelium with a large number of superficial "pavement" cells that serve a protective function and also provide most of the available glycogen. It is on their surface that the microridges are found and to which the bacteria, normal or pathogenic, adhere.

Lack of estrogen results in an atrophic condition wherein the protective superficial cells and their contained glycogen are both lacking. A more subtle change takes place when these estrogen effects are moderated by a relative dominance of progesterone. Pregnancy, lactation, and the use of oral contraceptives are examples of this progesterone-dominant state. Although they are quantitatively different, they are qualitatively similar, resulting in a relative decrease in the number of glycogen-containing superficial cells. The importance of glycogen in the vagina lies in its use as a substrate for a series of enzymatic and fermentative processes that result in the production of lactic and acetic acid. The metabolism of glycogen may be influenced by a variety of host factors, but the most striking example is that of altered carbohydrate metabolism seen in diabetes mellitus, where, because of increased glycogenolysis and subsequent decrease of available glycogen in the epithelium, a relative lack of this important substrate results.

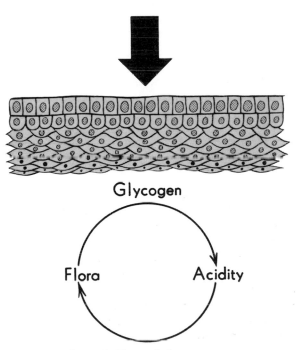

Figure 3. The vaginal ecosystem.

The flora that utilize this glycogen and its enzymatic breakdown products are migrants from the gut, and exist in a delicate and dynamic equilibrium. In the healthy vagina of the normal woman during her reproductive years, these flora consist largely of lactobacilli and acidogenic corynebacteria. Frequently, small numbers of *Candida* species are also present. These fungi are held in check by the overwhelming number of lactobacilli and corynebacteria. Both of these latter organisms produce lactic and acetic acid from glycogen and its breakdown products. The result of this symbiosis is a low vaginal pH, a milieu that is highly selective for bacterial growth and favors only the lactobacilli, corynebacteria, and candida organisms. Thus, while a wide variety of aerobic and anaerobic organisms can be cultured from the alkaline mucus of the endocervix, colonization of the vagina by these bacteria is greatly discouraged.

Nonetheless, in the presence of an overwhelming inoculum of foreign bacteria, the normal flora may lose the competition and, as they do so, the pH will rise, thus selectively favoring growth of the foreign invaders. Along these same lines, if the patient receives antibiotics for some unrelated disease process, the lactobacilli and corynebacteria are inhibited, and then the ever-present *Candida* species, freed from the competitive inhibition of the normal flora, proceed to overgrow within the acid milieu. The use of tetracycline for acne in teenagers taking oral contraceptives and the subsequent development of candidal vaginitis in these young women affords an ideal example of this phenomenon. In some women, as long as three months may be required before the vaginal flora spontaneously return to normal after an antibiotic insult.

At a low pH (3.5 to 4.1) normal flora predominate; but as the pH increases, various pathogens replace them. Knowing which pathogens occur in which pH ranges provides a valuable clue to the probable cause of any particular vaginitis (Fig. 4).

The acidity of the vagina, then, constitutes a protective mechanism produced, in large part, by the very flora whose growth and multiplication it encourages. This acidity itself may be influenced, in turn, by a number of other factors. Among these are an excessive amount of alkaline cervical mucus that might be expected to be produced by large eversions of the endocervix or by vaginal adenosis. During the normal menstrual period, the vagina is bathed with alkaline menstrual flow containing blood, an excellent growth enrichment factor for many bacteria. Therefore, the menstrual period constitutes another threat to the ecosystem and represents a time span in which any therapeutic measures directed at vaginitis become especially important. Failure to continue medication during the menstrual period is one of the most frequent reasons for failure of therapy.

Perhaps the commonest menace to the delicate balance of vaginal ecology is sexual intercourse. Masters and Johnson have demonstrated that the major vaginal lubricant is composed of a transudate that is "secreted" by the vaginal epithelium and is able to raise the vaginal pH. This lubricating fluid is present during all stages of sexual excitation, and a similar lubricant is present in increasing amounts throughout pregnancy. During intercourse, the deposition of the alkaline-buffered ejaculate raises the vaginal pH to a range of 6 to 7. This lasts for two hours after coitus, after which time it gradually returns to normal over an eight-hour period. Thus, frequently repeated coital acts keep the vagina in a constantly alkaline state. Such alkalinity is toxic to lactobacilli and coryne-

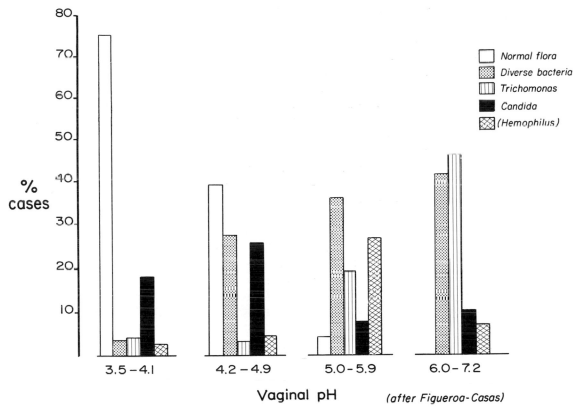

Normal flora
Diverse bacteria
Trichomonas
Candida
(Hemophilus)

% cases

Vaginal pH   (after Figueroa-Casas)

3.5 – 4.1   4.2 – 4.9   5.0 – 5.9   6.0 – 7.2

Figure 4. pH range of various organisms.

bacteria, but pathogens adapt quickly to the pH change and proceed to over-grow. Most women can easily tolerate this transient pH insult. But in some, the vaginal ecosystem is so delicately balanced that even a single episode of coitus is sufficient to tip the scales. They associate the subsequent symptoms with the partner and assume an infectious transmission from that source. But in fact, only a "dose" of buffer has been transmitted. Use of condoms or a simple douche soon after coitus will relieve this problem.

Candidal and atrophic vaginitis may occur in virgins, but other forms of vaginitis are generally found only in sexually active women. While a vaginal ecosystem may be rendered susceptible to colonization by foreign organisms, infection per se does not usually result unless those organisms are inoculated from an outside source. Fomites play only a minor role in the transmission of vaginitis, but trichomonas organisms have in fact been recovered from chlorinated swimming pools and hot tubs as well as wet towels and toilet seats. Neverthe-less, the usual source of infection, be it trichomonas, gardnerella, gonorrhea, condylomata, or herpes, is the sexual partner. Although therapy is available for the partner, the diagnostic methods are not as specific nor as successful when applied to a male consort. Then too, male infection may frequently present as a "carrier" state so that signs and symptoms will not be apparent. Nonetheless, in the face of stubborn or recurrent female infections, male involvement should be presumed even though documentation may not be possible. The temporary

13

use of a condom during the vaginitis treatment period, and continued use for a short time thereafter, will help to break the vicious circle of partner-to-partner reinfection. Some women become irritated by the lubricating solution in which condoms are packaged. If condoms cause such distress, they should simply be rinsed in plain water prior to use.

In a practical sense, it is sometimes unwise to overemphasize the venereal nature of these infections to the concerned patient. It cannot usually be proven that any particular case arose from sexual contact. Other modes of transmission are possible and should not be negated. It requires the utmost of tact to inform such a patient of the necessity for partner precautions (condoms, male examination, danger of reinfection), while at the same time not implying to a faithful wife that she has unequivocal evidence of her husband's infidelity.

On the other hand, these diseases are most common among the young and promiscuous, who learn, to their dismay, that "love" is not entirely "free." It is these women who most need to understand the venereal aspect of their illness if they are to avoid reinfection and further transmission. Such infections may occur singly, but are often found in combination. Therefore, the presence of one sexually transmitted disease should alert the physician to the possible coexistence of others in the same patient. Thus a diagnosis of condylomata mandates a culture for gonorrhea and a careful search for concomitant gardnerella, trichomonas, herpes, molluscum, etc.

DOUCHING

Douching of the vagina is one of the oldest medical procedures known. Detailed instructions are given in the Ebers papyrus, which dates from 1500 B.C. The Greeks knew that milk douches were beneficial and used them to treat vaginal infection.

Douching is not harmful per se when proper solutions are used on an occasional basis, or when douching is used in a therapeutic program. Overuse, however, particularly with hypotonic solutions such as tap water, may dilute the normal flora of the vagina. A list of common solutions and their specific indications is presented in Table 2.

Table 2. Douche Solutions

INGREDIENT	INDICATION
Normal saline	General use
White vinegar	General use
Alkaline powder	Mucolytic
Potassium sorbate "medicated"	Antifungal
Hydrogen peroxide	Antigardnerella
20% saline	Antitrichomonas
Sweet acidophilus milk	
Yogurt	Re-colonization and restoration of normal flora
Lactobacillus solution	
Buttermilk	Elimination of odor from vaginal fistulae

For routine cleansing, a dilute acetic acid solution composed of one tablespoon of vinegar per quart of water, or a physiologic saline solution made from one or two teaspoons of table salt per quart of water is ideal. Enema equipment should not be used for vaginal douching because of the danger of cross contamination. Bulb syringes are unsatisfactory, since excessive pressures may be created during the forceful flushing of the vagina, and the douche solution has little opportunity to contact all of the vaginal surfaces. Instead, a simple vinyl or rubber bag of one-quart capacity fitted with tubing and a douche tip is preferred. Douching should be done while reclining in a bathtub. The thighs should be flexed and the knees bent. The tip is then inserted into the vagina with slight downward pressure until the fornix is reached. At this point, the junction of the tip and the tubing is usually at the introitus. Using the fingers of one hand, the labia are now gently but firmly pressed together, squeezing the vagina closed around the douche tip and preventing the egress of fluid. The other hand then opens the valve, allowing the solution to flow into the vagina from the reservoir bag suspended at shoulder height. As the vagina fills with fluid (it will usually hold about ½ pint), a sensation of fullness will be felt. At this point the supply valve is closed, but the labia should be held together for a minute or so afterward to allow the solution to contact all the folds and crevices of the distended vaginal mucosa. The fluid is then allowed to run out and the process is repeated until the bag is empty.

Instructions, along with suitable diagrams, are usually packaged with the douche equipment. Some drug companies provide pads of preprinted instructions in leaflet form. For problems that require therapeutic douching, the instruction leaflet can be easily clipped to the prescription. Not only does this save time in the office, but the patient can refer back to the instructions if questions arise later.

CANDIDA

Candida species certainly rank as the commonest cause of vaginitis. Small numbers of these organisms are frequently present in the normal vagina, but their growth is checked by the competitive metabolism of the lactobacilli and corynebacteria, as well as by the specific fungal inhibitory factors they produce. Therefore, many candidal infections are not dependent on introduction from an external source. The organisms are opportunists, requiring only the lack of competitive inhibition by the normal flora to gain the upper hand. While candidal infections may be frequent, recurrent, and stubborn, their reputation may be somewhat worse than they deserve. Since these organisms are so ubiquitous, they are often the cause of a woman's first episode of vaginitis. With the initial attack, the patient will almost invariably seek a physician's help. She will then be told that she has "yeast infection," and will receive some form of therapy that will more or less eradicate the infection. But from that point onward, every time she experiences severe pruritus or vaginal discharge, she harkens back to her initial experience and assumes that she has another "yeast infection." Of course, she may be right; it could be candida again. But on the other hand, the current episode may be due to a completely different cause for which the leftover cream from the previous infection is ineffective. She then calls her physician on the phone and states that she has a recurrence of her "yeast infection." This usually results in a prescription telephoned to a pharmacy for a different fungicidal cream, which also fails to relieve her symptoms. It takes only a few such experiences to convince the physician that he is dealing with a very stubborn fungal species. Meanwhile, the patient has compiled a long shopping list of drugs that she has tried and that she knows from experience are worthless for her "yeast infection." For this reason, drug manufacturers' claims for effectiveness are not always borne out by clinical experience. Drug studies are carefully controlled with numerous cultures and "in vitro" sensitivity data; clinical experience is sometimes based on little more than the patient's own guess as to the causative agent. Again, this is why the "fresh look approach" is so essential for effective management of vaginitis from whatever cause, and office examination is necessary for each and every episode. The telephone is neither a diagnostic nor therapeutic tool, and the temptation to use it as such should be resisted.

If, indeed, the vaginitis is due to an overgrowth of candida organisms, the patient will probably present with pruritus as the major complaint. She may have noticed a curdlike discharge, either white or yellow in color, but the discharge is not the most prominent feature. Often the onset of symptoms will coincide with a recent menstrual period or episode of coitus. Early pregnancy, anemia, undiagnosed diabetes mellitus, and recent exposure to antibiotics, steroids, and cytotoxic agents are other predisposing conditions that may be associated with candidal infection. Whether or not the use of oral contraceptives constitutes such a factor remains a controversial point.

On speculum examination, the vaginal walls will have a dull but definite erythema. The classic patches of "thrush" adherent to the mucosa are pathognomonic findings for *C. albicans* infection, but usually the discharge is more diffuse with a less dramatic but certainly three-dimensional appearance, confined to the vaginal walls, and moderately adherent. It is relatively thick and dry and may be scraped off the surface with a speculum blade or Pap smear spatula. The pH of the lateral vaginal wall is often below 5.0, well within the normal range. Representative samples of discharge should be examined by wet smears using both KOH and fresh saline. It is possible to be misled on clinical appearance alone, and mixed infections may be present. The saline smear provides the opportunity to find other pathogens such as trichomonas while the smear is still fresh. Clusters of candida can be recognized on a saline smear (Fig. 5), but their presence is often obscured by adherent cellular material. The KOH prep, however, will lyse the vaginal epithelial cells, inflammatory leukocytes, and debris. Against this clear background, the branched and budding pseudohyphae of the fungus will stand out clearly (Fig. 6). Don't expect to see the organism in every field. It requires patience to carefully search the slide, but the rewards are worth the effort.

In 1978, the organism formerly known as *Torulopsis glabrata* was officially transferred by the International Association of Microbiological Societies to the genus *Candida* and is now properly called *Candida glabrata*. This is the second most common fungal pathogen found in the human vagina. In some parts of the world, it is twice as common as *C. albicans,* but in North America, *C. glabrata* accounts only for about 5 per cent of the cases of fungal vaginitis.

Candida glabrata causes a relatively mild inflammation of the mucosa without the formation of appreciable discharge. The patient may complain of burning, and this is one of the conditions that must be ruled out in the woman with vulvar pain who complains of "burning." But more often, the symptoms are

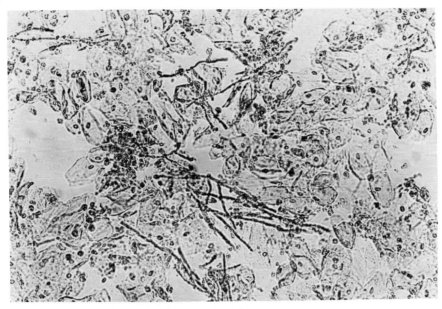

Figure 5. Saline smear with candida present.

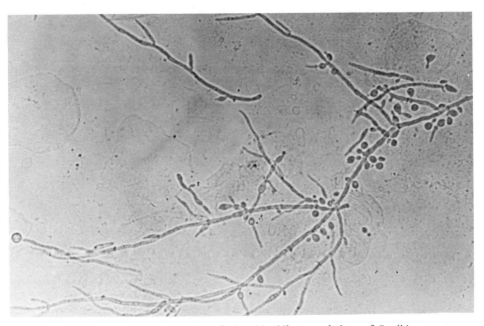

Figure 6. KOH smear shows branched and budding morphology of *C. albicans*.

usually mild. The pH is low (4 to 4.5); on saline wet smear, one sees only spores of varying sizes and shapes (2 to 8 microns) without filaments or branches. The spores are usually ovoid and often grouped together (Fig. 7). Large spores may resemble red cells but lack the characteristic central indentation of erythrocytes (Fig. 8). To confirm the diagnosis, a routine vaginal culture for fungus may be sent, but the request form should specifically state that *C. glabrata* is suspected.

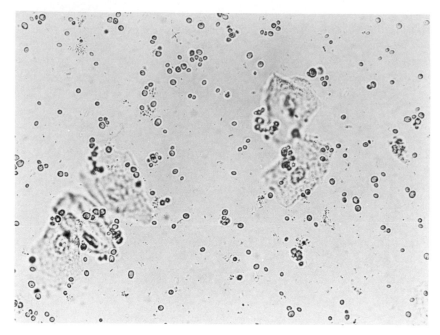

Figure 7. Candida glabrata (formerly *Torulopsis*). Clumped ovoid spores; compare with epithelial cells.

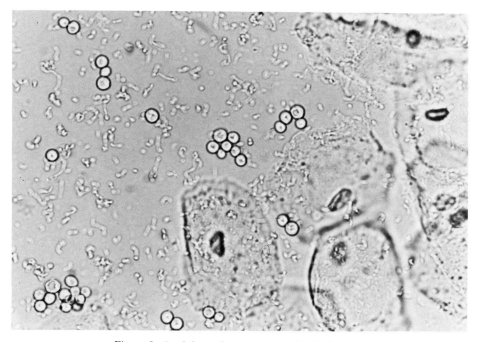

Figure 8. C. glabrata large spores under high power.

All fungi will respond equally well to topical gentian violet, and a 1 per cent aqueous solution of this dye should be considered as the primary drug of choice for candidal vaginitis regardless of the species. The gross colonies of fungus should be wiped from the vagina. This mechanically decreases the size of the pathogenic inoculum. The cervix and vaginal surfaces are then "painted" with the dye, using a large cotton swab. The anterior and posterior vaginal walls are, of course, covered by the blades when the speculum is fully inserted. Therefore, the partially opened speculum must be rotated both to the left and to the right in order to expose all of the vaginal surface. Once the entire vagina has been coated with gentian violet, the speculum may be reinserted and left open for a few minutes, allowing the vagina to dry. Absorb any residual liquid with a dry swab. This minimizes the staining caused by an excess of dye running out of the vagina when the patient stands upright. It is best to routinely paint the introitus and inner vulva with this same solution, even though grossly there is no sign of involvement, since culture of these areas will often be positive. The patient is then given a perineal pad, in order to prevent staining of her undergarments. A better than 95 per cent cure rate should be expected with the use of gentian violet, applied by the physician, using a 1 per cent aqueous solution. Other forms of gentian violet, impregnated in tampons or combined with a base as vaginal inserts, are not as effective.

There are only two drawbacks to the use of this therapy. Gentian violet has, reportedly, produced contact reactions resulting in local irritation, and it should not be used in patients who give a history of irritation following previous application. The incidence of this side effect is extremely low, however, if dilute solutions (1 per cent or less) are used at infrequent intervals (once a week). The second drawback is the undeserved reputation that gentian violet is messy. Rarely will a patient voice this complaint. Whatever inconvenience she experiences seems to be outweighed by the rapid relief of symptoms. If too much solution is applied and allowed to run over the perineum and down the patient's legs, then indeed it is messy. Should the patient have intercourse shortly after treatment, the male partner will note staining of the penis. But the patient should not be having intercourse during the treatment period, and if she does, a condom should be mandatory. In short, gentian violet can be made quite tolerable for the patient by using care in the application, giving the patient a perineal pad for immediate use, and asking her to wear her older underwear for a time, rather than risk staining a brand new pair. Physicians who are unaccustomed to wearing gloves for speculum examination will find gentian violet inconvenient, and run the risk of staining their hands. Others note that when plain cotton balls are used as swabs, the dye may spatter onto the clothing or shoes. Use of the preformed large cotton swabs, not overly saturated, does away with this problem. Aromatic spirits of ammonia and alcohol partially remove gentian violet from the skin and clothing, but the stain is a stubborn one that is best avoided by careful application.

After painting, the patient is sent home with fungicidal creams or tablets to be inserted vaginally for the next week, regardless of symptomatology and regardless of menstrual period. It is best to have the patient return one week after the initial treatment to assess the need for a second application of gentian violet. This can be repeated at weekly intervals if necessary, although one or two paintings are usually sufficient.

The imidazole drugs (clotrimazole, miconazole) are extremely effective as topical agents against *Candida albicans*. Clotrimazole has even been shown to be partially effective against trichomonas. But efficacy has not been shown against *Candida glabrata*. Used as vaginal creams or inserts, 14-day, 7-day, and 3-day regimens will all result in resolution of symptomatology in uncomplicated cases of *C. albicans* infection. Vehicle and dosage schedule can be individualized, but in general, the lowest recurrence rates over time are noted with the longer treatment schedules and higher total doses. This is especially true in pregnancy.

In stubborn, resistant, or recurrent cases of candidal vaginitis, many factors may be responsible. Oral-genital contact accounts for some of these. In all patients with recurrent infections, diabetes should be suspected and ruled out by appropriate tests. The immune system plays a definite role in candidal infection. Transitory immune deficiencies can be produced by a variety of factors including pregnancy, oral contraceptives, and even stress. For example, recurrent candidal vaginitis is more common among student populations during the weeks of final examination.

Knowing the importance of the intestinal reservoir of the organism, it is helpful to decrease the size of the candidal population in the gastrointestinal tract by the use of oral nystatin. This medication is not systemically absorbed, and does nothing for the vaginal infection directly. However, by eliminating fungal colonies within the intestine, the inoculum of organisms present on the anal skin after defecation is appreciably reduced. Many women with recurrent candidal vaginitis have never been aware that wiping the anus from back to front can carry *Candida* organisms to the vagina. A three-month course of t.i.d. oral nystatin is given, along with proper hygienic instruction. Oral nystatin can also be used to "cover" the administration of broad-spectrum antibiotics when they are given for an unrelated indication. Finally, the male partner should be checked for possible surface infection of the penis, especially if he is a diabetic. If present, candidal balanitis can easily be treated with the same vaginal cream containing clotrimazole or miconazole, or else with a preparation of 5 per cent boric acid in lanolin (Borofax). Vaginal inserts consisting of gelatin capsules containing 600 mg of boric acid powder given h.s. $\times$ 2 weeks are helpful for female infections as well.

Potassium sorbate is a food preservative used to retard mold in many dairy products. Clinical trials have shown that a 3 per cent aqueous solution works equally well in retarding the growth of vaginal candida. It may be likened to a synthetic version of the fungal inhibitory factor produced by the normal flora. Pharmacies can purchase potassium sorbate NF as a powder and make up concentrated stock solutions that the patient then dilutes at home, but the wholesale drug is difficult to find. Some brands of proprietary hygiene products contain potassium sorbate, available both as a douche and as suppositories. These products are advertised only as "medicated" and identifiable as containing potassium sorbate only if one looks at the fine print on the label. Once recognized, such products are both easily obtained and convenient. They are best used just before and during the menses, after coitus, or whenever the patient notes the vagina is most susceptible to candidal overgrowth, and when supplementation of inhibitory factor may prevent another recurrent infection.

Ketoconazole is a potent antifungal drug, given orally and absorbed systemically. It has been effective in treating widespread mucocutaneous candidiasis and candidal septicemia, but its hepatotoxic side effects limit its use for simple vaginal infections.

GARDNERELLA

The most frequent bacterial pathogen affecting the vagina is the facultative anaerobe *Gardnerella vaginalis*. This organism has been officially named after Herman L. Gardner, M.D., who was the first to establish its role as a common cause of vaginitis and who performed the original studies that fulfilled Koch's postulates.

Herman L. Gardner was born in Fort Worth, Texas, and attended the University of Texas and its School of Medicine, graduating in 1937. His postgraduate work in Obstetrics and Gynecology was completed at the University of Nebraska, and he entered private practice.

As a prominent obstetrician-gynecologist in Houston, Texas, Dr. Gardner was a clinical investigator. His careful observations contributed a great deal to the understanding of vaginitis, and it was he who first suggested that an international society be formed to study vulvovaginal diseases. Along with Dr. Raymond H. Kaufman, Dr. Gardner published the first American text since Taussig's dealing with diseases of the vulva and vagina. Both men served as president of the International Society for the Study of Vulvar Disease, and they have done much to expand and disseminate our knowledge in this area.

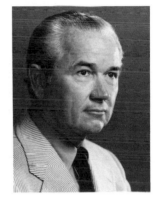
Herman L. Gardner, M.D.

Dr. Gardner achieved a rare distinction and well-deserved recognition when, in 1980, the International Journal of Systematic Bacteriology officially established a new genus for the organism he described. For many years it had been known as Hemophilus vaginalis *or* Corynebacterium vaginale, *but sophisticated bacteriologic studies showed that it lacked characteristics of both these genera and was, in fact, a unique organism. He did not care so much what the organism was called so long as the disease entity was recognized. He properly felt that the term "nonspecific" should not be used and worked until his retirement and death at his beloved Willow Springs, Texas, cattle ranch to achieve that goal.*

Gardnerella vaginalis vaginitis is a sexually transmitted disease that produces a characteristic odor often described as "fishy." As a rule, it is this feature of the infection that prompts the patient to seek advice. The odor is thought to be due to the presence of amines produced by anaerobic bacteria and released under alkaline conditions. Hence, the odor is usually first noted during coitus when buffered alkaline semen contacts the amines present in the vaginal pool. The same phenomenon may be noted by the clinician when gardnerella discharge is mixed with KOH for wet smear preparation.

On clinical examination, the vaginal pH will almost always be between 5 and 6. Any other pH reading practically rules out the diagnosis. The discharge is a gray homogeneous creamy material that wipes easily and cleanly from the vaginal walls. Erythema of the mucosa is not a prominent feature; in fact, this infection is associated with very little inflammatory response. Saline smears of this discharge show a paucity of white blood cells and a relatively clean background. Clusters of coccobacilli will often be found clinging to the surface of many of the desquamated epithelial cells. Such epithelial cells constitute "clue cells," and are characteristic of this particular vaginitis (Fig. 9).

21

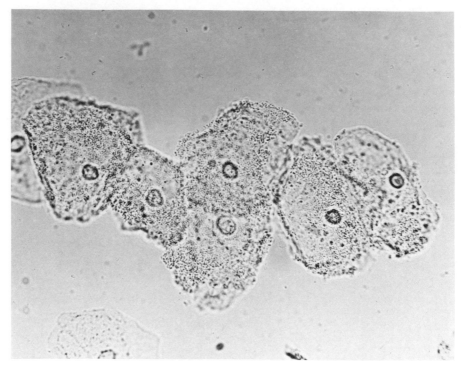

Figure 9. Saline smear of clue cells from *Gardnerella vaginalis* infection. Note clean background.

Laboratory confirmation of the diagnosis can be obtained by special culture of a vaginal swab specimen. However, the finding of clue cells in a gray discharge with a pH of 5 to 6 from a malodorous patient is sufficient to make the diagnosis of *Gardnerella vaginalis* infection, and further diagnostic study is generally unnecessary.

Therapy consists in the use of oral metronidazole 500 mg twice daily for five to seven days. In recurrent cases, the male partner should be treated simultaneously in a similar fashion, for, like trichomonas, the disease may be entirely asymptomatic in the male carrier. Although not impressive against gardnerella in vitro, metronidazole is effective clinically. This is probably due to the formation of an "hydroxy" metabolite that is formed by the oxidative metabolism of metronidazole and appears in effective concentrations in both the semen and the vagina after oral administration of the basic drug. In addition, this drug is active against other anaerobes that may be associated with the basic gardnerella infection. Ampicillin, 500 mg q.i.d. for five to seven days, has also been used with success. Cephradine, 500 mg q.i.d. for five to seven days, is reserved as the last line of defense to be used when all else fails. Given simultaneously to both partners, it is highly effective. *Gardnerella vaginalis* is very sensitive to hydrogen peroxide, which, when used in a dilute solution as a douche, can be a helpful adjunct to specific therapy.

TRICHOMONAS

Trichomonas vaginalis infection was formerly much more prevalent than it is today. Even so, as many as one in five American women may acquire this disease. The causative organisms are flagellated protozoa that may live quiescently in the paraurethral glands, and from this nidus of infestation cause overt infection in the susceptible vagina. *Trichomonas vaginalis* has been shown to survive for up to 24 hours in tap water at 20° to 30°C as well as in hot tubs, chlorinated swimming pools, and even dilute soap solutions. But the usual etiologic sequence begins with the deposit of a large inoculum of organisms contained in the buffered alkaline media of the semen at the time of sexual intercourse.

The primary complaint is that of a copious discharge, which may require the wearing of a perineal pad. Pruritus is another symptom frequently mentioned, but generally is a less prominent feature than with candidal infection. On examination, the vaginal epithelium is often intensely hyperemic. An abundant discharge is present that may sometimes have a frothy character, due to the presence of numerous small bubbles of carbon dioxide gas formed by the organism. There may be a greenish tint to the discharge, but generally it is an opaque grayish-white color, with a pH between 5 and 7. Discharge with a pH less than 5 is hardly ever associated with an active trichomonas infection, since the protozoa use glycogen at such a rapid rate there is little left to support normal acidogenic flora.

The classic "strawberry" appearance of the vaginal and cervical epithelium is a most unusual finding, noted in fewer than 5 per cent of infected women, most of whom are pregnant. When present, it is caused by small, papular, subepithelial abscesses that stand out as bright red granules or islets in a sea of thin discharge. It is from such an infection that the rare vaginitis emphysematosa may develop, as subepithelial bubbles of carbon dioxide from trichomonal metabolism coalesce into blebs.

A saline wet smear will show numerous motile organisms that have an ovoid

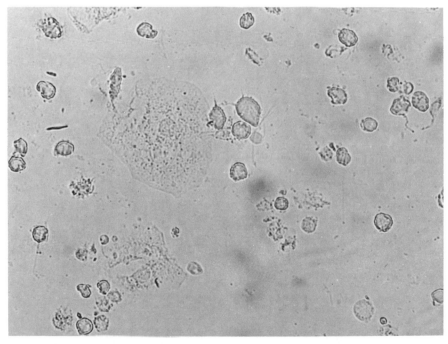

Figure 10. Saline smear with motile trichomonads in the center and nonviable forms mixed with white blood cells around the periphery.

or teardrop shape, and move independently of the fluid flow beneath the cover-slip (Fig. 10). On high dry magnification, tiny propellerlike motion is generally visible at one pole of the organism when the examiner focuses up and down. The whiplike flagellum may move slowly or rapidly at the other pole. The background will often show numerous white cells, since these organisms produce a vigorous inflammatory reaction. If the slide has dried or if the saline solution has become slightly hypertonic through evaporation, the organisms may appear spherical and lose much of their motility. Under these circumstances, differentiation from white blood cells or small intermediate cells of the vaginal epithelium can be difficult, but sometimes it is possible with careful focusing to see the reddish central inclusion in the trichomonads. The finding of greater than 10 WBC per high-power (40×) field on the wet prep is statistically associated with trichomoniasis even if the organisms cannot be positively identified.

Prior to the advent of the imidazole drugs (metronidazole, flunidazole, and nitrimidazine), therapeutic efforts were directed mainly at restoration of vaginal acidity in the hope that this change itself would be lethal to trichomonads. Micronized alum, free iodine liberators such as diiodohydroxyquin, and arsenical powders were used along with vinegar douches. However, no douche solution can produce more than a transient alteration in vaginal pH. Specific treatment is necessary and metronidazole has been consistently effective. "Resistant" cases are most often the result of reinfection, but strains of trichomonads with lowered susceptibility to metronidazole have been identified in the United States, and patients on antiepileptic medication metabolize the drug at an increased rate and so are relatively "resistant." An ordinarily effective dose of the drug (1 gm every 12h. × 2) is insufficient for these cases, which may require as much as 1 gm b.i.d. for up to 10 days. As a rule, a dosage schedule of 1 gm (4 tablets) in the A.M. and 1 gm P.M. in a single day produces both excellent trichomonacidal effect and a high level of patient compliance. Another successful regimen is the use of 500 mg q.12h. × 5 days.

The routine use of these drugs in the unexamined sexual partner is a controversial point. Unless reinfection occurs or chronic infection is established in the prostate or seminal vesicles, spontaneous decolonization of uncomplicated trichomonas infestation of the lower male urinary tract can be expected after three weeks. Many physicians routinely prescribe metronidazole for the coital consort in all cases; others point out a potential risk in prescribing drugs to treat an illness in a patient who has not been examined nor been shown to have the disease. Perhaps such use is best reserved for those cases in which the disease is recurrent and unresponsive to a single course of therapy, or in which trichomonads have been found in the male urine specimen. Nausea has been reported as a side effect during metronidazole therapy and may be aggravated by the simultaneous ingestion of alcoholic beverages. One old and effective remedy that is rarely used nowadays but that may be quite helpful in stubborn or frequently recurrent cases is the use of nightly douches with 20 to 25 per cent salt solutions. One cup of table salt stirred vigorously into four cups of water, and used as a douche, produces a transient hypertonic milieu that is lethal for trichomonads. In addition, the fungicide clotrimazole used as a vaginal cream for 10 days has been shown to be effective in eradicating trichomonads in over half of the cases investigated and may be an alternative to consider when metronidazole cannot be used, especially during the first trimester of pregnancy.

While specialized culture techniques are now available, routine vaginal swabs sent to a bacteriology laboratory in transfer media should not be expected to show trichomonads, even in cases of overwhelming infection. When the Pap smear is used as the only diagnostic method for trichomonas, both false-positive and false-negative results occur, giving an error rate of nearly 50 per cent. The saline wet smear, then, remains the primary diagnostic method for detection of clinical infection. Properly performed, this test alone can be used to determine the need for therapy.

ATROPHIC

The word "atrophic" is not synonymous with senile. Literally translated, it means "without nourishment" and, in this sense, is an accurate term for this group of patients. Throughout the premenarchal years and again after the menopause, the vaginal epithelium lacks the stimulation or "nourishment" of estrogen. As a result, the squamous cells proliferate at a slower rate, and differentiation into mature glycogen-containing forms does not take place. Consequently, the acidogenic flora are not present and the pH is high (6.5 to 7.5). Streptococci and coliform bacteria become more common in such an environment, while lactobacilli and corynebacteria are diminished. Fewer cell layers are present, so the epithelium is more susceptible to infection by a variety of different bacteria. Such conditions may prevail in the vagina during the physiologic states of childhood, pregnancy, lactation, and menopause. In addition, they may be produced by radiation or to a lesser and transient extent by oral contraceptives, clomiphene citrate, and danazol.

In children, foreign bodies may serve to carry *E. coli* and *Staphylococcus* and *Streptococcus* species to the susceptible vagina. Gut anaerobes may also be present, and sometimes the gonococcus may be transferred from an older sister by means of a wet towel or washcloth. But such infections are most often due to tiny fragments of feces-contaminated toilet paper that have been too zealously rubbed past the hymenal ring. The discharge is usually purulent and may have a distinctly foul odor if anaerobic infection is present. Visualization and culture of the vagina is not always necessary and may not be worth the potential emotional trauma. Instead, using only the force of gravity, room temperature physiologic saline is allowed to run from an IV bottle through the tubing of an intravenous administration set ending in the soft rubber connector that is held against the vulva by a nurse. This therapeutic "douche" is not uncomfortable and is frequently effective by itself, as the small bits of paper are rinsed out.

In recurrent cases, cotton swab culture and wet smear can almost always be obtained, even from the most uncooperative child. But a more thorough examination is necessary to rule out the presence of foreign bodies, if there is any blood present in the vaginal discharge or noted in the history. The gentle insertion of a long nasal speculum or veterinary (large animal) otoscope, combined with verbal anesthesia, will sometimes result in adequate visualization of the vaginal barrel. Otherwise, general anesthesia is necessary for complete examination and removal of all foreign objects.

Continued recurrence may be managed by stimulation of the vaginal epithelium with topical estrogen creams on a once-a-week basis until a more resistant membrane is produced. Instillation of conjugated estrogen cream directly from the tube is easily accomplished using a rectal tip applicator. Such administration should be discontinued after one or two months, however, since appreciable quantities of estrogen can be absorbed.

Pinworms (*Enterobius vermicularis*) are not uncommon in children and may result in a vaginitis when an adult worm migrates from the anus to the vagina. Such infection is usually accompanied by intense pruritus and rubbing, often most noticeable at nighttime. Presence of these parasites is easily confirmed by means of a cellophane tape slide preparation for ova. The sticky side of the tape is brought into contact with the perineal and perianal area and then placed adhesive side down on a microscopic slide. The large, double-walled eggs are quite characteristic (Fig. 11). A single dose of pyrantel pamoate suspension is generally sufficient to eradicate pinworm infestation, but attention must be given to the other family members as well. Mebendazole is similarly effective: a single chewable tablet is the recommended dose for adults and all children over the age of two. Cure rates of over 95 per cent are reported, but the drug is contraindicated during pregnancy.

During pregnancy, there is an abundance of vaginal glycogen and the pH is generally stable, although relatively alkaline. Parabasal cells are more common, and the overall balance is that of relative estrogen lack. The same is true during lactation, when many women notice irritation with coitus. This can be relieved by the twice-a-week use of conjugated estrogen vaginal cream throughout the period of breastfeeding.

Atrophic vaginitis is even more common at the opposite end of the age spectrum. After the cessation of ovarian function, the vaginal epithelium returns

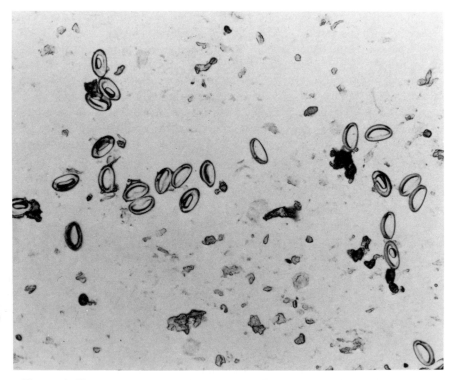

Figure 11. Pinworm ova on cellophane tape. Imprint from the perineum. Low power.

to the premenarchal state. The membrane is thin and composed of fewer cell layers, so there will be a paucity of well-differentiated glycogen-containing superficial cells. In far advanced years, only basal cells may be present. Under these circumstances, normal acidogenic flora will be absent, and the pH will be in the range of 6.5 to 7.5. Such an environment will support infection by a number of bacteria, and coliform bacilli, gut anaerobes, and the pyogenic cocci are the most frequent isolates. Trichomonas and candida infections are unlikely in the absence of estrogen replacement.

Because the epithelium is so thin and friable, inflammatory denudation frequently results in a rupture of the surface blood vessels; a pinkish or blood-tinged discharge is the result. The presence of bleeding from the vulvovaginal area after menopause is an alarming symptom and is generally the cause for seeking consultation.

On clinical examination, the vagina will have a pasty, pale appearance, and adhesion formation, with resultant agglutination of the fornices, may be noted. Such synechiae bleed easily when traumatized by the tip of the speculum blade or the examining finger. The discharge will show a relatively basic pH reaction. The character of this discharge is generally thin, scant, and yellowish in color. A Pap smear of the vagina and cervix is mandatory to rule out the presence of an unsuspected carcinoma—which alone could be the cause of an inflammatory exudate, resulting from secondary bacterial infection of a necrotic nidus of tumor. Wet smear examination shows numerous red blood cells, large numbers of inflammatory white cells, and the round or oval parabasal cells of the epithelium,

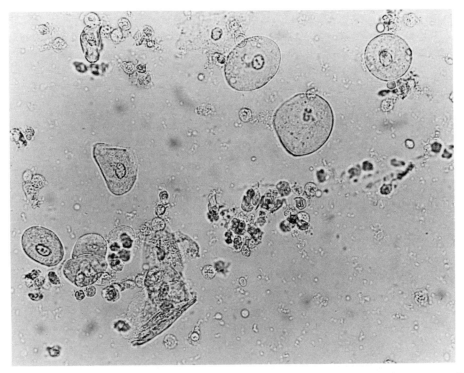

Figure 12. Saline smear of parabasal cells, red blood cells, and white blood cells from an atrophic vaginitis.

which have a relatively low nuclear-cytoplasmic ratio (Fig. 12). A bacterial culture will often result in the delineation of one or two predominant organisms.

Specific topical antibiotic therapy consists in the use of sulfa-containing creams, but their effectiveness will be greatly enhanced by the addition of topical estrogen. Once the initial infection is under control, future episodes can be prevented by the continued use of estrogen-containing creams on a twice-weekly basis. This may be necessary despite the use of oral estrogens. Some physicians use the vaginal maturation index as a guide to oral estrogen therapy. Nevertheless, there are patients whose vagina remains atrophic despite high doses of oral estrogen. Therefore, if vaginal differentiation is desired, topical therapy is the treatment of choice. Do not transpose this knowledge of vaginal pathophysiology to the vulva, which may also be the site of an atrophic change in this age group. The patient should be instructed not to use the estrogen-containing cream on the "outside" vulvar tissues, where it may slowly act to produce a paradoxical atrophy.

Douches are of little value in these women, and the douche nozzle can mechanically traumatize the delicate vaginal membrane. In the absence of an estrinized glycogen-containing epithelium on which the acidogenic bacteria may colonize, there is little that will permanently alter the pH.

OTHER CAUSES

Discharge not caused by candida, gardnerella, or trichomonas organisms, and not secondary to lack of estrogen stimulation, may be due to a variety of causes that we may conveniently call "other." Within this group there is little similarity; each specific cause has its own diagnostic criteria and its own therapy. To successfully treat such a patient, the cause of discharge must be correctly defined. The older literature used the term "nonspecific" when referring to this group but, as Gardner stressed so well, this is a misnomer. These causes are very specific; they are simply more difficult to isolate and recognize.

Physiologic discharge. Sensitized to the presence of infection from previous bouts of vaginitis, many women are alarmed by the presence of vaginal discharge despite the absence of other symptoms. A white opaque discharge, without itching or odor, associated with a normal pH and wet smear examination is "physiologic" and results from a mixture of cervical mucus and vaginal epithelial cells. The mucus may be more copious if a large cervical eversion is present or if oral contraceptives are used. The vaginal cells are shed in greater abundance under periods of emotional stress. At different times in a woman's life, more or less of this discharge may be present and each woman has her own threshold level at which point she finds it objectionable.

When the normalcy of all this is carefully explained, most women are able to cope with this phenomenon and adjust to it using panty liners to absorb the excess discharge. Tampons should not be used for this purpose. An alkaline douche may be helpful from time to time because it is mucolytic and acts to decrease slightly the population of lactobacilli, which in superabundance are said to cause an increased rate of cytolysis. The worst possible result occurs when the physiologic discharge is not accurately recognized and is treated as an infection. The normal flora are diminished by the therapy, ecological imbalance is produced, and a true vaginitis may result.

An iatrogenic discharge is produced after cryocautery or laser vaporization of the cervix. Such discharge may last for many weeks, but the patient may be reassured that it will cease and does not represent specific infection. By reducing the surface area of the eversion, such treatment may actually decrease the amount of physiologic discharge.

Human papilloma virus (*HPV*) causes *condylomata acuminata,* one of the genitotropic diseases seen with increasing frequency in sexually active patients. As a general rule, the patient will present with vulvar "bumps" or "warts," but vaginal and cervical involvement may be present independently. In fact, when the presence of koilocytotic atypia in routine Pap smears is used as the diagnostic criterion, the incidence of such infections on the cervix is relatively high. Frequently, these lesions are associated with a specific vaginitis, and the signs and symptoms of such an infection will be superimposed on the presence of small, papillomalike, warty growths, seen to be protruding from the surface of the vaginal or cervical squamous epithelium. At other times, only a fine granularity of the epithelium may be noted, or the lesions may be flat and circumscribed. A poorly understood symbiosis occurs between the virus and vaginal pathogens such that, with proper treatment of the vaginitis, the internal vaginal and cervical condylomata often regress spontaneously. On the other hand, the presence of pregnancy, the use of oral contraceptives, or other immunosuppressive influences will enhance the growth of these tumors and render almost any therapy of little value.

Topical caustics such as podophyllin or the halogenated acetic acids have no place in the treatment of vaginal and cervical condylomata. It is impossible for the patient to adequately neutralize the caustic compounds in these locations. When extensive intravaginal condylomata have been ill-advisedly treated with podophyllin, a severe desquamative vaginitis results and sytemic absorption of the drug, with subsequent neurotoxic effects, has been reported. Such patients need extensive irrigation of the vagina, with removal of as much caustic material and necrotic tissue as possible. The vagina must then be packed with a corticosteroid cream, and oral analgesia given as needed. Such dramatic sequelae can be avoided if the specific vaginitis is treated first and the stimulating causes eliminated, if possible. The use of sulfa-containing creams and suppositories is sometimes helpful, and, in the presence of pregnancy, these substances may retard the growth rate of the condylomata even if they do not produce complete eradication of the lesions. Destruction by laser beam, electrodesiccation, or surgical excision may be necessary.

Herpes simplex virus (*HSV*) *type II* infection, when confined to the cervix or vagina, is often asymptomatic. A thin watery discharge, of normal pH, may be present in cases of herpes vaginocervicitis, and with very careful inspection of the vaginal walls, small ulcers may be noted in the mucous membrane. Such ulcers are shallow and generally will have a pale yellow center surrounded by a bright red border. These lesions may be best appreciated through a low-powered colposcope and may be found anywhere from the squamocolumnar junction of the cervix down to the hymenal ring. Such lesions are rare, however, and "asymptomatic shedding" is more common.

In practice, therefore, the diagnosis is generally dependent on a viral culture or a Pap smear obtained from the cervix and vaginal pool, which demonstrates the cytopathic effect of the virus: clusters of "ground glass" nuclei, or multinucleated cells with eosinophilic intranuclear inclusion bodies. When such cells are noted by the cytopathologist, they may be reported on the Pap smear record as "atypical due to viral changes." Such a report should alert the clinician to the probable presence of herpes infection. Occasionally with herpes, a dramatic necrosis of the portio vaginalis of the cervix is seen, grossly resembling invasive carcinoma. However, both Pap smear and biopsy of such a lesion will show only necrotic debris, inflammatory cells, and sparse viral atypicalities. This finding has great clinical significance during pregnancy. If noted within one or two weeks of delivery, provided the membranes are intact, many obstetricians would elect to perform cesarean section rather than risk possible neonatal infection.

The virus can be inactivated with the use of 10 per cent povidone-iodine solutions painted on the cervix and vaginal walls during the office examination. The patient should continue the therapy at home with the use of twice daily douches of the same compound. Thymol solutions produce a similar result. Regardless, the active infection is self-limiting and the lesions resolve spontaneously within two or three weeks. Shedding of infectious virus then usually ceases, but asymptomatic shedding may recur at a later date. Since herpes infection is thought to play a possible cocarcinogenic role in cancer of the cervix, such patients are at higher risk for the development of squamous neoplasia and deserve close follow-up observation.

Purulent vaginitis is a description rather than a distinct disease. A persistent yellowish discharge is noted with an abnormally high pH. The saline smear shows abundant leucocytes, no protozoa, and no hyphae. Lactobacilli are absent but cocci are numerous. Cultures of such a discharge usually grow streptococci, and other bacteria may be present as well. The cause of this condition is frequently obscure. Management consists first in the eradication of pathogenic bacteria using both systemic and local antibiotics. Either povidone-iodine preparations or sulfa-containing creams are used locally each day for one or two weeks. In the office, the vagina is then examined and thoroughly cleansed prior to the application of an estrogen-containing cream. Beginning the following day, and throughout the next week, the patient douches daily with a lactobacillus culture using sweet acidophilus milk, plain yogurt, or dissolved granules in order to replace the normal flora and establish anew a healthy microenvironment. The milk is available in most markets and health food stores, and must be kept refrigerated. A pint at a time is then allowed to come to room temperature before use.

Psychosomatic vaginitis is a real entity, but fortunately it is rare. The complaints of vaginal pain, burning, and discharge usually suffice to neutralize any unwanted sexual advances. Unconsciously, these same complaints may form a defense mechanism when coitus is not desired. Such psychodynamics may be suspected in the patient whose complaints do not correlate with the normal physical findings. Usually these women have seen multiple physicians, report themselves "allergic" to most vaginal medication, and exhibit signs of severe emotional lability. Extensive counseling can often be of great benefit to these patients, but many resist the suggestion that their symptoms may be without organic cause.

Tampon-related problems rarely cause discharge but are important aspects of vaginal disease. Literally billions of tampons have been used by women without ill effect since their introduction by Dr. Earle C. Haas of Denver in 1933. Only recently have problems related to these products been identified. Large ulcers of the vagina, usually seen in one of the lateral fornices, are rare, but when present are most commonly caused by tampons. Such ulcers have a clean granulation tissue base with smooth, rolled edges of healing mucosa (Fig. 13). Treatment consists of the simple discontinuance of tampons. Minor mucosal alterations can be seen with a colposcope immediately after tampon removal. Areas of drying, layering, or peeling of the epithelium and microulceration have been reported. Such changes are transient and seem to have little clinical significance. Certain species of *Staphylococcus aureus* are capable of causing toxic shock syndrome. This disease has occurred in men, children, and nonmenstruating women and has been associated with vaginal diaphragms and sea sponges as well as postsurgical and postpartum infections. But the majority of cases occur during a menstrual period in women who use tampons. The tampon is probably inoculated with bacteria from the labia during the process of insertion. The cellulose fibers impregnated with menstrual exudate support the bacterial growth in the vaginal incubator. If toxin is produced and absorbed, a severe multisystem illness may result that is sometimes fatal. It is characterized by high fever, progressive hypotension, and a "sunburnlike" body rash. A purulent ulcerative

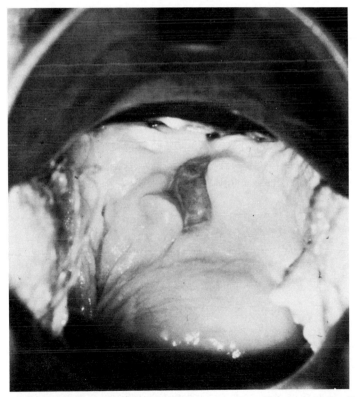

Figure 13. Tampon-related vaginal ulcer in anterior fornix. (From Friedrich, E.G.: Tampon effects on vaginal health. Clin. Obstet. Gynecol. 24:395, 1981.)

vaginitis is frequently found. Cultures of the discharge in these patients yield *Staphylococcus aureus,* which is penicillin-resistant. As an early step in management, the vagina should be thoroughly and completely cleansed and rinsed with a mild antiseptic. Fluid support, careful monitoring, and the use of β-lactamase–resistant penicillins are all indicated. Patients who recover report desquamation of their palmar skin within two or three weeks after onset of the disease.

Both minor mucosal alterations and toxic shock syndrome were statistically more frequent when superabsorbent fibers were used in the tampon. Once this was recognized, most manufacturers discontinued the use of such fibers in their tampons, and the incidence of both problems has now declined.

Every field of medicine has its boring and routine aspects, and office gynecology is no exception. However, there is no reason for failure to properly work up cases of vaginitis, no matter how common such complaints may be. When Dr. J. Marion Sims first inserted a bent spoon into the vagina of a patient in the knee-chest position, he was amazed by all that could be seen! He stated that he felt like ". . . an explorer in medicine who first views a new and important territory. . . ." We must try to rekindle some of that excitement. The use of pH paper and wet smears, combined with occasional cultures and cytologic studies, will result in a specific and accurate diagnosis in almost every case; and will enable the physician to prescribe intelligent and effective therapy. The frequency of iatrogenic vaginitis in the super-douched, overanxious, and poorly treated patient can be greatly reduced if such a protocol is followed. Once the vagina has been properly evaluated and the secondary effects of its diseases have been neutralized, attention can then be focused on the primary vulvar disease.

FURTHER READING

ECOLOGY

Hafez, E.S.E., and Evans, T.N.: The Human Vagina. Amsterdam, North-Holland Publishing Company, 1978.
> *A multi-authored collection of scholarly monographs on various aspects of vaginal physiology and pathology.*

Larsen, B., and Galask, R.P.: Vaginal microbial flora composition and influences of host physiology. Ann. Int. Med. 96:926–930, 1982.
> *A comprehensive discussion of the vaginal ecosystem.*

CANDIDA

Boquet-Jimenez, E., and San Cristobal, A.A.: Cytologic and microbiologic aspects of vaginal torulopsis. Acta Cytol. 22:331–334, 1978.
> *A rare paper with an excellent discussion and photographs of this condition* (Candida glabrata) *that deserves wider recognition.*

Rein, M.F.: Current therapy of vulvovaginitis. Sexually Transmitted Dis. 8:316–320, 1981.
> *A succinct presentation of therapeutic regimens available for candida, gardnerella, and trichomonas infections.*

Syverson, R.E., Buckley, H., Gibian, J., et al.: Cellular and humoral immune status in women with chronic candida vaginitis. Am. J. Obstet. Gynecol. 134:624–627, 1979.
> *This study suggests a lack of immune response in women with chronic candidal infection and documents the importance of the intestinal reservoir.*

GARDNERELLA

Gardner, H.L., and Dukes, C.D.: Haemophilus vaginalis vaginitis. Am. J. Obstet. Gynecol. 69:962–976, 1955.
The landmark study of this condition that fulfilled Koch's postulates and established the entity.
Osborne, N.G., Grubin, L., and Pratson, L.: Vaginitis in sexually active women: relationship to nine sexually transmitted organisms. Am. J. Obstet. Gynecol. 142:962–967, 1982.
An excellent study of the relative prevalence of these common pathogens in a middle-class population.
Vontver, L.A., and Eschenbach, D.A.: The role of gardnerella vaginalis in nonspecific vaginitis. Clin. Obstet. Gynecol. 24:439–460, 1981.
A thorough discussion of all aspects of this entity.

TRICHOMONAS

Andrew, D.E., Bumstead, E., and Kempton, A.G.: The role of fomites in the transmission of vaginitis. Can. Med. Assoc. J. 112:1181–1183, 1975.
A unique study of bathroom fixtures and washrooms, showing their lack of importance in the spread of disease.
Fleury, F.J.: Adult vaginitis. Clin. Obstet. Gynecol. 24:407–438, 1981.
A thoughtful analysis of over 20,000 cases of vaginitis, with many practical suggestions for diagnosis and therapy.
McLellan, R., Spence, M.R., Brockman, M., et al.: The clinical diagnosis of trichomonas. Obstet. Gynecol. 60:30–34, 1982.
Demonstration of the significance of high white cell count in abnormal discharge; contains excellent historic references.
Santler, R., and Thurner, J.: Contagiousness of trichomonas vaginalis. Wien. Klin. Wochenschr. 86:40–49, 1974.
This German article carefully documented the ability of trichomonads to survive at low temperatures, in tap water, in chlorinated swimming pools, and even in soap solutions.
Weston, T.E.T., and Nicol, C.S.: Natural history of trichomonal infection in males. Brit. J. Vener. Dis. 39:251–257, 1963.
A landmark study showing risk of infection and spontaneous remission rate in male consorts.

ATROPHY

Huffman, J.W., Dewhurst, C.J., and Capraro, V.J.: Premenarchial vulvovaginitis. Chapter 6. In: The Gynecology of Childhood and Adolescence. 2nd ed. W. B. Saunders Company, Philadelphia, 1981.
A complete and authoritative discussion of all pediatric aspects of vaginitis.

TAMPON EFFECTS

Friedrich, E.G., Jr.: Tampon effects on vaginal health. Clin. Obstet. Gynecol. 24:395–406, 1981.
A summary of the known changes associated with tampon use.

OTHER

Roy, M., Meisels, A., Fortier, M., et al.: Vaginal condylomata: a human papillomavirus infection. Clin. Obstet. Gynecol. 24:461–483, 1981.
A comprehensive introduction to the newer aspects of this old disease.

3

DIAGNOSIS AND THERAPY

HISTORY AND INSPECTION

PHOTOGRAPHY

TOLUIDINE BLUE TEST

SMEARS

CULTURES

SEROLOGIC TESTS

TOPICAL DRUGS

IMMUNOTHERAPY

All physicians and surgeons are familiar with the basic principles of diagnosis and therapy, and these are applied to vulvar diseases as to the diseases of any other organ. But the diagnosis of vulvar disease is not always straightforward and cannot be based on gross appearance alone. With practice and experience, certain features of some disorders become familiar and are readily recognized, but most involve a differential diagnosis. Fortunately, special techniques are available that will aid in this task.

Most vulvar diseases are managed with the same therapy applicable to other areas of medicine and there is no need to repeat those here. But some disorders of the vulva respond to specialized methods of treatment not familiar to all clinicians. These require explanation and discussion if they are to be used effectively and with understanding.

HISTORY

A truly complete medical history is a teaching exercise for students, usually supplanted in clinical practice by the preprinted form or computerized questionnaire. Each specialty emphasizes its own system review. But vulvovaginal diseases overlap a number of specialities, so the programmed history requires augmentation.

A familial background of diabetes, atopy, cancer, psoriasis, or other skin disease indicates a propensity for similar problems in the present case. Has the patient herself ever had cancer? Breast, genital, and gastrointestinal cancers may all be associated with separate and seemingly unrelated cutaneous manifestations on the vulva.

The method of contraception, coital frequency, and number of sexual partners all relate to vaginitis and the genitotropic diseases. Some afflictions of the vulva and vagina have a definite relationship to the menstrual cycle. The possible existence of an early pregnancy, indicated by a delay in menses, may limit the use of a great many drugs. For these reasons, a menstrual history should always be obtained.

The presence of known allergies should alert the examiner to the potentiality of reaction to soaps, deodorants, underwear fabrics, bleaches, or perfumed toilet paper. Even without an atopic background, these materials may act as irritants to sensitive individuals. A woman who was raised on a farm may have directly handled arsenical insecticides and after voiding in the field, she is likely to have used chemical-coated vegetation in lieu of toilet paper. Such chronic exposure to arsenicals has resulted in keratoses and carcinomata many years later.

The success or failure of previous therapeutic efforts is important. If the complaint is a subjective one, like pruritus or burning, the patient has probably noted what actions seem to relieve or aggravate the condition. Some women experience pruritus only after eating "acid" foods such as tomatoes or citrus fruits, and simple antacid tablets occasionally result in complete relief. Others note that their symptoms vary with their emotional state and regress in the absence of anxiety.

Few women will volunteer the symptoms of urinary incontinence or chronic diarrhea. Yet these conditions may result in a secondary vulvar reaction that clears only after correction of the primary problem. Direct questions regarding bowel and bladder function may therefore provide valuable clues.

With experience, each physician will find certain historical hints that have significance for his or her practice. Where hay fever is common, vulvar edema may be the presenting sign; a high rate of drug abuse brings an increase in the number of sexually transmitted diseases. Once identified, such local correlations can greatly improve diagnostic efficiency.

INSPECTION

Heading the list of diagnostic equipment is a pair of patient and well-trained eyes. Look at the vulva! Separate the crural folds and expose the intertriginous areas between the vulva and the thighs. Take note of the skin surfaces on the hair-covered mons and labia majora by parting the hairs with the examining hand. Separate the labia and expose the interlabial sulci. Look at both lateral and medial surfaces of the labia minora. Strip back the prepuce and expose the glans of the clitoris. Finally, observe the vestibule up to the hymenal ring. With a little experience, all of this takes less time to do than it does to read.

Many lesions are quite small; others cause subtle surface changes. Magnification is therefore essential to a thorough examination. Since the total average area of the vulva is approximately 200 sq cm, examination under excessive magnification would require an inordinate amount of time. For this reason, the colposcope is of relatively little value in the overall diagnosis of vulvar disease. But a simple 2× or 4× magnifying glass of at least three inches diameter permits rapid screening of the entire area under sufficient, but not inefficient, magnification. Such an instrument is an invaluable asset that should be kept handy in the examining table drawer. Examined in this way under good lighting conditions, very little vulvar pathology will go unrecognized. For larger clinics, the ideal instrument combines both a fluorescent light source and a magnifying lens at the end of a universal arm, and the entire unit is mounted on a rolling stand (Fig. 14). Such an instrument constitutes a "colposcope" for the vulva and greatly facilitates swift and accurate examination.

Colposcopy itself is not helpful for routine vulvar screening. The keratinized vulvar surface does not display characteristic vascular patterns. But once a lesion is identified, colposcopy is helpful for serial observation. The differentiation of vestibular papillae from early condylomata can be accomplished with the colposcope. Finally, pubic lice or nits or both are readily identifiable in situ under colposcopic magnification and no additional tests are required.

A Wood's light is a desirable, although not essential, piece of office equipment that can be helpful in vulvar diagnosis. Inexpensive hand-held models are available at most medical supply firms and contain one or two black light tubes. These bulbs emit a long-wave ultraviolet light above 3200 Å and are safe for producing diagnostic fluorescence.

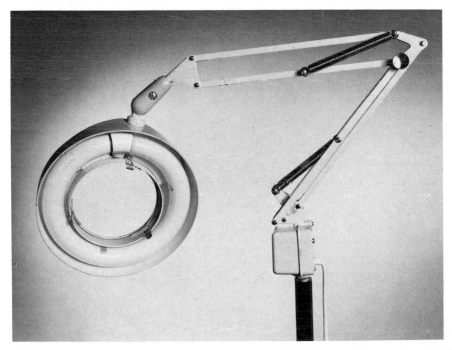

Figure 14. A fluorescent lamp encircling a low power magnifying lens provides excellent visibility for vulvar examination.

Diffuse irritating erythema of the vulva can result from a wide variety of causes. One of these is a superficial infection due to *Corynebacterium minutissimum*. Such infection is known as erythrasma, and while it is rare, it can be quickly recognized by its peculiar coral-red fluorescence under Wood's light. The organism produces porphyrins as part of its metabolism, and it is these compounds that exhibit fluorescence. Formerly, the tetracycline-induced fluorescence test (TIFT) was used in the diagnosis of neoplasia and required Wood's light inspection after tetracycline injection. Because of a lack of accuracy and repeatability, it is no longer recommended.

PHOTOGRAPHY

One diagnostic method often overlooked amidst the battery of laboratory studies is the simple observation of the natural course of the lesion. The life history of many diseases is unique and, while a nonspecific-looking ulcer or mass may be present at the first visit, the morphologic changes that take place during the ensuing weeks (or even months) can help to clarify the true nature of the lesion. A photographic record of the serial observations is therefore most helpful. This is especially true when following an untreated patient with carcinoma in situ, when treating vulvar dystrophies over a long period of time, and when trying to accurately evaluate the effect of therapy on any lesion. The longer the interval between successive observations, the more important this becomes. Few physicians are sufficiently gifted as artists to sketch an accurate picture in the office chart. But a simple color photograph preserves the subtleties of size and clinical appearance. If the photograph is then clipped to the chart, a permanent record is available for comparison at the next visit. Such documentation assumes particular significance in cases of trauma associated either with rape cases or with the battered child syndrome.

Simplicity and unobtrusiveness are the keys to success in patient cooperation and consent. Very few patients will object to photography of the vulva if it is simply explained, in a matter-of-fact way, that a routine photograph is necessary for documentation of clinical appearance. When this explanation is followed by the simple click of a shutter and a brief flash of light, little if any patient resistance is encountered.

In clinical practice, those cameras that produce an immediate color print are the most useful. For research and publication, color slides are preferred. A wide range of photographic apparatus is available, and the choice is largely dictated by budgetary limitations. Cameras can be plain or fancy, but should be able to function within a range of 2 to 18 inches. This range of focus allows for documentation of diffuse processes (involving the vulva, inner thighs, and buttocks), as well as small, isolated lesions (with fine subtleties of shade and hue). The total apparatus should be as simple as possible to operate. This spares both the physician and the patient the embarrassment of much fumbling around with lenses, rangefinders, adapters, and light meters. A foolproof and relatively inexpensive outfit can be obtained through most camera stores, utilizing the "Instatech" additions to the Kodak system.* This set has attachable close-up lenses

---

*Distributed by Lester A. Dine Company, Farmingdale, New York.

of varied fixed-focus distances. The attachments are designed to allow only the proper amount of light from the flashcube to reach the exposure area. One has only to place the focus frame on the lesion and click the shutter to obtain satisfactory results, in either the slide or print format. Polaroid outfits with close-up attachments are also well suited to this purpose and give acceptable color prints within a few seconds for immediate inclusion into the chart. A running record of which negative goes with which patient, or the use of numbered labels, is therefore unnecessary.

If clinical photography is beyond the scope of the physician, or is so infrequently used that its cost is not justifiable, then at least a crude sketch in the patient's chart should be made at the time of initial visit. Along with descriptive comments, such documentation is extremely valuable when following the natural course of a given disease.

TOLUIDINE BLUE TEST

The toluidine blue dye test was first used on the uterine cervix by Richart and later modified for vulvar use at the New Orleans clinic of Dr. Conrad Collins. It has become an extremely valuable diagnostic aid used to delineate suspicious skin areas for biopsy.

Conrad G. Collins, M.D., was born in 1907 and raised in Louisiana. He received his medical training and M.D. degree at Tulane University and completed his postgraduate work in obstetrics and gynecology at various hospitals in New Orleans. He remained in that city, becoming Chairman and Professor of the Department of Obstetrics and Gynecology at Tulane University, a post he held until his death in 1971.

He initiated the idea of a vulvar clinic in 1947 to organize the work-up, treatment, and follow-up of oncology patients. In 1950, the service expanded to include all vulvar diseases, and dermatologists, pathologists, and internists were present each week. This multidisciplinary approach was unique and provided an exceptional opportunity for mutual education at all levels.

Data were collected and published, new approaches were evaluated, and new ideas developed. The application of the toluidine blue test to the vulva is but one example. During his lifetime, Dr. Collins contributed a great deal to the understanding and appreciation of vulvar disease, and his clinic served as a model for those that followed.

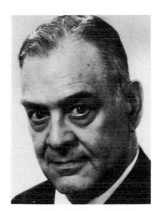

Conrad G. Collins, M.D.

Toluidine blue dye is a nuclear stain, and when applied in vivo it becomes fixed to cell nuclei. Dilute acetic acid decolorizes any dye that is not bound to nuclear material. In a normal keratin layer there are no surface nuclei; therefore, when used on a normal skin surface, the dye stains the skin and is then decolorized and washed away with dilute acetic acid. Nuclear material is present on the surface whenever there is a break in the continuity of the epidermis, as in an ulcer, or when nucleated squames are present in the uppermost epithelial layers. This latter condition is known as parakeratosis and constitutes an abnormality of squamous cell maturation (Fig. 15).

Parakeratosis alone does not denote cancer—it may also be found in benign conditions in which there is a rapid turnover of cells, e.g., condylomata acuminata. Nonetheless, where there is one hallmark of abnormal squamous matura-

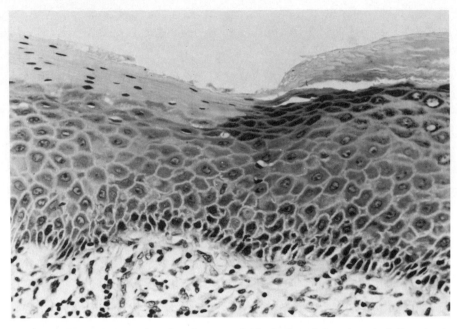

Figure 15. Parakeratosis (retention of nuclear material in the keratin layer) on the left contrasts with hyperkeratosis (a thick but acellular keratin layer) on the right.

tion, there may be others. Thus, parakeratosis can serve as a surface clue to an underlying epithelial atypicality of more severe degree.

It is unfortunate that many clinicians have little regard for this simple and important test. Failing to understand its basic method of action, they look upon it as a test for cancer and are understandably disappointed at the high number of "false-positives." There is really no such thing as a "false-positive" toluidine blue test. The test simply indicates the presence of superficial nuclei. The presence or absence of cancer can be confirmed only with biopsy. When confronted with a diffuse vulvar abnormality, then, the toluidine blue dye test may be used to direct biopsies, such that the most suspicious areas are sampled. This is the same advantage that makes the colposcope such a helpful instrument for cervical diagnosis; it directs the biopsy to the area most likely to contain an abnormality.

Another aspect of this test, which is rarely appreciated, derives from colposcopy, in which acetic acid by itself is used to dehydrate cells such that areas of increased density and atypia appear opaque and white. On the vulva, even when there is no retention of toluidine blue, areas of carcinoma in situ or cellular atypia may take on a white appearance and become more obvious because of this same phenomenon.

When performing this test, make certain that the vulvar skin is free of ointment, lubricant, or powder. Such vehicles mask areas of superficial nuclei by interposing a layer of foreign material impervious to the water-dye solution, much like a raincoat. A 1 per cent aqueous solution of toluidine blue is applied to the vulva with a large cotton swab. This is allowed to dry for one or two minutes, during which time excess solution can be absorbed with a dry sponge. Next, the entire vulva is rinsed gently with a 1 per cent aqueous solution of acetic acid.

Once again, the excess can be wiped away, but this action should not be vigorous or forceful. The skin has now been decolorized and a normally keratinized surface will show essentially no areas of adherent stain. With a little practice, spurious concentrations of dye, in smegma beneath the prepuce or in the interlabial folds, become obvious and these areas can then be ignored. Any other blue area, however, should be carefully inspected under a good light and preferably with some magnification.

With the exception of some basal cell cancers, most early squamous neoplasms exhibit a surface layer of either hyperkeratosis or parakeratosis. Ulcerated areas, even though they will stain a deep royal blue, are therefore not as suspicious as are areas of intact skin that have a bluish tinge. Often the depth of the blue color is not dramatic; still, this is an indication of parakeratosis and such an area should be biopsied. The vagina and the vestibular portion of the vulva are lined by squamous epithelium of the nonkeratinizing type wherein the uppermost layer of cells consists of nucleated squames. These structures should then be expected to take a light blue stain in the normal situation (Fig. 16).

Do not be confined by the toluidine blue test. All cancer is not parakeratotic—all parakeratosis is not cancer. Biopsy any area that looks suspicious whether it is white, gray, red, dark, raised, or flat. Choose a mature site, one where the process seems to have fully developed. Avoid the edges of a lesion where the change may be equivocal, and avoid areas of obvious necrosis and infection. But given a relatively homogeneous and extensive change, biopsy what seems to be a typical site and use the toluidine blue test to identify foci of parakeratosis.

SMEARS

The Papanicolaou (Pap) smear technique, applied to the cervix and vagina, has become a routine part of the pelvic examination and may reveal important clues that can be of great assistance in vulvar diagnosis. For example, if carcinoma is found to be present on the cervix, one should be particularly alert to the possibility of concomitant carcinoma in situ of the vulva. Diagnosis by exfoliative cytology depends on the shedding of cells whose morphology suggests the parent histology. Intact skin, however, including that of the vulva, is keratinized and so nucleated squamous cells are not shed from the superficial layers. For this reason, Pap smear of a vulvar lesion covered with intact epithelium is generally a futile exercise. Some cases of vulvar Paget's disease have shed diagnostic cells from the red "open" areas. Similarly, some cases of vulvar carcinoma in situ and invasive carcinoma are relatively nonkeratinized and may yield adequate cellular material. But in both diseases, biopsy is necessary for diagnosis; exfoliative cytology plays a limited role in diagnosis, but may be helpful in follow-up.

Ulcers, however, constitute breaks in the keratinized surface. Smears, then, can be of value in the differential diagnosis of ulcerative lesions: herpes, granuloma inguinale, and syphilis.

Herpes simplex virus (*HSV*) infections begin as fluid-filled vesicles that later erupt into shallow ulcers. Confirmation of the diagnosis of HSV can be made by viral isolation culture techniques or by cytology noting the cytopathic viral effect in desquamated cells aspirated from the vesicular fluid or smeared from

41

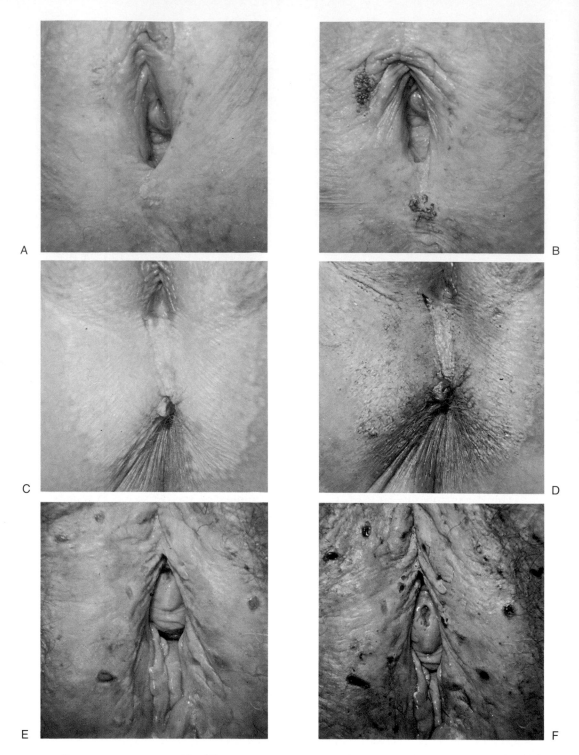

Figure 16. A and *B,* In this diffuse dystrophy, two areas of parakeratosis are revealed by the tolui-dine blue stain. *C* and *D,* A "butterfly" pattern of dystrophy showing no areas of dye concentration. *E* and *F,* Excoriated dystrophy with secondary ulcerations shows expected dye uptake in ulcerated areas.

Illustration continued on opposite page.

42

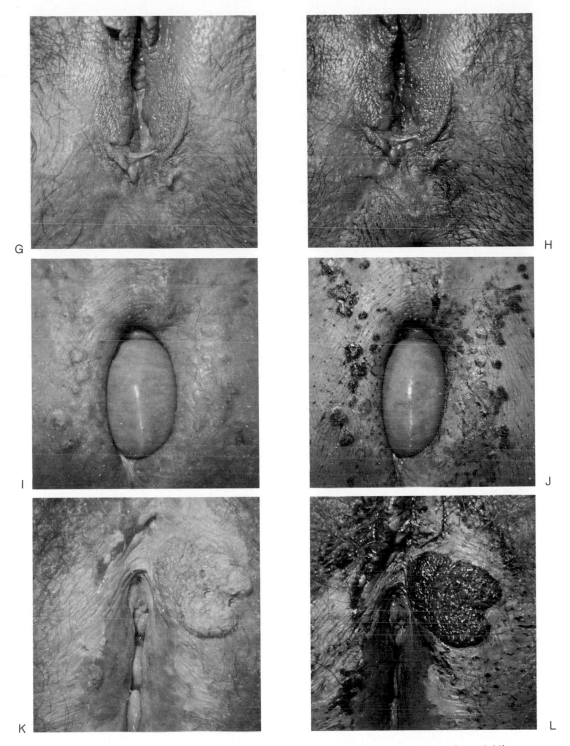

Figure 16. Continued. G and *H,* Perineal focus of carcinoma in situ clearly visible after toluidine blue. *I* and *J,* Pink papules in a post-vulvectomy patient represent parakeratotic sites of carcinoma in situ. *K* and *L,* Exophytic mass of invasive carcinoma stains deeply with toluidine blue.

the ulcer base. Scraping the ulcers with a wooden spatula is painful. But adequate material can be comfortably obtained with an "imprint technique," using the fully frosted Dakin-type slide or the frosted end of a common Pap slide. Frosted glass enhances the adhesion of cells that are suspended only in serum and lack the sticky mucus of cervical specimens. The frosted surface is simply pressed firmly against the ulcer. With only the barest suggestion of a wiping motion, the slide is removed and placed immediately in fixative solution. The accompanying laboratory slip should note if only the frosted end has been imprinted and that viral atypia is suspected. Thus forewarned, the cytotechnologist who stains and screens the slide will not reject it as a "blank" nor overlook the sometimes unfamiliar change of multinucleation, ground glass appearance, or intranuclear inclusion bodies characteristic of viral effect. Once this procedure has been established with the cytology laboratory, technical errors are infrequent and a reasonable degree of diagnostic accuracy is possible. Cytologic smears for HSV are not as sensitive as viral culture methods, and false-negative results do occur, but smears possess the advantages of speed, simplicity, and wide availability, and immunofluorescent methods increase the accuracy. Both smears and cultures are most reliable when performed on vesicular fluid. Once ulceration has occurred, the accuracy of both techniques drops sharply after three days and continues to decline thereafter.

Granuloma inguinale is caused by *Calymmatobacterium granulomatis*—an obligate intracellular organism. Serologic tests are not available for this disease. Smears and biopsies, therefore, represent the only methods of identification that are currently practical. When granuloma inguinale is suspected, a deep biopsy should be done from the growing edge of a cleaned lesion. In addition to the routine hematoxylin and eosin, both Giemsa and silver stains should be made of the tissue in order to recognize the pathognomonic macrophage cell with its "safety pin," bipolar-staining, cytoplasmic inclusions (Donovan bodies). Diagnostic accuracy in this disease is improved by the preparation of deep tissue smears made from the base of the excised tissue specimen and from the depth of the biopsy defect. Many such smears should be made on frosted and plain glass slides. Some should be air dried and others fixed, and submitted to both the microbiology and cytology laboratories. Wright's, Giemsa, and Gram's stain of these smears should be done and a patient, painstaking search is necessary if the elusive organisms are to be identified. Even a partial and inadequate amount of antibiotic therapy may result in complete disappearance of the Donovan bodies from an otherwise typical lesion. Failure to demonstrate their presence, therefore, should not preclude treatment instituted on the basis of the presumptive diagnosis.

Syphilis may mimic a wide variety of diseases. In the past, the dark-field examination of ulcer exudate was relied upon for diagnosis. But in many centers, this technique has become a lost art and has been replaced by the fluorescent-antibody dark-field test (FADF). In performing this test, the crust must be removed from the suspect lesion. The surface is abraded using a saline-soaked gauze sponge followed by a dry sponge until slight bleeding ensues. Do not use any soap or antiseptics, for these interfere with the test. Once light bleeding is established, the lesion is blotted until only clear serum exudes. A glass microscopic slide is then pressed against this serum such that the serum adheres to an area of about 1 cm diameter. The slide is allowed to air dry without a coverslip and is then sent to the laboratory in a closed container. The laboratory technician will incubate the slide with a fluorescent-labeled, antitreponemal globulin and examine it under a dark field. *Treponema pallidum* organisms, although non-motile, will be identified by their adherent fluorescence. Although this test is quite specific, sources of error are introduced by the multiplicity of steps in the process and the necessity for fresh, properly prepared fluorescent conjugate. Like the old dark-field examination, this test is only as good as the quality of the serous exudate obtained by the clinician.

Herpes simplex viral infections may be confirmed using a similar technique. Lesional smears are *AIR–DRIED*, not fixed, and sent to the laboratory for application of commercially available fluorescent antisera that is type specific.

Fungal smears are made and interpreted in the office. When a skin fungus is suspected, sample the active advancing edge of the lesion. Surface cells are scraped onto a glass slide using a scalpel blade. The scrapings are then pushed to one end of the slide and a drop or two of 10 per cent KOH solution is placed over them and covered with a coverslip. Gentle heating with a match or lighter speeds the action of KOH. While the slide cools, the keratin, cells, and debris will be hydrolyzed. Under high dry magnification, with the iris diaphragm partially closed, hyphae and spores will stand out against a relatively clear background (Fig. 17).

Parasitic smears for *Phthirus pubis* and *Sarcoptes scabiei* require some practice before the technique becomes routine. Both of these parasites can be detached from the skin by probing or teasing with a hypodermic needle. This should be done under a drop of mineral oil or small amount of surgical lubricant placed on the skin surface. This will prevent accidental loss of the tiny specimen caused by resilient hairs or room air currents. Once on a glass slide and under a

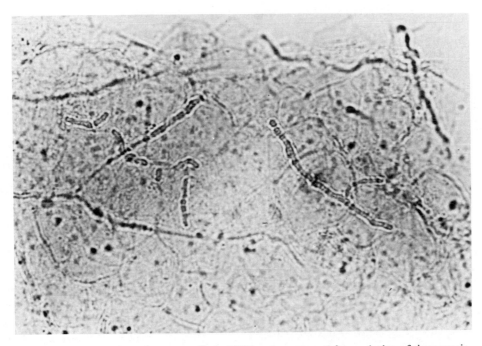

Figure 17. Trichophyton rubrum mycelia in KOH smear prepared from a lesion of tinea cruris.

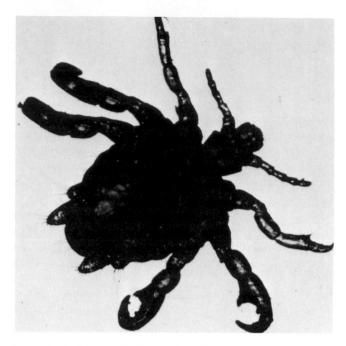

Figure 18. Crab louse (*Phthirus pubis*)—low power microscopic view.

coverslip, the parasite can be securely transported to the microscope. With the 10× objective, the pubic louse will be seen to have a rounded body with three pairs of crablike legs terminating in circular claws that are used to grasp the hair shafts (Fig. 18). The blood-filled digestive tract, shaped like a horseshoe or wishbone, is generally visible through the plated, transparent body. The scabies mite is similar in size and general body shape, but it lacks the lateral legs and claws. Instead, two triangular hairy buds are seen on either side of the anterior mouth parts.

But it is rarely necessary to go to such lengths for confirmation. The colposcope is sufficient for positive identification of the pubic louse in situ, and the burrow ink test readily identifies scabies. With this latter test, an inexpensive fountain pen is used to allow ink to run over a suspect site. The ink that runs down the burrow of a mite will not wipe away with alcohol but, rather, outlines the burrow and directs a shallow shave biopsy, which is then examined like a smear for evidence of scabies.

CULTURE

Swabbing a vulvar lesion with a cotton-tip applicator and submitting this for routine culture is a complete waste of time. Skin bacteria will be found and reported, but no special attempt will be made to isolate or identify any of the special fungal species, viruses, or bacteria that especially pertain to vulvar disease unless the laboratory is previously alerted. Special media and techniques are required to isolate such organisms. It is not necessary for the clinician to know all the details of such isolations, but an appreciation of the complexities involved is helpful in assessing the value of a negative report.

When esoteric fungal species are suspected, laboratory culture on Sabouraud's slants should be requested. In vitro growth is slow, however, and reports may not be available for two or three weeks. A reliable method for the in-office differential diagnosis of trichophyta and candida by culture is the use of DTM (dermatophyte test medium). Commercially supplied by Pfizer Diagnostics, small bottles of this medium are easily stored in an office refrigerator. The medium contains a mold inhibitor, two antibacterial antibiotics, and a pH indicator. Suspicious lesions should be cleansed with 70 per cent alcohol. Surface scrapings are then inoculated into the vials and incubated at room temperature for one or two weeks. Care must be taken not to twist the cap tightly closed, since this would result in the exclusion of air and prevent proper growth of the organisms. The growth of a dermatophyte changes the medium color from yellow to red, and produces a characteristic whitish colony. Saprophytic contaminants from the skin will not produce a color change. *Candida albicans* produces a growth with easily recognizable morphology even though the yellow medium may sometimes turn red. For vulvar use, this test allows for rapid differential diagnosis between a cutaneous candidal infection and the more unusual tinea cruris infections caused by dermatophytes.

Positive identification of *herpes simplex virus* (HSV) can often be made on the basis of cytologic smear, but false-negative results are not uncommon, especially when the ulcers have been open for more than three days. Viral isolation culture techniques also become progressively less reliable as the lesions mature, but in general, culture is more sensitive. The material should be harvested from the lesion using a prepackaged swab-medium combination or an ordinary swab, which is then immersed in a viral transport medium. Once at the laboratory, these swabs will be used to inoculate cell culture monolayers made from locally obtained fibroblasts or commercially prepared culture kits. Cells infected by virus round up and detach from the layer in a characteristic fashion. If there is an average population of virions present, the results will be obvious in 24 to 48 hours. Up to one week is required to be certain of negativity, however. Culture techniques are not microbiologic miracles and will not substitute for a clinical assessment and the use of simpler methods. They are a part of the diagnostic chain that must be used with understanding and perspective and, in this manner, may yield valuable information.

SEROLOGIC TESTS

Serologic tests require only samples of the patient's blood and are helpful in the diagnosis of syphilis, herpes simplex (HSV), and lymphogranuloma venereum (LGV).

Syphilis detection has relied on serologic reactions for many years. The Venereal Disease Research Laboratories (VDRL) reaction measures the reactivity of a patient's serum to an antigen prepared from beef heart (reagin). If positive, this reaction can be quantified and is reported as either 1+ to 4+, or in terms of dilution, i.e., 1 dil. to 4 dil. Positive reactions, in the presence of suspicious clinical findings, are highly indicative of syphilitic infection, past or present. In the absence of clinical suspicion, however, a reactive VDRL must be verified. Both temporary and chronic biologic false-positives occur, often associated with "autoimmune" disease such as lupus erythematosus, chronic active hepatitis, and rheumatoid arthritis, as well as with heroin addiction, pregnancy, LGV, and conditions involving active tissue regeneration. Therefore, the serologic result does not give a definite answer regarding the presence of syphilis. It simply provides one piece of evidence that must be interpreted as a part of the entire clinical picture.

A serologic card test, based on the same reagin reaction, is now used in many centers. The rapid plasma reagin (RPR) card tests require unheated serum or plasma, or can use blood from a finger puncture, and are helpful in large-scale screening. But the card test and the VDRL are both nonspecific and, if positive, require further investigation with specific treponeme-based test.

The fluorescent treponemal antibody absorption (FTA–ABS) test is the most widely used and reliable of these. In the laboratory, nonviable *T. pallidum* organisms are mixed with the patient's serum. Antibody globulins present in the serum of syphilitics coat these spirochetes. After removal of substances that might react to *T. pallidum* in a nonspecific manner, fluorescent-tagged antihuman globulin is then added to the slide. The presence of fluorescent organisms indicates *T. pallidum* antibody production by the patient. Quantitation is again possible; a rising titer indicates active disease, while a falling titer is associated with successful therapy. While sporadic false-positive results have been reported in patients with elevated or abnormal immunoglobulins, these reactions are rare and the FTA–ABS test is often relied on to determine whether a reactive VDRL is due to latent syphilis or is a biologic false-positive result. The FTA–ABS is sensitive in both the very early and the very late stages of syphilis, and usually remains positive for a long time after treatment. Over 70 per cent of cases with a syphilitic chancre will show serologic reactivity when first examined because of both patient and physician delay. The VDRL and FTA–ABS tests should, therefore, be obtained in all suspected cases of primary syphilis and, if negative, they should be repeated in four to six weeks. Virtually 100 per cent of those with secondary syphilis will show a positive reaction.

Herpes simplex virus infections may also be confirmed with serologic methods. Complement fixation (CF) tests are delicate, indirect measurements of the ability of a patient's serum to undergo reaction with a known antigen and bind complement in the process. Unbound complement is measured in a second step by means of a hemolytic reaction to sensitized erythrocytes. The more hemolysis seen, the more unbound complement is present and the less the specific antibody titer in the patient to the specific antigen being measured. All the necessary reagents are available from commercial sources for the detection of herpes simplex antibodies by means of complement fixation tests, and most laboratories are equipped to perform these procedures.

The first commercial herpes antigens required the use of paired sera from the patient and a positive reaction was based on the difference between the acute and convalescent phase samples. Current tests make use of other antigens and are capable of detecting infection with a single blood sample. They are especially helpful later in the course of the disease when cultures and smears are no longer reliable.

Lymphogranuloma venereum is a difficult disease to identify with certainty and a positive CF test is the only means of confirmation, since the intradermal Frei test was discontinued. Paired serum samples are requested, and a fourfold rise in titer occurring in a patient with clinical evidence of the disease is considered to be positive. Patients with LGV, however, rarely present early in the course of the disease, as the initial lesion is often asymptomatic and evanescent. Therefore, a high CF titer (1:64 or greater) is frequently present by the time the patient is first seen and should be considered as positive evidence of infection. Only rarely is a fourfold increase observed. Nor is the physician usually willing to wait two or three weeks with a patient with enlarging inguinal nodes before beginning therapy, in order to get the maximum antibody response. On the other hand, if the patient received any antibiotic therapy shortly after infection, she might never develop antibody to the LGV chlamydia, and the CF tests would remain negative despite the presence of infection. A single CF test should therefore be sent at the time of initial consultation. Treatment can then be started empirically on the basis of the clinical diagnosis.

TOPICAL DRUGS

Successful management of many vulvar diseases depends on mastery of the art of topical therapy. An axiom of dermatology states that the more acute, exudative, or ulcerative the lesion, the gentler should be the therapy. A topical application consists of an active drug suspended in a vehicle. In order of decreasing gentleness, the common vehicles include: wet dressings, lotions, creams and ointments, and pastes.

Wet dressings are helpful in acute ulcerative diseases like herpes infections, during the initial phase of post electrosurgical and laser healing, and in groin wound separation occurring after radical vulvectomy. In each of these instances, an aqueous solution is applied by means of a saturated piece of fabric or by immersion. If fabric is used, fine mesh gauze or batiste is the best material, but an old piece of cotton bedsheet or a well-worn washcloth serves almost as well. Wet dressings are, paradoxically, drying agents. The evaporative process that occurs on the surface of the dressing removes moisture from the lesion and gives a cooling, soothing sensation.

Creams and ointments are both emulsions that differ in the proportion of water to oil that each contains. A cream is a suspension of oil in water, while an ointment is a suspension of water in oil. Creams are more easily removed and are generally preferable for use on delicate tissues like the vulva. Ointments are difficult to remove, cause heat retention, and by trapping moisture beneath the oily layer, their use may result in maceration. Nevertheless, some compounds like testosterone propionate are most effectively absorbed from an ointment vehicle, which therefore cannot be avoided.

Pure mineral oil is an excellent vulvar cleanser and may be confidently recommended in place of soap for routine vulvar washing. Mineral oil is a soothing, gentle solvent for the skin oils and their contained debris. It is particularly beneficial when other cleansing agents have caused irritation.

Pastes are combinations of powders and ointments and lie at the opposite extreme from wet dressings. They are used to coat or protect the vulvar skin from irritating external moisture. Patients with urinary incontinence, recalcitrant vaginal discharge, intestinal fistulae, or draining sinuses may all benefit. Common formulas for protective pastes usually include equal parts of white petrolatum and a powder containing approximately half-and-half of zinc oxide and starch.

As noted, some drugs are best suited to specific vehicles. Those effective on the vulva can be divided into the aqueous solutions, the steroids, and the cytotoxic agents.

Aqueous Solutions

Burow's solution is one of the commonest active agents used in wet dressings. It is a dilute aqueous solution of 5 per cent aluminum acetate, and is both an astringent and an antiseptic. As such, it is useful for the initial therapy of any weeping ulcerative disorder, especially herpes (HSV-2) infections and acute excoriations secondary to pruritus from whatever cause. Pharmacists will dispense bottles of Burow's solution, but the transport of large volumes may be a problem for the patient. Alternatively, Domeboro tablets or powder packets of premixed dry chemicals are available. These are simply added to a volume of water at home according to the supplied directions. Burow's solution is not used full strength but rather diluted 1:10, 1:20, etc. Evaporation of the wet compress results in concentration of the chemical, so it is best to begin with a higher dilution. One tablet or powder packet in one pint of water gives a 1:40 Burow's solution. If the dilute solution is kept in a refrigerator, the cold wet dressing will be even more soothing. A rectangular strip of gauze or cloth, large enough to cover the vulva, is soaked in a bowl of the solution and laid gently on the affected area. The patient may place a thick towel under her buttocks to absorb any excess solution. During the 30 minutes or so that the dressing is in place, more solution can be added with an irrigating syringe or a simple tablespoon, but the compress should not be allowed to become completely dry.

Natural or artificial sea water produces a similar effect. A prepackaged powder of sodium chloride, magnesium sulfate, and other salts is obtainable under a variety of brand names at stores that sell aquarium supplies. Dilution directions are given by the gallon, which is ideal for a tub large enough for vulvar immersion. Sea-water soaks relieve the pain after laser and electrosurgical procedures and aid in healing.

Silver nitrate in a 0.25 per cent solution is another astringent and antiseptic, which in addition promotes the development of granulation tissue. It is of greatest use in the continuous wet pack therapy of wound separations—particularly those that occur in the groin after radical vulvectomy. In the early stages of treatment, a single layer of fine mesh gauze should be applied to the necrotic areas and soaked with the silver nitrate solution. Evaporation is then allowed to take place and the dressings are removed when dry. Minor débridement is thus achieved. Once the areas are clean and free of all necrotic tissue, multiple layers of gauze are applied and kept constantly moist with the solution. This will stimulate a profuse granulation tissue response that will have a bright pink cobblestone appearance. Such tissue rapidly fills in the defect caused by the separation. Once flush with the surface epithelium, the growing edge of the epidermis will re-cover the defect. Silver nitrate will tint the surrounding normal skin to a brownish-black color, but this effect is temporary and disappears soon after stopping the compresses. During therapy, the silver ions will form salts with the patient's chloride. The serum electrolytes must therefore be monitored and replaced as necessary with supplemental sodium and potassium chloride.

Steroids

Corticosteroids are anti-inflammatory, promote healing, and produce atrophic effects on the skin. They are therefore useful on a short-term basis to assist the healing of many ulcerative disorders and reduce the inflammatory aspects of acute reactive vulvitis and some superficial infections. They are used over a somewhat longer period in cases of hyperplastic dystrophy, in which their atrophy-producing properties become an asset instead of a liability. To an extent, the more potent the steroidal compound, the shorter the treatment time. Plain 1 per cent hydrocortisone cream, for example, may require months to achieve what a more potent steroid can accomplish in a matter of days or weeks. In decreasing order of potency, the common drugs in use include: halcinonide (Halog), fluocinonide (Lidex), triamcinolone acetonide (Aristocort, Kenalog), fluocinolone acetonide (Synalar), betamethasone valerate (Valisone), and hydrocortisone (Cortdome). Each of these is available in a variety of concentrations and vehicles for specialized used. In general, any steroid is more potent in an ointment base and somewhat less so as a cream. In most cases, it makes little difference which of these preparations is chosen, but it is wise to choose one and become thoroughly familiar with its performance. Only when you know what to expect from one compound can you evaluate others by comparison.

Itching is a major feature of most vulvar lesions amenable to topical corticosteroid therapy. Relief from this symptom can be accomplished by using steroids alone, but the antipruritic effect will be greatly enhanced if crotamiton (Eurax) is added to the mixture. A cream containing 7 parts of betamethasone valerate (Valisone) and 3 parts Eurax works particularly well for hyperplastic dystrophies and is also helpful in seborrheic dermatitis. Applied twice daily, morning and bedtime, results can be expected in about two weeks. Continuation of therapy after that time depends on the particular lesion. Very thick hyperplastic lesions may require many weeks of treatment unless occlusive dressings are used, and these are difficult to apply to the vulva. Once the skin has been restored to normal, however, the treatment should be stopped. Chronic use of unopposed topical corticosteroids can result in atrophy and, in the long run, lead into more difficult problems than the original disease. When these compounds are used only on the vulva area, over a short period of time, and without occlusive dressing, systemic absorption with subsequent adrenal suppression does not become clinically significant, and secondary cutaneous atrophy or striae have not been observed.

R_x Valisone   7 parts ⎱
      Eurax   3 parts ⎰ cream
      DISP: 4 oz (120 gm)
      SIG: Apply b.i.d.
      Will last approximately four weeks.

Testosterone is the main trophic hormone for skin. It is unopposed androgen that accounts for the thicker, more hairy, and more oily skin of the male; whereas these effects in the female are offset by the presence of estrogen. Estrogen has a mild atrophic effect on skin, hence its use in common cosmetics to decrease sebum production and hair growth and give a fine smooth texture to the skin.

Skin disorders that are characterized by lack of growth, such as lichen sclerosus dystrophy, should therefore be stimulated with testosterone. It is a common misconception, particularly among gynecologists, that since estrogen is the trophic "female" hormone, it must have a positive effect on the vulvar skin. In fact, the opposite is true; since the vulva is composed of skin, estrogen will only antagonize whatever endogenous androgens may be present and the result is even further atrophy. Evidence for this can be seen in cases of XY individuals with androgen insensitivity (testicular feminization syndrome). The vulvae of such patients are relatively lacking in hair and sebaceous glands, and the epithelium is quite thin and fragile. The fact that the in utero exposure of a female fetus to androgens results in genital masculinization suggested the presence of receptor sites for androgens in vulvar tissue even before they were demonstrated in dermal fibroblasts from the labia majora. In addition, the effects of various steroids on the metabolism of aging skin have been well studied and lend further support to the rationale for the use of testosterone in lichen sclerosus. A number of well-controlled studies have now been published on the effectiveness of testosterone and its metabolites in the treatment of lichen sclerosus vulvar dystrophy, and all confirm its effectiveness over long periods of time and in many parts of the globe.

At present, there are no commercially manufactured preparations of topical testosterone. Each prescription must be compounded by the local pharmacist. Two per cent testosterone propionate in white petrolatum should be used. The testosterone propionate is available in sesame oil for injection and can be obtained from wholesale drug houses in multiple dose vials containing up to 100 mg/ml. Three vials (30 ml) of this hormone, thoroughly mixed into 120 gm of white petrolatum USP, provide 4 oz of medication, enough to last eight weeks. An ointment vehicle is necessary to potentiate this steroid, since the hormone is not sufficiently absorbed into the dermis from water-soluble bases. Only a small amount is required at each application and should be thoroughly massaged into the affected skin. Since lichen sclerosus results in loss of the epithelial rete pegs, vigorous or rough massage can cause ecchymoses. The application must, therefore, be gentle but thorough. A mass of ointment about the size of a kidney bean (0.5 gm) is sufficient to cover the entire labia majora, minora, and prepuce, and contains about 8 to 10 mg of testosterone. This application is performed two or three times daily in the first six weeks of treatment and can be decreased thereafter once an effect has been observed.

Maintenance therapy is mandatory. Unlike corticosteroids, testosterone must continue to be used or else the signs and symptoms will recur. Most cases of lichen sclerosus dystrophy can eventually be controlled for an unlimited time by applying testosterone only once or twice a week. The initial phase of the treatment, however, usually requires four to six months. The macerating tendency of ointments has already been mentioned. If ulceration occurs with the use of testosterone in petrolatum, the drug should be discontinued until the ulcers heal. (A week or so of corticosteroid cream will usually bring this about.) Testosterone is then reinstituted on alternate days only, with corticosteroid cream used on the days testosterone is not applied. These two medications are, to some extent, antagonistic. But over a period of 12 to 24 months, the trophic effect of the testosterone will prevail. In the meantime, the patient is free of symptoms and the vulvar skin is slowly returning to a more normal state. Clitoral hypertrophy, increased libido, and aggravation of pre-existing facial hair growth are sometimes observed as undesirable side effects of this therapy. Serial measurements of plasma testosterone levels, however, have failed to show significant systemic absorption. Libido increase can be particularly troublesome for elderly women who have no opportunity for sexual contact. They may be frightened and distressed by the reactivation of these dormant thoughts and desires. Masturbation may be sought as an outlet, and if guilt and anxiety occur, it may be necessary to discontinue the drug. Similarly, testosterone is unsuitable for use in young children because of the masculinizing effects.

> R_x Testosterone propionate 2 per cent in white petrolatum.
> DISP: 4 oz (120 gm)
> SIG: Apply gently with fingertip as directed, b.i.d.
> Amount will last approximately eight weeks.

Progesterone has been used successfully in those cases of dystrophy unresponsive or unsuited to testosterone. It is helpful in the treatment of childhood lichen sclerosus when applied twice a day, and also for those few adult women who develop intolerable testosterone side effects. Again, there is no commercial preparation that can be purchased and the pharmacist must compound it on an individual basis using progesterone in oil, 100 mg per 1 oz (30 gm) of hydrophilic ointment or cream.

It is probable that since progesterone is the parent compound for the other steroids, the drug is locally converted to both cortisone and testosterone before exerting its final effect. Such a mechanism would also explain the clinical observation that topical progesterone works much more slowly than do the other steroids.

> R_x Progesterone in oil 400 mg in 4 oz Aquaphor
> DISP: 4 oz (120 gm)
> SIG: Apply b.i.d.
> Amount will last four to six weeks.

Cytotoxic Agents

Podophyllin is not a single compound but rather denotes a resinous mixture of extracts from the horizontal root (rhizome) of the mandrake or mayapple plant (podophyllum peltatum). Podophyllotoxin is one of the active compounds in this resin, which was used as a per oral cathartic many years ago. If significant quantities are absorbed systemically, neurotoxicity and even death can result. Teratogenic effects and vascular compromise of the decidua can occur with systemic absorption during pregnancy. Use of this drug is therefore contraindicated during gestation. Podophyllin should not be applied to the cervix or vagina, since the patient cannot easily remove it from these areas and both systemic absorption and tissue necrosis may result. The drug has a colchicine-like effect, especially evident in rapidly growing tissue. Although it is of little value in the treatment of any other condition, even other warts, it is effective in causing regression of some venereal warts (condylomata acuminata). New growths, tiny seedling lesions, and the white, filiform, frondy papillomas are most likely to regress after podophyllin. Flat, pigmented, older lesions generally exhibit little response.

Failures of podophyllin therapy usually result from expecting too much from this topical drug. It is not a panacea and cases should be carefully selected. It should never be applied for diagnosis with the idea that if it works, the disease must be condylomata, and if it does not, then perhaps it is carcinoma. Susceptible lesions on the external vulvar surfaces will often disappear after two or three applications of podophyllin no more than a week apart. Large lesions on the skin, those on the vagina and cervix, and those occurring during pregnancy are better treated by other means. For appropriate cases, a 25 per cent solution of podophyllin in compound tincture of benzoin should be applied with a cotton-tip applicator. At least two coats of solution are used. The first application is allowed to dry and form a sticky base before the next coat is applied.

Podophyllin works over a period of time, exerting its effect primarily on dividing cells. It is a potent drug, and exposure times should be carefully regulated. It should be left in place for no more than four to five hours and then deactivated with soap and water; this prevents damage to normal adjacent skin. Used in this manner, it is unnecessary to protect the surrounding area with petrolatum. Such protection may even be self-defeating, since the ointment may contact the wart and prevent proper absorption of drug.

Podophyllin in alcohol is a solution that cannot be accurately confined to diseased tissue. The same objection pertains to preparations of podophyllin in petrolatum or mineral oil. These vehicles are difficult to control when trying to achieve precise application and localization, and their removal is often incomplete, with resultant overexposure and tissue necrosis. The benzoin vehicle, however, is sticky and adheres to the surface of the condyloma without running over onto large areas of normal skin. If the saturated cotton applicator tip is rotated into the wart, the material will get into all the crevices of the filiform lesion and penetrate better into the epithelium. The adhesive qualities of the benzoin can be undesirable if the coated lesion adheres to an unaffected area when the patient's legs are brought together. This can be avoided by lightly powdering the treated lesion with talc before allowing the patient to get up from the examining table. Podophyllin application should be done only in the office, under direct vision. Preparations of podophyllin should never be given to a patient for self-application at home.

Podophyllin "burns" result from overexposure. They are quite painful and require immediate attention. After thorough washing of the lesion, wet dressings of cold 1:40 Burow's solution are applied two or three times a day. After drying, the area should be covered with a corticosteroid anti-inflammatory cream or lotion, preferably containing an antimicrobial compound. Oral analgesics may be necessary, but such treatment will usually afford prompt relief of pain, stop further necrosis and slough, and promote uncomplicated healing.

The histologic effects of podophyllin have been well described and may mimic some of the atypical changes seen with carcinoma in situ. Formation of corps ronds, abundant mitoses, and large pale cells with chromatin grains ("podophyllin cells") may all be seen. A correct interpretation of condyloma biopsies is therefore more difficult if the lesion has been recently exposed to podophyllin. These effects diminish with time but may last six weeks or more. For this reason, the drug should not be used for one to two months prior to contemplated biopsy, and the information slip that accompanies a tissue specimen should indicate the date on which the drug was last used.

Halogenated acetic acid has been used by dermatologists for many years to destroy cutaneous lesions. Like nitric acid, the drug denatures whatever protein it contacts. The gray-white change produced indicates the extent of destruction. Use of this compound on vulvar condylomata requires careful application to avoid a caustic spill. Large lesions will require a "layered" treatment schedule for complete eradication and the recurrence rate is no different from that with podophyllin. The package insert includes the admonition that the treated area be kept dry for at least 12 hours. Frequent contact with urine and vaginal discharge makes this a difficult task. But the liberal use of talc or starch powder applied before leaving the office will help.

5-Fluorouracil (5-FU) is a pyrimidine analogue that acts by interfering with the metabolism of thymidilic acid, preventing synthesis of normal DNA. It is used systemically in tumor chemotherapy, but since only 6 per cent of a topical dose is absorbed through the skin, it can also be used for skin surface lesions without significant systemic effect. Because its action is primarily on rapidly dividing tissue, 5-FU has been used, on an experimental basis, in the treatment for condylomata acuminata, vulvar carcinomata in situ, and localized recurrent areas of vulvar Paget's disease. Since long-term studies of its effectiveness are not yet available, this drug should not be used unless both the physician and the patient understand the lack of data on distant side effects and recurrence rates.

The drug is commercially available in topical form as a 5 per cent cream (Efudex) and can be self-applied by the patient. Use of disposable vinyl gloves for application is not absolutely necessary but constitutes an added safety precaution.

When employed for extensive condylomata acuminata, the cream is applied once daily at bedtime. Removal is not necessary other than normal bathing routine, and the patient is followed at weekly intervals. As with podophyllin, young early lesions that are rapidly growing show the best response. Some will disappear completely in two or three weeks. Others will undergo a marked regression in size, making them suitable for electrosurgical or excisional therapy. If no effect is seen after two or three weeks, however, the lesions are not likely to respond to increased doses. Increasing the frequency of application may result in ulceration and sloughing of the normal vulvar skin.

R_x 5 per cent 5-fluorouracil cream
DISP: 1 tube (30 gm)
SIG: Apply h.s. as described
Amount will last two weeks.

5-FU has also been used in the topical treatment for vulvar carcinoma in situ and recurrent Paget's disease of the vulva. It is now recognized that unless a given lesion is treated intensively, two or three times daily for an uninterrupted six weeks, recurrence often takes place. Unless the disease is confined to a very small area, a complete course of therapy can rarely be given to a vulvar lesion. After two weeks of three times daily application, a severe inflammatory reaction occurs, and at four weeks, severe necrosis and sloughing with ulceration begins. These reactions are accompanied by a burning painful sensation that most patients find intolerable in the vulvar area. In order to be effective, however, the therapy must be continued for an additional two weeks or longer until all evidence of the lesion has disappeared. Only then can the drug be discontinued and the epithelium allowed to heal.

Topical 5-FU has not been proven as effective for lesions that are heavily keratinized, due to their decreased absorption of the drug. Its effectiveness in recurrent cases of Paget's disease has been variable, but some lesions have shown marked regression. Topical 5-FU will probably not become a major mode of therapy for vulvar intraepithelial neoplasia. In a collected series of published cases, the overall response rate was only 50 per cent. However, for localized lesions of carcinoma in situ or recurrent Paget's disease that are not markedly hyperkeratotic, in a patient willing to persevere through the painful ulcerative phases of the treatment, 5-FU offers an alternative to surgical excision. Informed consent should always be obtained and careful long-term follow-up is mandatory.

Acyclovir and other nucleoside analogues are activated by herpesvirus-produced enzymes and in their active form inhibit cellular and viral DNA replication. The drugs are therefore cytotoxic to all cells, but much less so to uninfected cells. They are commercially available in topical vehicles for use in herpes simplex infections.

An amount sufficient to cover all lesions should be applied every three hours throughout the day, i.e., six times daily for one week. Used in this way, the drugs have been shown to decrease the duration of viral shedding and reduce the amount of pain in immunocompromised patients and in some of those with primary herpetic attacks. There is little clinical benefit when used topically in those women with recurrent disease who are otherwise normal. Resistant viral strains have already been reported, so the topical preparations should not be used casually when there is little hope of effect. Oral preparations of these drugs are proving to be much more effective over a wider clinical spectrum.

Retinoids are a group of vitamin A acid analogues that are at least temporarily helpful in a wide variety of dermatologic conditions. Topical vitamin A acid is useful in the treatment of molluscum contagiosum and, when combined with corticosteroids, in psoriasis and Fox-Fordyce disease as well. The drug greatly diminishes keloid formation, and this group of compounds may prove to be beneficial in other proliferative disorders of the skin. However, the risk of significant side effects may limit their application.

IMMUNOTHERAPY

Autogenous vaccines and the induction of specific sensitivity are two immunotherapeutic techniques with vulvar application.

Vaccines can be prepared from condylomata acuminata and administered therapeutically rather than for prophylaxis. It may be that the HPV virus is protected by the condyloma it produces and is thus able to avoid contact with antibody-producing cells and others of the lymphoid system. To disrupt the tissue envelope and expose the cell-free extract by injection is the aim of autogenous vaccination. The oncogenic potential of the HPV virus is known. How, if at all, this potential might be exerted after systemic exposure by vaccination is unknown.

Before attempting this technique, the physician should be familiar with the literature cited under *Further Reading* and the informed consent of the patient should be obtained. Vaccination during pregnancy, or in a woman using oral contraceptives, should be avoided. Patients with collagen vascular disease or cancer, as well as transplant recipients, may all be on immunosuppressive therapy and these women are poor candidates for vaccinotherapy.

The vulvar lesions should be free of secondary infection. A surgical scrub of the area, followed by thorough rinsing, is advisable prior to excision. Under local anesthesia, approximately five grams of condylomata are sharply excised. A representative lesion should be sent for routine histologic confirmation. The tissue specimens are then trimmed to remove as much normal skin as possible. If the vaccine is to be prepared on the immediate premises, the condylomata are placed in sterile saline and taken promptly to the laboratory. If a distant laboratory is to be used, the specimens are dropped into liquid nitrogen for quick freezing, then packed in dry ice and speedily shipped to the preparation facility. Using sterile technique, the tissue is then homogenized in a blender and subjected to a series of freeze-thaw cycles that ruptures the individual cells. After centrifugation and heat inactivation procedures have been completed, the supernatant fluid is further clarified by filtration and its bacteriologic sterility is ascertained. The clear, sterile liquid is then either stored, frozen, or lyophilized until used by the clinician.

About 0.25 ml of vaccine fluid is first administered to the patient as an intradermal skin test. The vaccine may contain antigenic substances to which the patient is already sensitive. If a reaction develops at the test site within 48 hours after such injection, the vaccine should not be used. In the absence of any delayed hypersensitivity reaction, 0.5 to 1.0 ml of the vaccine may then be given subcutaneously at weekly intervals. The usual course requires six injections, after which disappearance of the condylomata may be expected. If progression of the lesions is noted two to four weeks after initial injection or if the lesions become stationary at eight to ten weeks even though some initial regression occurred, the therapy should be abandoned and the patient considered unsuitable for further trial. Follow-up is mandatory; at least one patient has been reported in which carcinoma in situ developed after successful vaccinotherapy. A double-blind controlled study compared autogenous vaccine with placebo and found no difference in responses. Others, however, have reported good results when all else has failed.

2, 4-Dinitrochlorobenzene (DNCB) sensitization is another form of immunotherapy in which cell-mediated immunity plays a major role. A number of chemicals, among them DNCB, are strong sensitizing agents. Ninety-five per cent of normal subjects will become sensitized to this compound after topical exposure of a 2 sq. cm area of skin to 2 mg of DNCB dissolved in acetone. Once sensitivity has been established, further cutaneous exposure to even small amounts of the same agent produces an immune reaction characterized initially by erythema, edema, and vesiculation followed by erosion, exudation, and necrosis. This reaction occurs in tumor tissue at dose ranges below those that incite a similar reaction in normal tissue. Therefore, if the agent is selectively applied either topically or by intralesional injection to a superficial neoplasm such as carcinoma in situ, destruction of the tumor will take place.

This technique has been employed in the treatment of vulvar atypia and carcinoma in situ with satisfactory results, but recurrence rates after therapy remain unknown. Not enough cases have been reported to accurately assess the response rate. But enough have been documented to identify the technique as one to be considered in the treatment of carcinoma in situ of the vulva. A familiarity with the literature is necessary prior to using or recommending DNCB. Untoward immune reactions including arthralgias have been associated with this technique. The DNCB itself must be handled with great care by the physician and office personnel, who must assiduously avoid contact with the chemical. But despite these drawbacks, the method has merit and deserves conscientious consideration.

FURTHER READING

PHOTOGRAPHY

Olmstead, C.B.: Instant color print photography in dermatology. Cutis 29:585–587, 1982.
The author compares the available equipment and discusses office use techniques, record keeping, and medicolegal aspects.

TOLUIDINE BLUE TEST

Collins, C.G., Hansen, L.H., and Theriot, E.: A clinical stain for use in selecting biopsy sites in patients with vulvar disease. Obstet. Gynecol. 28:158–163, 1966.
The introduction of the toluidine blue dye technique, as first applied to vulvar disease at the famous New Orleans clinic.

SMEARS

Nauth, H.F., and Schilke, E.: Cytology of the exfoliative layer in normal and diseased vulvar skin: correlation with histology. Acta Cytol. (Baltimore) 26:269–283, 1982.
An analysis of cytologic findings in 464 patients. Fifty per cent of malignant tumors show positive cytology.
Woodley, D., and Saurat, J.H.: The burrow ink test and the scabies mite. J. Am. Acad. Dermatol. 4:715–722, 1981.
A wonderful article that reads like a novel and is full of history as well as information on the technique of using a fountain pen for diagnosis.

SEROLOGIC TESTS

Felman, Y.M., and Nikitas, J.A.: Syphilis serology today. Arch. Dermatol. 116:84–89, 1980.
This excellent review emphasizes the applications and limitations of available techniques.
Moseley, R.C., Corey, L., Benjamin, D., et al.: Comparison of viral isolation, direct immunofluorescence and indirect immunoperoxidase techniques for detection of genital herpes simplex virus infection. J. Clin. Microbiol. 13:913–918, 1981.
This study applied three techniques in the diagnosis of 76 patients. The merits and drawbacks of each are discussed.

TOPICAL DRUGS

Corey, L., Nahmias, A.J., Guinan, M.E., et al.: A trial of topical acyclovir in genital herpes simplex virus infection. N. Engl. J. Med. 306:1313–1319, 1982.
A placebo-controlled study demonstrating decreased length of shedding and accelerated healing in some infections with little effect in others.
Krupp, P.J., and Bohm, J.W.: 5-Fluorouracil topical treatment of in situ vulvar cancer. Obstet. Gynecol. 51:702–706, 1978.
This report from Dr. Collin's successor describes the technique and illustrates the course of therapy.
Papa, C.M., and Kligman, A.M.: The effect of topical steroids on the aged human axilla. Chapter 6. In: Advances in Biology of the Skin (W. Montagna et al.), Vol. 6—Aging. New York, Pergamon Press, 1965.
A landmark paper that has had great influence, since axillary and vulvar tissues are quite similar.
Slater, G.E., Rumack, B.H., and Peterson, R.G.: Podophyllin poisoning—systemic toxicity following cutaneous application. Obstet. Gynecol. 52:94–96, 1978.
A case report and discussion that emphasizes the danger and reviews the literature.

Thomas, J.R., and Doyle, J.A.: The therapeutic uses of topical vitamin A acid. J. Am. Acad. Dermatol. 4:505–513, 1981.
A concise but complete review of the topical experience with this drug in a variety of conditions.

Von Krogh, G.: Podophyllotoxin for condylomata acuminata eradication. Acta. Dermatovener. Suppl. 98:1981.
A magnificent piece of work that reports extensively on the author's clinical and experimental studies comparing podophyllum extracts, colchicine, and 5-FU preparations.

Williams, G.A., Richardson, A.C., and Hathcock, E.W.: Topical testosterone in dystrophic diseases of the vulva. Am. J. Obstet. Gynecol. 96:21–30, 1966.
A landmark paper that reported on 57 cases with good long-term follow-up data and stimulated others to advance the work.

IMMUNOTHERAPY

Abcarian, H., and Sharon, N.: The effectiveness of immunotherapy in the treatment of anal condyloma acuminatum. J. Surg. Res. 22:231–236, 1977.
Contains a detailed description of vaccine preparation techniques and describes their successful use.

Foster, D.C., and Woodruff, J.D.: The use of dinitrochlorobenzene in the treatment of vulvar carcinoma in situ. Gynecol. Oncol. 11:330–339, 1981.
This article details the techniques used and reports a series of successful applications.

Madison, M.D., Morris, R., and Jones, L.W.: Autogenous vaccine therapy for condyloma acuminatum —a double blind controlled study. Brit. J. Vener. Dis. 58:62–65, 1982.
A unique investigation that found wart vaccine no more effective than placebo prepared from the patient's normal skin.

Powell, L.C.: Condyloma acuminatum: recent advances in development, carcinogenesis and treatment. Clin. Obstet. Gynecol. 21:1061–1079, 1978.
A master of the subject reviews all aspects and details the use of autogenous vaccination.

SURGICAL PROCEDURES

4

BIOPSY
MARSUPIALIZATION
WORD CATHETERIZATION
ALCOHOL INJECTION
CORTICOSTEROID INJECTION
ELECTROSURGERY
LASER
CRYOSURGERY
WIDE EXCISION
PARTIAL VULVECTOMY
TOTAL VULVECTOMY
RADICAL VULVECTOMY

The special nature of vulvar disease requires equally special knowledge and skill in diagnostic and therapeutic procedures. Many of these are surgical—some straightforward, others complex. But all are important, and the office techniques should be mastered by every physician who proposes to offer vulvar care. The more extensive procedures that require an operating room and general anesthesia lie within the scope of any trained gynecologist, while radical vulvectomy and lymphadenectomy properly belong in the hands of trained surgical oncologists who perform them regularly.

We are still ignorant in many areas of vulvar physiology. The subtleties of sexual function include the patient's perception of her appearance as well as the actual anatomic realities that pertain. Realizing with Professor Ross Baldessarini that "surgery is basically a subtractive process," the goal should always be to preserve as much normal structure and function as possible. Cosmetic appearance is important to all patients but is achieved only with painstaking and time-consuming techniques. Nerve injury and repair sometimes lead to intractable pain and may arise after a surgical procedure that, in retrospect, was not worth

61

the sequelae and was best left not performed. So it is always important to reflect on the need for the procedure selected. Maloccurrences and complications will continue as long as surgery is practiced. They are acceptable to both the informed patient and the surgeon, providing the procedure is carefully performed and consistent with the disease being treated.

Procedures themselves seem to have a life cycle of their own. They come into fashion, are advocated by prominent figures, and then gradually are replaced by newer techniques practiced by the next generation. The problem, of course, is that what is new is not necessarily better than the procedure it replaces. In this chapter are detailed those procedures, old and new, that have been helpful in current practice.

Nothing is really too basic. The simplest operations are also the ones that are done most frequently and that will affect the largest number of patients. Therefore, even the most elementary procedures are included for illustration and discussion.

BIOPSY

Vulvar biopsy is not a major procedure. It does not require hospitalization, general anesthesia, or a scrub nurse. Special consent procedures are no more necessary for vulvar biopsy than they are for cervical or endometrial biopsies. Most physicians regard these latter procedures as part of their routine office examination whenever their performance seems indicated by historical or physical findings. The same attitude should apply to the vulvar biopsy. It is an axiom of gynecology that one cannot differentiate benign from malignant cervical conditions on the basis of gross inspection alone. Similarly, the gross appearance of a vulvar lesion is not always indicative of its histologic character. Office biopsies, which should be rapid, simple, and painless, are necessary for accurate evaluation.

The vulva differs from the cervix and endometrium in that some anesthesia is necessary before biopsy can be performed. To ignore the nerve endings present in this sensitive anatomical area is overly callous if not actually barbaric. But more important, if a simple diagnostic procedure causes significant pain, the patient is unlikely to return for follow-up and proper therapy, no matter what the histologic result.

Anesthesia is therefore essential and may be accomplished by either local infiltration or pudendal nerve block. For diagnostic biopsies, local infiltration is quite sufficient. A 1 per cent solution of lidocaine is injected subepidermally with a fine 25-gauge needle. The addition of epinephrine prolongs the anesthetic effect and promotes vasoconstrictive hemostasis. Because of the rich vascular and lymphatic supply of the vulva, small amounts of anesthetic may be quickly dissipated. This can be avoided if a generous volume of solution is used at the outset, i.e., 5 to 8 ml per site. The local swelling this causes actually facilitates the biopsy and produces some vasoconstriction, thus minimizing blood loss. But when multiple biopsies are done, the total milligrams of drug may become excessive. For single biopsies then, a generous amount of plain lidocaine is ideal. When multiple sites are to be sampled, smaller amounts of solution containing epinephrine may be used instead.

Whether the anesthetic is simply injected at the biopsy site or placed in an

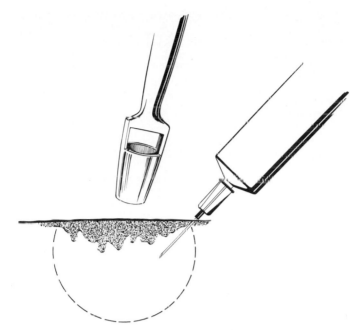

Figure 19. Simple local infiltration for punch biopsy.

encircling wall around the lesion to produce a true "fieldblock" depends entirely on the size of the lesion and the type of biopsy contemplated. Most sampling biopsies require only a single injection (Fig. 19), while large excisional biopsies are better done using a fieldblock technique (Fig. 20).

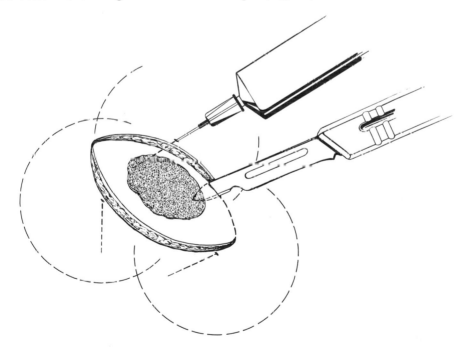

Figure 20. Field block infiltration for elliptical excision biopsy.

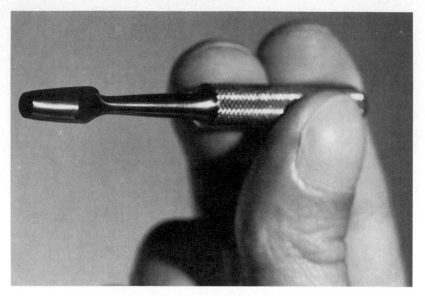

Figure 21. The Keyes cutaneous biopsy punch.

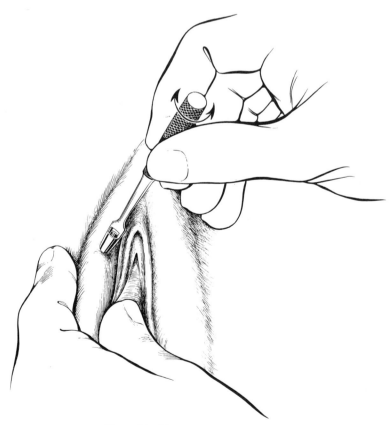

Figure 22. Diagnostic punch biopsy.

Regional anesthetic techniques (pudendal nerve block) are also available, but when a procedure is contemplated that requires an extensive field of anesthesia, it usually means increased blood loss, operative time, and infection risk. Such operations are better performed in a hospital surgical suite.

As soon as anesthesia is established (within 60 seconds of injection), the biopsy can be performed. Surgical skin preparation is not necessary, as the vulvar skin is remarkably resistant to its own local flora. For most lesions that require biopsy, the pubic and vulvar hair is not a problem. If hair growth obstructs the biopsy site, it can be easily snipped away with a small scissors. The formal "shave and prep" is both unnecessary and time-consuming.

The Keyes cutaneous punch is a dermatologic instrument used to core out a small circular plug of skin (Fig. 21). It works on the same principle as a corkborer and comes in diameters ranging from 2 to 12 mm. The 4-mm and 5-mm diameters are the most practical for vulvar use and result in a pellet-shaped specimen that is easily oriented and has sufficient surface to allow adequate sectioning. The instrument can be obtained from most surgical supply houses and a disposable variety is also available. If kept sharp by periodic use of a pencil-shaped whetstone, these instruments cleanly incise the skin with only light pressure and a simple twisting motion. The circular biopsy incision may be carried as deeply as desired by maintaining the pressure and rotation until the subcutaneous tissue is reached (Fig. 22). If the physician is unfamiliar with this instrument, a few minutes of practice with both an orange and a tomato will accurately simulate most clinical conditions. The depth of the biopsy will vary with the lesion, depending on epidermal thickness. There is a vague sensation of decreased resistance when the dermis is reached, and this can be appreciated after only a few procedures. Making the incision too deep results in cutting the deeper and larger blood vessels and inviting more blood loss than is necessary. Too shallow a cut results in a fragmented specimen on which no accurate diagnosis is possible.

Once the incision is made, the punch is laid aside. The specimen is grasped beneath the epithelium with an Adson mousetooth forceps, and the dermal tissue cut across with a small scissors. A clean circular or elliptical defect results, which is sometimes almost avascular (Fig. 23). In the presence of slight bleeding, a silver nitrate stick or drop of Monsel's solution is sufficient for hemostasis. Such is often the case in the relatively avascular dystrophic lesion when the 4-mm punch is used. Stubborn bleeding sites, or those made with the 5-mm instrument, are best handled with a single figure-of-8 stitch using 3–0 chromic gut suture swaged on a small curved cutting needle. Plain gut allows the defect to open at home before primary healing has occurred. The polyglycolic acid sutures are retained too long and annoy patients unnecessarily. With a minimum of planning, it is possible to have all of the instruments and materials prepared and sterilized ahead of time in a vulvar biopsy set (Fig. 24) containing anesthetic, a syringe and needles, Keyes punch, pick-up forceps, a scissors, and a small needle holder. For convenience, sponges and suture material can be taped to the pack after sterilizing or kept separately in a handy location.

Punch biopsies are ideal for obtaining representative samples of suspicious areas and, when used with the toluidine blue test as a guide, accurate diagnoses can be consistently obtained. By contrast, snippets of skin taken with cervical biopsy instruments or "shave biopsies" done with a knife blade held parallel to

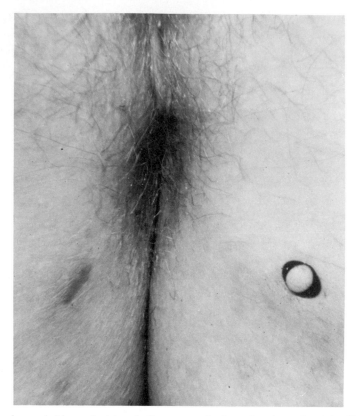

Figure 23. Fresh punch biopsy incision (before removal of specimen) on the right. Healing punch biopsy incision (one week after chromic suture closure) on the left.

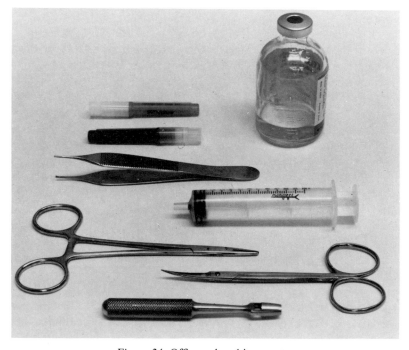

Figure 24. Office vulvar biopsy set.

the skin surface almost invariably result in confusing diagnoses from inadequate and poorly oriented sections.

Excisional biopsy is generally employed for circumscribed lesions (nevi, individual cysts, or papules) where complete removal is desired. The Keyes punch instrument is not suited for this purpose. Instead, the incision should be made with a No. 15 knife blade held at right angles to the skin surface. Whenever possible, an ellipse or diamond should be inscribed and a shallow wedge of subcutaneous tissue below the lesion should be included in the excision. The long axis of the excision should be placed in a dorsoventral direction if the lesion is located on the labia. On the perineum, a horizontal axis is preferred, while in the introitus or lower vagina, the ellipse should parallel the vaginal axis. Attention to placement of the long axis of the ellipse will result in a linear scar under minimal tension. Upon completion of the healing process, such excision sites are virtually invisible.

The edges of the defect should be closed without tension, in a linear fashion, using interrupted figure-of-8 stitches of 3–0 chromic gut suture material. Cutting needles are a must, since some skin areas are very resistant and tapered needles are liable to bend or break.

When a large excisional biopsy is performed, secondary edema may result. This can be minimized by the use of an ice pack. Ask the patient to fill a plastic sandwich bag with crushed ice when she arrives home and to wear this like a pad during the rest of the day. Thereafter, daily warm baths help to assure complete absorption of the suture material along with rapid and uncomplicated healing. Little if any scarring results from these procedures, and the biopsy sites are almost invisible within two or three weeks. Whatever discomfort is present during the healing period is minimal and requires nothing more than simple, over-the-counter analgesics.

As a rule, the total procedure of vulvar biopsy can be accomplished in less than five minutes. The site is infiltrated, the incision is made, the specimen excised, and the defect closed. It is rapid, simple, and except for the initial stick of the anesthetic needle, painless. The patient tolerates such a biopsy extremely well and is not reluctant to have the procedure repeated, if need be, at a later date.

The most elegant biopsy, however, is completely worthless if it fails to yield an accurate pathologic diagnosis. It is not possible for a pathologist to give a precise interpretation from tissue that is dried up, distorted, or tangentially oriented and cut. Thus the procedure of vulvar biopsy does not end with adequate hemostasis, but rather must include the proper handling of the tissue specimen. The excised tissue should be placed epidermal side upward on a small piece of absorbent cardboard (Fig. 25). While the biopsy site is being closed, enough serum will exude from the tissue to seep into the cardboard fibers, dry, and become adherent. Only then is the cardboard piece inverted gently into a small bottle of tissue fixative solution, and allowed to float on the surface with the adherent tissue specimen downwards. Rough handling of the specimen jars at this point may knock the tissue loose, and it will sink to the bottom of the bottle and curl up into an amorphous mass prior to fixation. Gentle handling, then, is essential so that fixation will take place while the specimen is still adherent. If later on it comes loose from the cardboard, it will make no difference; after flat fixation it will retain its shape and the pathologist can easily recognize the epithelial surface. At the pathology cutting table, the disc-shaped specimen is ori-

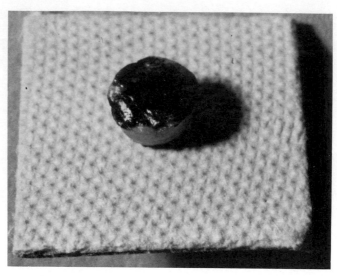

Figure 25. Five-mm punch biopsy from toluidine-blue-positive area, adherent to cardboard square.

ented with the epithelium upwards and hemisected with a fresh razor blade. The cut edges are then lightly stained for identification, and the tissue segments are wrapped in filter paper prior to being placed in the processing cassette. The laboratory technician who imbeds the sections in the paraffin block will recognize the stained edges and orient the tiny sections so that these edges are parallel to the cutting surface of the block. With this procedure, clear right-angle sections result and accurate histologic diagnoses can be made.

MARSUPIALIZATION

Incision and drainage of a Bartholin duct cyst or abscess may give immediate and dramatic results, but the recurrence rate after such a procedure is unacceptably high. As a result, "I & D" techniques are no longer recommended. While the mucous secretion of the Bartholin gland contributes little to vaginal lubrication during intercourse, it does help to maintain the moisture of the non-keratinized epithelium of the vestibule. Dryness of this introital tissue may result in difficulty during early intromission, and in prepubertal girls whose Bartholin glands have not begun to function, the formation of synechiae can occur. It is therefore desirable, though by no means crucial, to maintain the function of the gland whenever possible. Total excision of the duct and gland is rarely required and even deep biopsy should only be considered for enlargements of the Bartholin area in women over the age of 40 to rule out the rare carcinoma of the Bartholin gland. It is not a simple dissection and requires general anesthesia with careful attention to hemostasis in a highly vascular field. It may result in scarring and vulvar pain. As such it represents a form of therapeutic "overkill" for women with uncomplicated cysts of the gland duct.

It is, therefore, preferable to create an epithelialized tract from the vulvar vestibule to the lumen of the expanded duct. This results in the formation of an accessory duct that allows continued function of the gland, assures adequate drainage, and greatly reduces the possibility of recurrence. Such a tract can be

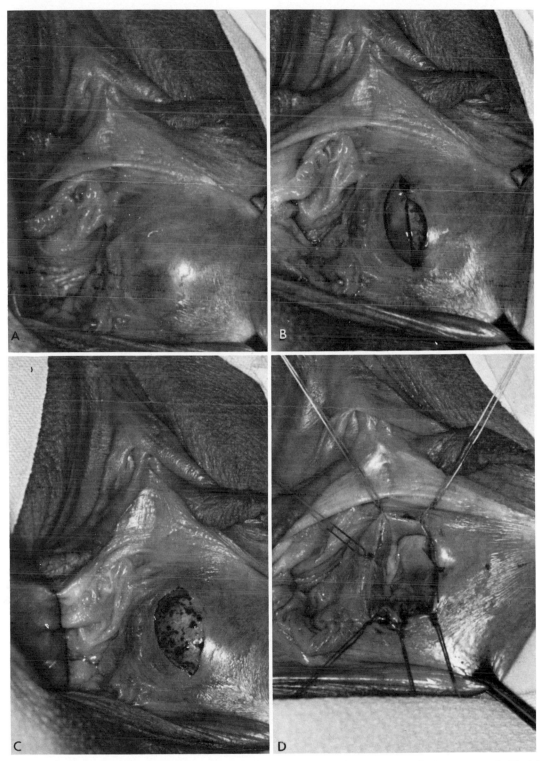

Figure 26 Marsupialization of Bartholin gland duct cyst: *A*, Exposure of overlying vestibular mucosa. *B*, Excision of mucosal ellipse. *C*, Cyst wall protrudes through defect. *D*, After cyst cavity is opened and rinsed, cyst wall is sewn to mucosal edges.

69

developed either by surgical "marsupialization" or by the insertion of a Word catheter.

Marsupialization involves the creation of a pouch by approximating the lining ductal epithelium of the cyst or abscess to the overlying introital epithelium. A unilateral pudendal block affords excellent anesthesia for this procedure but local infiltration of the introital mucosa and submuscosal tissues is also satisfactory. Rarely is a general anesthetic necessary, and marsupialization can be rapidly accomplished in the office or emergency room with little patient discomfort.

The operative technique of marsupialization is illustrated in Figure 26. A generous vertical ellipse of vestibular epithelium is excised. Some have advocated a single linear incision, but if an ellipse of skin is removed, there is less tendency to premature contraction and exposure of the cyst wall is facilitated. This initial incision should be made as close to the hymenal ring as possible and certainly within the vestibule, internal to the pigmented skin margin of the labium minus.

Once this incision is completed the ellipse of skin is removed and any intervening areolar tissue is bluntly dissected from the surface of the cyst wall. The cyst is then allowed to bulge through the skin defect and is incised. Most cysts contain purulent-looking material. Routine culture may be performed, but in the absence of other signs of acute inflammation, this fluid is generally sterile. The cyst cavity should be thoroughly evacuated and rinsed with sterile saline. If loculations are noted within the cavity, these should be broken up with blunt dissection.

The edges of the incision in the cyst wall are now sutured directly to the edges of the vestibular incision with interrupted, fine, absorbable sutures. Chromic gut (2–0) or fine polyglycolic acid sutures are ideal. If bleeding points appear along the incision lines, a figure-of-8 stitch usually suffices to achieve hemostasis. Warm sitz baths, twice daily during the week following surgery, encourage healing and result in greater patient comfort. The size of the defect will gradually diminish but a small opening will remain to represent the newly established duct orifice. Antibiotics are not routinely given unless acute gonorrheal infection is suspected, since, once drainage is established, any local edema and inflammation quickly subside.

WORD CATHETERIZATION

If an inert foreign body is placed between the wall of a cyst or abscess and the skin, and left in situ for a sufficient period of time, a fistulous tract will develop. It is this principle that Dr. Buford Word employed in the development of his catheter technique. The Word catheter is a short latex stem with an inflatable bulb at the distal end (Fig. 27).* It is similar to a very short pediatric Foley catheter without the central lumen.

In this technique (Fig. 28), local infiltration or even topical ethyl chloride spray suffices for anesthesia. A small stab wound is made *in a direction toward the operator* through the vestibular mucosa, as close as possible to the hymenal ring, and into the cyst or abscess. The size of this incision should be no greater

---

*These catheters are available individually packaged and presterilized from the American Latex Corporation, Sullivan, Indiana, 47882.

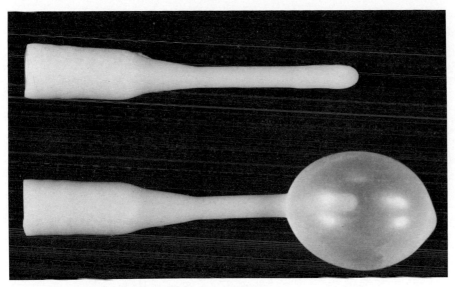

Figure 27. Word catheter ready for insertion, and after inflation.

than the width of the No. 15 knife blade, and care must be taken not to make the wound too large. After exploring and rinsing the cavity, the catheter is inserted. The fit should be snug. A small amount of water or saline is then injected using a very fine needle (23 or 24 gauge) in order to distend the balloon. The inflation should be just enough to keep the catheter in place. If the incision has been kept small, minimal distention is necessary. The stem of the catheter protrudes into the vestibule but can be angled upward along the vaginal canal where it does not seem to interfere with normal coital activity.

The only undesirable feature of this technique is the fact that for complete epithelialization of the new tract to occur, a wait of about 4 to 6 weeks is required. But this is not a problem for the patient if the procedure is performed properly so that the stem of the catheter lies easily within the vagina and does not protrude to catch on the underclothing. Patients who have kept a diary of their Word catheter experience report no discomfort or interference with routine activity. Coitus is easily accomplished, as is douching. External pads should be substituted for tampons, however, during the intervening menses.

ALCOHOL INJECTION

In rare cases, topical medical therapy may fail to provide relief of symptoms of vulvar dystrophy after months to years of conscientious trial. These unusual patients then become candidates for alcohol injection, which may be used to interrupt the sensory impulses coming from the vulvar skin. Although it is a radical form of therapy for benign disease, it is preferable to the even more radical procedures of total vulvectomy or surgical denervation (Mering procedure). Thorough histologic evaluation of the vulvar lesion must be performed to rule out foci of atypia or early neoplasia, since such cases would be more logically treated with vulvectomy. Patients whose primary complaint is one of "burning" or "pain" rather than "itching" should also be excluded. For reasons

71

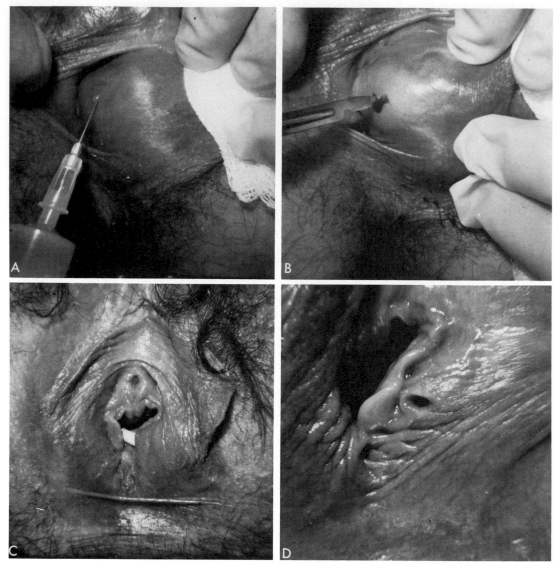

Figure 28. Word catheter insertion: *A,* Superficial anesthesia. *B,* Stab wound close to hymen directed towards operator. *C,* Catheter inserted and inflated, stem in vagina. *D,* At six weeks with accessory duct intact.

that are not clear, alcohol injection often fails to relieve painful and burning sensations and, in fact, may even aggravate them.

The procedure is performed under general anesthesia. The entire vulvar area from mons to anus is marked off, in grid fashion, into 1 cm squares using a cutaneous pencil. At each intersection of the lines, between 0.1 and 0.2 ml of absolute ethyl alcohol is injected into the subcutaneous tissue via a 25-gauge, ½-inch needle (Fig. 29). It often takes two assistants to keep the syringes ready with the premeasured solution. Injection into muscle or deep vasculature may result in extensive necrosis and slough, and the patient should be informed that this may occur. Therefore, while the alcohol should be deposited just beneath the dermis, deeper penetration must be avoided. It is best to start posteriorly

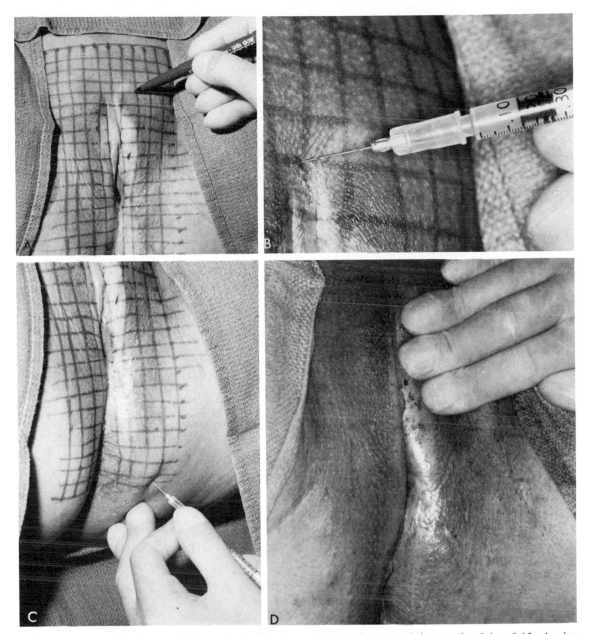

Figure 29. Alcohol injection: *A*, Vulva marked off in 1-cm grid. *B*, Inject at each intersection 0.1 to 0.15 ml using short needle. *C*, Begin injecting at bottom working upward. *D*, Massage gently but thoroughly to distribute alcohol.

and work toward the mons, since droplets of alcohol that exude from the injection sites run downward and blur the grid markings. Thin folds of labia minora should be injected only at their bases. Once all the injections have been made, the area should be firmly massaged in order to facilitate the radial spread of the alcohol outward from each injection site. Twice daily sitz baths are recommended for one week postoperatively along with analgesics as required. A localized edema develops rapidly and will be present for two to three weeks after the procedure. In some cases, this swelling persists beyond one month, but pruritus is almost always relieved. Recurrent symptoms, six months or more after therapy, have been reported and require additional treatment. The majority of patients, however, experience semipermanent relief to the extent that their pruritus can be controlled with topical agents alone. In some cases of hyperplastic dystrophy, histologic reversal to a more normal pattern has been shown to occur, along with improvement in the gross appearance of the vulva. If used only when indicated, the procedure of alcohol injection will be used infrequently. But for selected cases, it is a valuable therapeutic technique that produces gratifying results.

CORTICOSTEROID INJECTION

Corticosteroid injection is an office procedure that may be helpful in the treatment of vulvar pruritus resulting from biopsy-proven benign conditions. Some women with idiopathic pruritus or burning and no visible lesion may also be relieved. The duration of such relief is variable, but some women have remained symptom-free for many years after injection.

Essentially, the technique is the same as that used for alcohol injection, substituting corticosteroids for alcohol. The same subcutaneous depth should be reached, but general anesthesia is not necessary. If a visible area of surface change can be identified, that area alone may be treated. An injection solution that has given good results is triamcinolone acetonide (Kenalog) in a 10 mg/ml concentration. Three and one-half ml of this is mixed in the syringe with .5 ml of 2 per cent lidocaine. A long needle is used so that a large area may be injected through a single puncture site. The danger of tissue slough is minimized with the use of corticosteroids, but care should be taken to keep the needle in the subcutaneous plane. Intradermal injection is ineffective and may even be harmful, as is injection into the subcutaneous fat, which can result in necrosis and sterile abscess formation.

ELECTROSURGERY

High-frequency electrical wave energy in contact with tissue produces dehydration, coagulation, and mechanical disruption of the tissue cells. When combined with knife-blade curettage, electrosurgery is the most efficient of all treatment methods for condylomata acuminata. The overall treatment time is short and recurrence rates are low. Electrosurgery is also useful for laying open the sinus tracts of hidradenitis suppurativa as described by Duncan, in treating molluscum contagiosum and urethral caruncles, and in small skin tags. It can provide a means of achieving hemostatsis in small biopsy sites near the clitoris.

There are basically two types of electrosurgical apparatus; monopolar and bipolar. Monopolar instruments are for in-office use and do not require a large "indifferent" electrode plate in contact with the patient. These units are about the size of a cigar box. Reasonably priced models are manufactured by a variety of companies and may be inspected at most medical supply firms. Bipolar instruments are a good deal larger and contain both cutting and coagulation circuits. Useful in larger procedures, they form part of the standard equipment in most hospital surgical suites.

Monopolar office units are used for fulguration and desiccation. Fulguration derives from the Latin word for "lightning" and describes what happens when an electrode is held very close to but not in contact with a tissue surface. A spark of energy arcs across the gap, producing an area of pinpoint destruction. Desiccation (drying) is slightly different. If the electrode actually touches or is inserted into the tissue, the cells in the immediate area are dehydrated. In actual practice, both effects are achieved at virtually the same time.

Before operation, the proper current adjustment must be chosen. For vulvar use, this corresponds to roughly 40 per cent of the maximum output of most machines—enough to achieve a spark when the electrode tip is brought to within 1 mm of the tissue. (If an ordinary prescription blank is placed on a bar of hand soap, the proper strength current will barely etch the soap through the paper, leaving only pinpoint-size brown dots on the paper surface.) In a practical sense, the operator quickly acquires a "feel" for the unit, and power setting becomes a simple matter of trial and adjustment until the desired tissue effect is obtained.

A large selection of electrode tips is available, but the short angled point is the best choice. Anesthesia is necessary and, for in-office procedures, either local infiltration or pudendal block is satisfactory. Ethyl chloride spray is inflammable and should not be used for anesthesia in electrosurgical procedures. Alcohol preps are similarly hazardous. The only other note of caution concerns patients with cardiac pacemakers. Such devices can be inactivated by electrosurgical instruments.

When treating condylomata acuminata, the electrode tip is inserted directly into the center of the anesthetized lesion. The current is then applied until the lesion "bubbles." The tissue will blanch, puff up, and coagulate. The current flow is then stopped and the electrode removed. Necrotic tissue may adhere to the electrode point and should be wiped off or scraped away. The treated area is then stretched or pinched between the fingers such that a flat surface is presented. A No. 15 knife blade is used to scrape the surface, removing more necrotic debris and creating an extremely shallow ulceration or abrasion in the skin. Many times the physician will feel a firm rubbery "core" in the center of the lesion. This represents residual wart tissue and must be redesiccated and scraped until the base of the defect is absolutely smooth. Fulguration is then performed on the edges and surface of the defect with the electrode tip held close to but not touching the surface. This sparking effect produces hemostasis and contracture of the ulcer and leaves a dark eschar (Fig. 30). Hemostatic fulguration is useful in other situations as well. After the core of a molluscum contagiosum lesion has been removed, the crater can be fulgurated. When a superficial lesion has been sharply excised from the surface of the clitoris or urethral meatus, sutures often provoke additional bleeding, but fulguration seals the small vessels without further damage.

The bipolar instruments used in operating rooms are more powerful than office machines and produce both cutting and coagulation effects. Many surgeons prefer to coagulate minor bleeding points rather than tie them, and some prefer to make incisions with the cutting current of an electrical knife in place of a steel one. These same procedures are useful for the treatment of extensive condylomata acuminata. When a major portion of the vulvar skin surface is affected or when the lesions involve the urethral meatus, clitoris, or anal mucosa, a single procedure under general anesthesia is the most efficient therapy. To

75

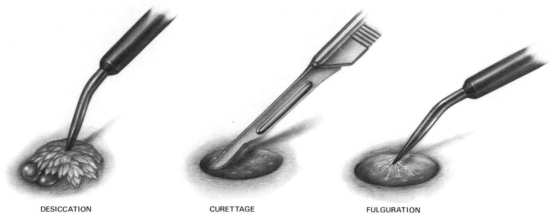

DESICCATION   CURETTAGE   FULGURATION

Figure 30. Monopolar office electrosurgery: steps in treatment of condyloma.

individually anesthetize and treat each lesion in the office would be too time-consuming and require excessive amounts of local anesthetic.

Both coagulation and cutting current adjustments must be made by the circulating nurse at the physician's direction once the tissue effects are observed. Wire loops of various diameters and a selection of pointed and flat electrode tips should be available. Again, avoid the use of volatile prep solutions when cleansing the skin. Cut, rather than shave, the pubic hair, since shaving can implant new condylomata if old ones are accidentally nicked.

Choose a wire loop of about 0.75 cm diameter and, using the cutting current, pass the loop beneath the wart (Fig. 31). At first the sensation will seem strange, like cutting through butter. The tendency is to cut too deeply and this is aggravated if a loop with too small a radius of curvature is used. Keep the cutting wire shallow so as to encompass the lesion but not destroy the adjacent normal skin. The ulcerative defect thus produced should extend into the dermis but not into the underlying fat. The particular architecture of each lesion determines which electrode tip is most suitable; i.e., those lesions not amenable to loop cutting are coagulated with the flat tip or tapered point. Vaginal and cervical warts and those on the anal/rectal mucosa can all be treated in similar fashion

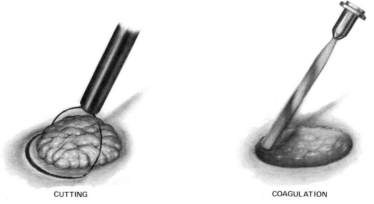

CUTTING   COAGULATION

Figure 31. Bipolar hospital electrosurgery: wire loop excision and flat blade desiccation.

using appropriate specula for exposure. Small blood vessels are immediately sealed by the cutting current. Coagulation current and pointed electrodes are used to achieve hemostasis if larger vessels are transected. Take the time to treat all visible lesions.

The ulcerated areas present after extensive electrosurgery should be covered with a burn dressing, and a transurethral or suprapubic catheter should be inserted to prevent voiding over the freshly treated region. Postoperative discomfort varies from negligible to severe and must be individually managed. The burn dressings are allowed to soak free during daily sitz baths. Once a serum crust has sealed the healing ulcers, the bladder catheter can be removed and the patient allowed to void. Corticosteroid creams, with or without antibiotic additives, aid in the final healing process, but the patient should not be discharged until she can void comfortably and manage her own perineal care.

Recurrent lesions may appear within a week or so after electrosurgery, so the initial postoperative office visit should not be delayed. As new lesions develop, they must be treated with in-office desiccation, curettage, and fulguration. Such recurrences do not represent failures of treatment. Rather, these are new warts caused by residual virus present in the skin at the time of initial electrosurgery. If each new lesion is promptly treated, in the absence of a fresh inoculum (reinfection), complete eradication can eventually be accomplished. Any case of condylomata acuminata can be managed with electrosurgery, but it is especially indicated in the treatment of immunosuppressed patients. During pregnancy, massive condylomata may fill the vaginal canal. Even though such lesions are friable, uncontrollable hemorrhage with vaginal delivery is a rare event. The real hazard posed by these lesions is that of newborn infection, and laryngeal papillomas may occur in infants thus exposed. Attempts at predelivery vaginal antisepsis are futile when confronted with a mass of secondarily infected condylomata. A variety of other infections may also be transmitted during pelvic delivery. Electrosurgery provides the only alternative to cesarean section for such patients, and a number of cases have been successfully managed by this method.

LASER

Laser (Light Amplification by Stimulated Emission of Radiation) energy was first developed for research and industrial use. The early laser relied on solid lasing media such as ruby crystals, which were excited by flashes of light from an external source. This excitation produced a new beam of light of nearly uniform wavelength propagating in parallel bundles rather than divergent rays. These two attributes, parallelism and wavelength uniformity, characterize *coherent* light. A laser, then, is a device that produces a coherent light beam of energy. Many substances have been found to act as lasing media when excited by appropriate energy. The beam produced when carbon dioxide gas is excited by high voltage electrical current or by radiofrequency has been found particularly useful in biologic systems.

The physical properties of the carbon dioxide laser beam are such that when it impacts on living tissue, an extremely rapid vaporization takes place. Intracellular temperatures of 100°C are produced almost instantaneously. In this process, the laser energy is absorbed so that deeper tissues, and those immediately adjacent to the impact area, are not affected. The depth and size of the vaporized area depends on the power density of the beam and the time of contact, and can be regulated over a wide range. Thus, the energy can be applied only to the most superficial cell layers, or, if desired, completely through the epidermis and into the dermal tissue. This precise degree of control affords an accuracy of destruction that cannot be obtained by any other means.

Because it is coherent, the laser energy is narrowly confined within the beam, which, in turn, is focused on a selected target area. Only the cells within the area of impact will be vaporized. Therefore, unlike other methods of destruction, there is essentially no surrounding zone of damaged tissue. The area of impact is no larger than one millimeter, but by moving the beam back and forth, larger areas can be quickly and completely covered (Fig. 32).

Laser vaporization can be used to destroy almost any surface lesion, such as condylomata acuminata and areas of hyperplastic atypia, etc. It is especially well suited to the treatment of vaginal and cervical condylomata acuminata that are easily visualized through the colposcope. Although the vagina and cervix can be laser treated without anesthesia, the vulvar skin cannot. Isolated vulvar lesions can be locally anesthetized, but the treatment of extensive areas of involvement requires either a pudendal block or general anesthetic. Among the vulvar diseases, recognized indications for the laser now include condylomata acuminata, hyperplastic dystrophies and atypias, and carcinoma in situ. In these disorders the laser can achieve results similar to those obtained with excision or fulguration and therefore constitutes simply an alternative instrument rather than a unique procedure. Scarring is minimal and postoperative pain can be controlled with frequent artificial sea-water sitz baths. These can be easily prepared using a powdered mix available at most pet stores that handle tropical fish. The real thing is, of course, widely available but not always at the desired temperature and location.

CRYOSURGERY

The destruction of tissue by means of extreme cold is based on the production of thermal injury largely through the formation of intracellular ice crystals and dehydration. Congelation and necrosis of animal tissue will occur at a temperature of $-20°C$ held for a period of 1 minute. In order to achieve this tissue temperature, an object much colder must be applied. Cryosurgical units therefore make use of liquid nitrogen ($-196°C$), nitrous oxide ($-85°C$), carbon dioxide ($-70°C$), or freon ($-60°C$) to cool an instrument tip.

Many dermatologists find cryosurgery useful and most prefer to use liquid nitrogen, which they keep handy in a small thermos bottle. But on the vulva there are few indications for cryosurgery. It has been used in the treatment of condylomata, but the process of producing a frozen tissue ice ball that includes the entire lesion, letting it thaw, and then re-freezing takes over 10 minutes per lesion. Anesthesia is not necessary, but the total time involved for multiple lesions is prohibitive. In addition, cold preserves the papilloma virus and there is an unacceptable rate of recurrence among condylomata treated with cold alone. That it works at all may be due to the destruction of wart tissue, which possibly exposes antigenic sites and stimulates a host immune response.

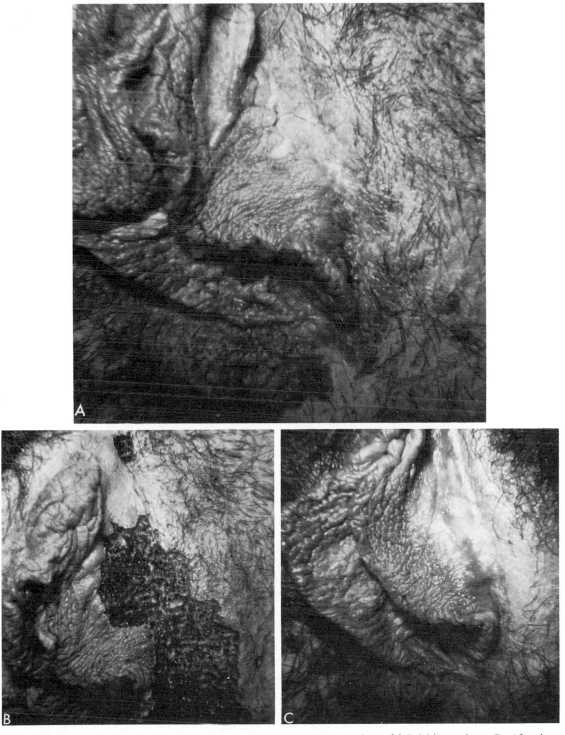

Figure 32. Laser vaporization: *A,* Hyperplastic dystrophy on lateral surface of left labium minus. *B,* After laser application to depth of 1 to 1.5 mm. *C,* Healed at eight weeks.

When very small tips are available, cryosurgery is excellent for the painless treatment of molluscum contagiosum. Even a single freeze is often curative, scarring is minimal, and pain is nonexistent.

The same unit many gynecologists maintain in the office for cervical use may be of great value in the treatment of urethral prolapse. The technique is painless and requires no anesthesia. The urethral lesion is contacted by the freezing probe and an ice ball is formed that includes all of the abnormal tissue. The probe is warmed and removed once the ice ball has spread to its desired extent. If a tip with a surface area equal to that of the lesion is chosen, a suitable ice ball will form after approximately three minutes of freezing. The tissue is then allowed to thaw and the freezing process is repeated. Dramatic regression of these benign urethral conditions can be achieved in this manner, just as is the case with benign cervical eversions.

Despite extensive thermal damage, cryosurgery has failed to destroy foci of carcinoma in situ and should not be used to treat vulvar neoplasia.

WIDE EXCISION

A wide local excision, carried down into the underlying fat and fascia is appropriate for the definitive treatment of unifocal or isolated multifocal areas of carcinoma in situ (Fig. 33). It is similarly useful for repeat excision of suspected residua following diagnostic removal of small superficial melanomas (level II or less). Areas of severe atypia and fields of repetitively infected epidermal cysts are additional indications.

In a modified form, this technique is highly effective used in the posterior midline to excise the web of fourchette skin that so often becomes the site of fissures resulting in dyspareunia. Woodruff has detailed and illustrated this latter procedure and described the technique of undermining the vaginal flap and bringing it downward to form a new estrogen-responsive coital platform.

The nature of the anesthesia needed will depend on the individual case. Similarly, the skin margin width will depend on the reason for excision as well as the geometry of the dissection. In order to achieve primary closure without tension, it is often necessary to make the defect longer, wider, or of a different shape than would be absolutely necessary based on diagnosis alone. Recognition of when this flexibility is required comes with experience, but often it is "made up as you go along." Using skin hooks (usually reserved for plastic surgeons) secure opposing edges of a given wound and bring them together as you would intend to suture them. See what tension, "dog ears," and unwanted folds this creates. You can then modify the margins until sham apposition with the hooks gives the desired result. Remember to close these defects with multiple layers of interrupted sutures. Not only will the deeper layers hold the wound secure, they should also relieve the tension on the skin layer so that the external sutures simply approximate the skin edges. Fine (3–0) polyglycolic acid sutures are ideal for the skin/skin or skin/mucosa approximation; and other than powder to keep the area dry, dressings are not necessary.

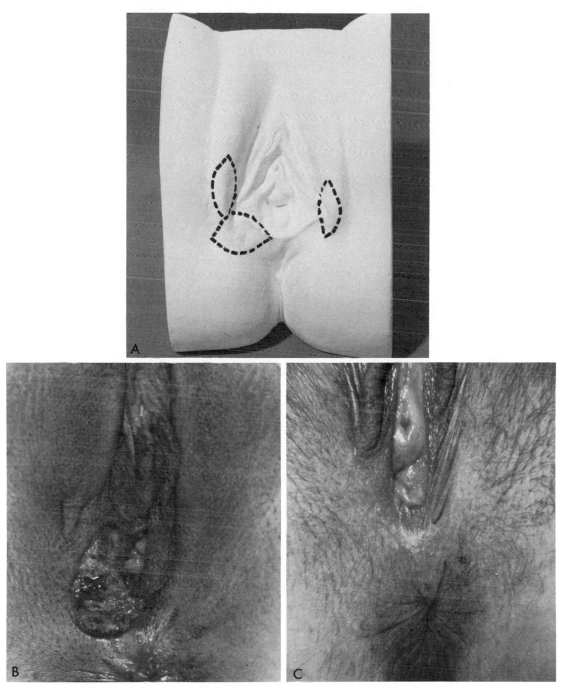

Figure 33. Wide excision: *A*, When possible, orientation of ellipse or diamond should follow skin lines. *B*, Lesion removal as deep as underlying fat. *C*, Cosmetic appearance at six weeks.

PARTIAL VULVECTOMY

Coalescent lesions of carcinoma in situ may involve large areas of the vulva. Extensive and stubborn areas of condylomata, as well as verrucous carcinoma and hidradenitis suppurativa, are all amenable to this technique. The latter conditions would of course require a much deeper dissection than in situ carcinoma or condylomata.

The intent of this procedure is to remove affected tissue and retain as much normal structure as possible. Often this requires more time than would a total vulvectomy, but it is time well spent if the clitoris, prepuce, or frenulum can be spared with normal function as a result (Fig. 34). And this is often the case, since in most patients the disease does not directly involve the clitoris and periclitoral structures. Keep in mind, too, that these diseases are not malignant and should they recur they will usually be obvious and may be re-excised. Thus, it seems prudent to retain as much normal-appearing tissue as possible.

The same plastic considerations apply here as in wide excision. The skin edges should be handled with hooks or sharp-tooth fine forceps and never crushed. Many common surgical tools are not sufficiently delicate for vulvar use and do not allow the surgeon to treat the tissue with the respect required.

When large areas of the vulva are superficially denuded, many bleeding points are exposed. Good healing requires meticulous hemostasis, and the electrocoagulation of small bleeders helps the procedure move along with a dry field. But take care not to use the instrument near the skin edge, where thermal injury would delay wound healing. Primary closure is almost always possible and should be attempted. Grafting adds time as well as a graft scar at the donor site and is rarely needed with this procedure.

Postoperative care should concentrate on keeping the wound dry with powders and air blowers. The traditional perineal heat lamp should be avoided at all costs. It spreads the perineum, puts tension on the sutures, and causes the vulva to sweat—all are undesirable consequences. Early ambulation and rapid restoration of bowel and bladder function should reduce the hospital stay to a minimum.

TOTAL VULVECTOMY

Known as simple vulvectomy, this procedure was once applied prophylactically to any patient suspected of having a premalignant disease. Its use now is limited to the treatment for widespread carcinoma in situ, Paget's disease, and severe cases of Crohn's disease or other destructive disorders that have become medically unresponsive. In none of these is the procedure simple, and again, the depth of dissection is dependent on the disease being treated (Fig. 35). Total vulvectomy for Paget's disease requires that the apocrine-bearing tissue of the majora be removed, and these glands extend to the subdermal fat. Carcinoma in situ warrants a more shallow dissection, but foci of possible microinvasion must always be considered.

The two incisions are circumscribed and connected at the desired depth. The dissection is made easier by the injection of 10 to 20 ml of saline or dilute epinephrine in the rectovaginal septum close to the perineum. This protects the rectum, which is otherwise easily entered near the perineum, and also assists in

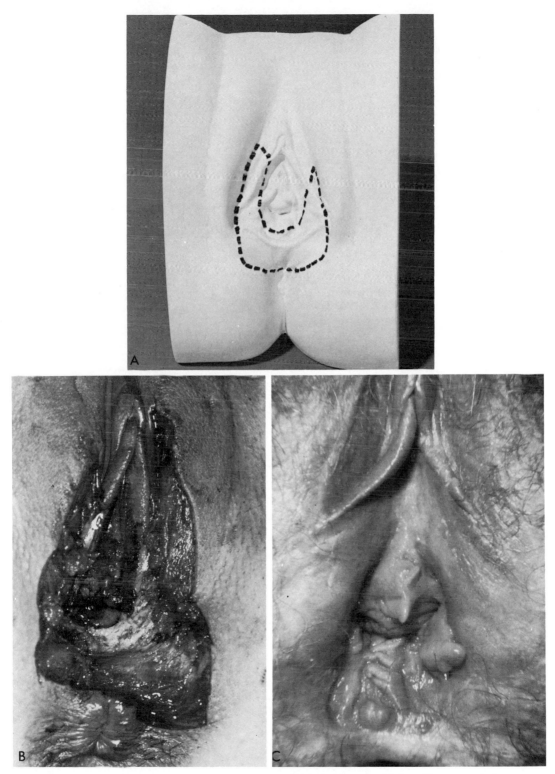

Figure 34. Partial vulvectomy: *A*, Incision encompasses all involved areas with 8 to 10 mm margin but spares unaffected tissue. *B*, Dissection shallow down to underlying fat. *C*, Final result shows good cosmetic appearance.

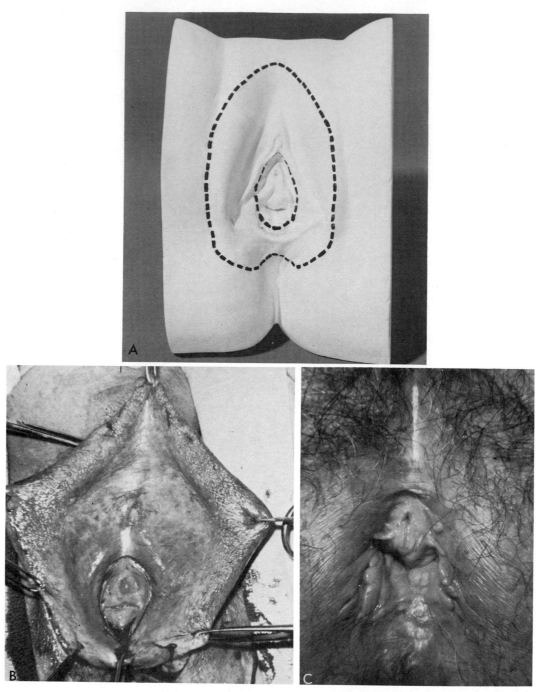

Figure 35. Total vulvectomy: *A,* Incisions circumscribe vulva and vestibule and encompass labia majora. *B,* Incisions are joined as underlying tissue is dissected to depth dependent on indication. *C,* Final appearance. Note urethra unobstructed and supported in midline.

the development of the vaginal flap. Incising the specimen in the midline through a disease-free area and dissecting each side separately is also helpful. There is little to be gained by submitting an intact specimen to pathology if it makes the procedure more difficult.

Primary closure is almost always possible if plastic techniques are employed. It is especially important to reconstruct the perineum and establish a bridge of tissue separating rectum from vagina. This step is cosmetically and anatomically essential in order to prevent vaginal infections, promote hygiene, and facilitate coitus. Another critical area concerns the urethra. The direction of the urine stream is dependent on fixation of the meatus by the vulvar tissues. When these are removed, the distal urethra must be resuspended and fixed to the surrounding tissue. If not present, such supportive tissue must be developed by flap graft. Closure of this area must be accomplished so that a hood of skin does not form in front of the exposed meatus and impair the urinary system.

Standard surgical texts omit the plastic techniques used in vulvar reconstruction after total vulvectomy. However, excellent descriptions of innovative methods have been published and are listed under *Further Reading*. The direct application of a split-thickness skin graft obviates the need for flap development. Nevertheless, a donor site scar is produced and is cosmetically unacceptable to a great many women.

Anectomy must often be added to the procedure of total vulvectomy. The squamous epithelium of the anal canal up to the dentate line is frequently involved by carcinoma in situ as well as Paget's and Crohn's diseases. Anal specula and retractors, along with biopsy forceps and rectal packs, should always be avilable and preoperative lower bowel preparation is advised.

RADICAL VULVECTOMY

Patients who are candidates for this operation are those with invasive malignancies of the vulva. Most are in the older-age high-risk group with compromised cardiopulmonary and vascular function, and require the facilities available in a tertiary level center.

For no other vulvar procedure are there so many variations on the theme. The surgical books of Mattingly, Uyttenbroeck, Way, Stening, Copenhaver, and Tovell each describe in detail a different technique. Each has advantages and disadvantages, and all work well in the hands of those who have used and developed them over the years. The particular operation used at any given center will depend on the training and background of the oncologic surgical team. The standard landmarks, however, include the anterior superior iliac crest and the apex of Hunter's canal in the groin marking the lower boundary of the femoral triangle (Fig. 36).

Some techniques depend more heavily on histologic accuracy of specimen evaluation than do others. Many units now xerox the specimen to provide a permanent record of the gross architecture and produce a "road map" for identification and removal of the lymph nodes. Reconstructive surgery using myocutaneous flaps developed from the inner thigh adds time to an already lengthy procedure, but improves the final appearance. Lesions that involve the rectum or bladder or both can still be successfully excised if exenterative procedures are simultaneously employed. And so radical surgery continues to evolve as new

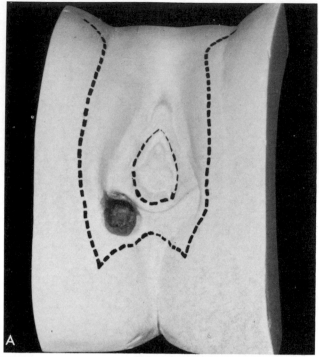

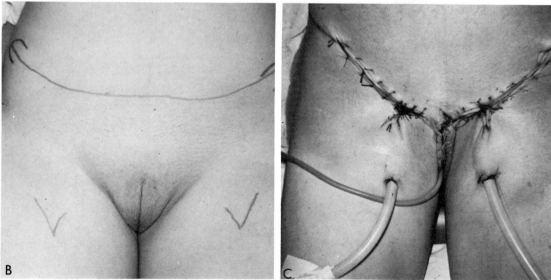

Figure 36. Radical vulvectomy: *A*, Outline of incision includes perineum. *B*, Landmarks for groin dissection incision are iliac crests and apices of Hunter's canal in legs. *C*, Postoperative, with Way drainage system.

approaches are tried incorporating unilateral dissections, abbreviated lymphadenectomies, and new combinations of surgery and radiotherapy.

Wound breakdown was once accepted as a frequent operative complication. Erosion of the denuded femoral artery by wound necrosis was responsible for some operative deaths and led to the sartorius muscle transplant to prevent this occurrence. But if the technique is designed to avoid undermining the skin edges, to allow for primary closure without tension, and to adequately and continuously drain the operative site, wound breakdown should not occur and muscle transplant may be unnecessary. Thrombosis of the deep veins of the legs with the resultant possibility of pulmonary emboli constitutes another postoperative hazard. Various techniques are available to reduce the incidence of this problem: prophylactic anticoagulation, the use of intensive physiotherapy for patients confined to bed, support stockings, and venous flow monitoring.

The most significant long-term complication is leg edema resulting from the groin dissection. Compromised drainage is inevitable when the saphenous vein is removed and collaterals are not always sufficient. Leg elevation and support hose are helpful but usually not completely effective. From both a functional and cosmetic viewpoint, new methods of management that eliminate or reduce this problem will be received with great enthusiasm.

FURTHER READING

SURGICAL TEXTS

Copenhaver, E.H.: Surgery of the Vulva and Vagina. W. B. Saunders Company, Philadelphia, 1981.
Mattingly, R.F.: TeLinde's Operative Gynecology. 5th ed. The Williams & Wilkins Company, Baltimore, 1979.
Stening, M.: Cancer and Related Lesions of the Vulva. ADIS Press, Australasia Pty, Ltd., Balgowlah, 1980.
Tovell, H.M.M., and Dank, L.D.: Gynecologic Operations. Harper and Row, Hagerstown, Md., 1979.
Uyttenbroeck, F.: Gynecologic Surgery. Masson Publishing USA, Inc., New York, 1980.
Way, S.: Malignant Disease of the Vulva. Churchill-Livingstone, Edinburgh, 1982.

BIOPSY

Pinkus, H.: Skin biopsy: a field of interaction between clinician and pathologist. Cutis 20:609–614, 1977.
An excellent and detailed discussion.

MARSUPIALIZATION

Jacobsen, P.: Marsupialization of vulvovaginal (Bartholin) cysts. Am. J. Obstet. Gynecol. 79:73–78, 1960.
A well-illustrated and well-discussed article on this subject.

WORD CATHETER

Word, B.: Office treatment of cyst and abscess of Bartholin's gland duct. South. Med. J. 61:514–518, 1968.
An excellent account of the history, anatomy, and pathophysiology of the duct, with use of the Word catheter described by its inventor.

ALCOHOL INJECTION

Woodruff, J.D., and Babaknia, A.: Local alcohol injection of the vulva: discussion of 35 cases. Obstet. Gynecol. 54:512–514, 1979.
Presents 20 years of experience with this technique and discusses patient selection, the procedure, and the results.

ELECTROSURGERY

Duncan, W.C.: Surgical treatment of hidradenitis suppurativa. J. Derm. Surg. 2:153–157, 1976.
A well-written and illustrated article demonstrating use of electrosurgery for unroofing and cauterizing the cysts and sinus tract.

Graber, E.A., Barber, H.R.K., and O'Rourke, J.J.: Simple surgical treatment for condyloma acuminatum of the vulva. Obstet. Gynecol. 29:247–250, 1967.
The classic description of fulguration and curettage.

LASER

Baggish, M.S., and Dorsey, J.H.: CO_2 laser for the treatment of vulvar carcinoma in situ. Obstet. Gynecol. 57:371–376, 1981.
A responsible report of laser performance for this disease, which describes the use of the instrument, illustrates results, lists complications, and proposes sea-water baths.

PLASTIC TECHNIQUES

Chafe, W., Fowler, W.C., Walton, L.A., and Currie, J.L.: Radical vulvectomy with use of tensor fascia lata myocutaneous flap. Am. J. Obstet. Gynecol. 145:207–213, 1983.
A detailed description of vulvar reconstruction with excellent illustrations of the operative technique.

Graves, K.L., Wilson, E.A., and Greene, J.W.: Surgical technique for clitoral reduction. Obstet. Gynecol 59:758–760, 1982.
An elegant procedure that preserves function and restores appearance in cases of ambiguous genitalia is illustrated and described.

Julian, C.G., Callison, J., and Woodruff, J.D.: Plastic management of extensive vulvar defects. Obstet. Gynecol. 38:193–198, 1971.
The design and construction of local flap grafts are well illustrated in this excellent "how to do it" article.

Körlof, B., Nylen, B., Tillinger, K.G., and Tjernberg, B.: Different methods of reconstruction after vulvectomies for cancer of the vulva. Acta Obstet. Gynecol. Scand. 54:411–415, 1975.
Beautifully outlines and diagrams methods of flap-plasty for use with partial or total vulvectomies. These direct suture techniques gave better cosmetic and functional results than did grafts.

Schultz, B.C., and Roenigk, H.H., Jr.: The double scalpel and double punch excision of skin tumors. J. Am. Acad. Dermatol. 7:495–499, 1982.
An interesting technique for the evaluation of surgical margins that allows for plastic closure.

Strauss, R.J., and Fazio, V.W.: Bowen's disease of the anal and perinanal area. Am. J. Surg. 137:231–234, 1979.
The importance of anal involvement and the technique of anal biopsy and anectomy are described.

Trelford, J.D., and Silverton, J.S.: Successful plastic procedures of the perineum. Gynecol. Oncol. 7:239–247, 1979.
Step by step, three innovative methods that will find frequent application are described.

Weiss, A., Kapetansky, D.I., and Pierce, A.K.: A new method of perineal reconstruction following vulvectomy. Plastic and Reconst. Surg. 65:824–827, 1980.
Remarkable use of a vaginal flap for external reconstruction.

Wheeless, C.R., McGibbon, B., Dorsey, J.H., and Maxwell, G.P.: Gracilis mycutaneous flap in reconstruction of the vulva and female perineum. Obstet. Gynecol. 54:97–102, 1979.
Excellent surgical drawings complement this report of a series of Baltimore cases.

Woodruff, J.D., Genadry, R., and Poliakoff, S.: Treatment of dyspareunia and vaginal outlet distortions by perineoplasty. Obstet. Gynecol. 57:750–754, 1981.
An extremely valuable technique to be used again and again. A must for mastery by all surgeons who see and treat vulvar disease.

5

MANAGEMENT OF NEOPLASIA

All clinicians should be familiar with the general concepts involved in the management of the patient with vulvar malignancy. The nomenclature and staging of tumors, the current method of therapy, and the essentials of pretreatment evaluation and follow-up care constitute the basic principles of oncology. With these in mind, the primary physician can function as a uniquely trusted source of information for the patient, advising her as to the exact nature of her disease, its prognosis, and its meaning to her overall life and setting the stage for successful future therapy. Such referring physicians also act as peer reviewers for their colleagues; since they are able to recognize sound and proper management, they can make certain that their patients obtain it. The purpose of this chapter then, is to present the contemporary concepts of vulvar neoplasia. The final outcome of any therapeutic program is directly proportional to the accuracy of pretreatment evaluation and the quality of follow-up care. In these crucial areas, every physician should be an expert.

The detection of cancer during the initial phases of its development is one of the most important responsibilities of any physician, and although the routine screening of asymptomatic patients may sometimes be tedious work, when the search results in the recognition of an early and completely treatable malignancy, the task is well rewarded. The discovery of such lesions requires a high index of suspicion and the frequent use of in-office biopsy procedures. All large and advanced tumors were at one time small and subtle. An alert clinician, at tuned to the possibility of their occurrence, acquainted with their gross appearance, and willing to obtain tissue for histologic confirmation could have prevented their progression.

Intraepithelial disease requires individualization of therapy. All patients need careful pretreatment evaluation and long-term follow-up care. Treatment possibilities range from simple observation to extensive dissection and plastic repair that may involve bowel surgery. The treatment of patients with invasive disease is best accomplished in a regional oncology unit. No generalist, occupied with the cares and problems of a busy varied practice, can keep truly current with the rapidly changing field of oncology. No surgeon can maintain peak proficiency with a radical procedure if it is performed only on rare occasions. The patient, therefore, is best served if her malignant disease is primarily treated in an oncologic center where advanced therapeutic techniques can be applied and where specialized surgical teams reinforce their skills with frequent use.

Clinical neoplasia is the result of a cellular phenomenon, determined by an oncogenic stimulus and modified by the host reaction. Deep in the DNA of an epithelial cell, a genetic event occurs that alters the chromosomal make-up of that cell, endowing it with new properties that eventuate in uncontrolled replication. Such genetically altered cells may remain silent and obscure for many years before they are histologically recognizable as abnormal. Even then, their potential for harm is dependent on the host defense mechanisms that may reject the foreign cells, hold them confined, or become ineffective and allow growth. This change in cellular genetics may affect a single cell from which a clone of identical cells may be developed or it may affect a number of different cells more or less simultaneously. Investigative techniques are now available to measure and characterize this change. The total DNA present within a cell nucleus can be characterized and quantified. Histograms can be constructed to reflect the karyotype of a given lesion. Aneuploid lesions show abnormal amounts of nuclear DNA, which indicates lack of normal cell division and replication processes. Euploid and polyploid lesions, on the other hand, show even multiples of 2n chromosomal DNA and represent controlled cell replication. It is possible to further characterize individual DNA strands. In some carcinomas, bits and pieces of viral DNA sequences have been identified from both condyloma virus (HPV) and herpes virus (HSV).

Once the affected cells are manifest by their altered histologic appearance, and provided these cells are found to be confined to the epithelial layer without invasion of the subjacent stroma, intraepithelial neoplasia exists. When this process occurs in the squamous cells of the vulvar epidermis and is confined to that layer, the result is known as vulvar carcinoma in situ.

CARCINOMA IN SITU

In the early part of this century, physicians began to notice localized areas of cutaneous abnormality. Some of these lesions were red, some were brown, some were white. Their histologic appearance was similarly variable, although a predominance of certain atypicalities were seen more often in some lesions than in others. For this reason, each variety was thought to represent a different disease and various names were attached to them, usually that of the physician who first called attention to the illness.

Historically, then, three varieties of intraepithelial neoplasia of the vulvar skin were recognized. But we now know that when they occur on the vulva, "Bowen's disease," "erythroplasia of Queyrat," and "carcinoma simplex" exhibit such marked biologic similarities that they should be grouped under the single heading of "carcinoma in situ." A fourth variety of more recent description, *Bowenoid papulosis* is histologically identical and must be considered to represent the same disease.

One of the first investigators to thoughtfully consider this disease was Richard Knight, M.D., of New York. In 1943, he reviewed the published literature in all languages and added six personal cases, concluding that the condition represented a slowly progressive epithelioma, that the term precancer was not applicable, and that the treatment of choice should be wide local excision. From our present perspective he was completely right. But at the time he was not able to offset the clamor of those who, then and since, pointed to the presence of in situ lesions at the border of some invasive tumors. From this "guilt by association," they concluded that prophylactic removal of the entire vulva was justified whenever a focus of intraepithelial disease was found. We now know that this approach is no longer justified.

Carcinoma in situ of the vulva is characterized by the histologic criteria of disorientation and a loss of epithelial architecture that extends throughout the full thickness of the epithelium (not including the most superficial layers in tissue from keratinized surfaces). Giant cells, multinucleated cells, abnormalities of nuclear/cytoplasmic ratio, dyskeratosis, individual cell keratinization, corps rond formation, abnormal mitoses, mitotic figures above the basal layer, and an increased density of cell population may all be seen in varying degrees (Fig. 37). Less commonly, full-thickness change is not present, but intraepithelial squamous "pearls" are present at the tips of the rete pegs associated with loss of the normal basal layer (Fig. 38).

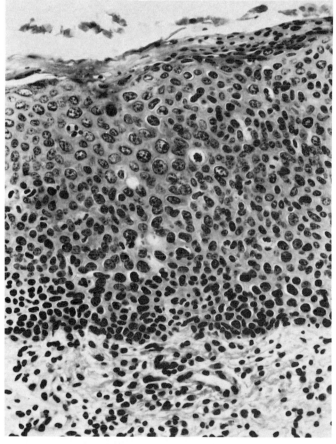

Figure 37. Carcinoma in situ. Full-thickness replacement of the epithelium. Corps ronds, mitotic figures, nuclear pleomorphism, increased cellular density, and parakeratosis are all present.

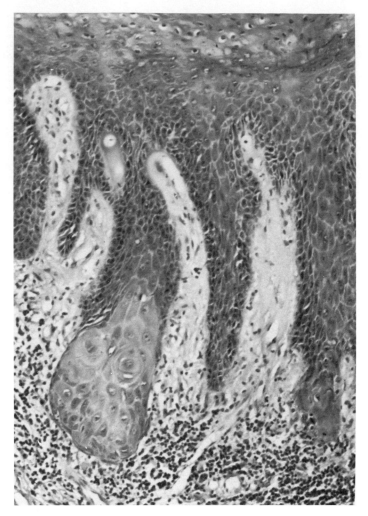

Figure 38. "Pearl" of abnormally mature squamous cells occupies tip of rete ridge, a truly preinvasive lesion.

The clinical appearance of these lesions is highly variable. They are multifocal in approximately 70 per cent of patients and unifocal in the remainder. They may be red, pink, white, dark, eczematous, dry, or moist. They not infrequently resemble condyloma acuminatum, with which they are frequently associated. Almost all of these lesions are raised above the level of the surrounding skin and may therefore be characterized as papular. Somewhat over half of the lesions will exhibit superficial parakeratosis and so will retain topically applied 1 per cent toluidine blue dye. Finally, one third of the patients with this disease exhibit hyperpigmented lesions with sharp borders. These clinical hallmarks are summarized in Figure 39.

The incidence of this disease is increasing and it is being found in younger and younger patients. Whereas once the disease was only looked for in the elderly, the average age at onset is now in the third and fourth decades and it is not an uncommon finding even in teenagers. There is a high degree of association with sexually transmitted diseases. In one study, 60 per cent of the patients

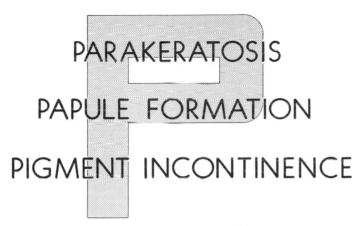

PARAKERATOSIS

PAPULE FORMATION

PIGMENT INCONTINENCE

Figure 39. Clinical hallmarks of carcinoma in situ.

exhibited at least one venereal disease by history or examination. The most commonly associated disease was that of condyloma acuminatum. There is one case report of apparent venereal transmission of the carcinoma in situ between sexual partners. Carcinoma in situ of the cervix is another frequent associate and has been found in up to 20 per cent of patients with vulvar in situ disease. Arsenical insecticides have been implicated in six cases occurring in farm workers, and immunosuppression, from whatever cause, increases the risk of development of the disease. A familial tendency has not been documented, but there is at least one case of the disease occurring simultaneously in identical twins. All of these areas should therefore be investigated in the initial history and evaluation of the patient.

Such evaluations must include cytology and colposcopy of the cervix and vagina to rule out concomitant neoplasia of these areas. Sexually transmitted diseases must be looked for and, if available, tests of immunocompetence should be performed.

About half of the women with vulvar carcinoma in situ have no complaints, and the disease is only found after careful screening examination. The remainder notice pruritus or the presence of a surface irregularity. Contiguous structures may be superficially involved (Fig. 40). Of these, the anus is the most frequent site of involvement. For this reason the anal canal must be thoroughly evaluated

Figure 40. Frequency of involvement of contiguous structures by carcinoma in situ.

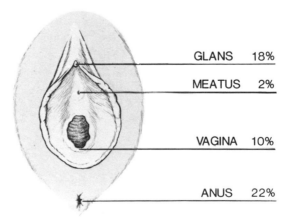

GLANS 18%

MEATUS 2%

VAGINA 10%

ANUS 22%

93

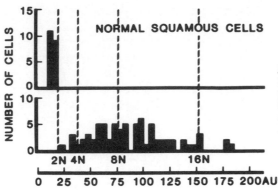

Figure 41. DNA histogram of a cell from a lesion of carcinoma in situ (bottom) compared with patient's normal squamous cells (top). (From Friedrich, et al.: Carcinoma in situ of the vulva: a continuing challenge. Am. J. Obstet. Gynecol. 136:830, 1980.)

in each case with anoscopy and biopsy of any suspicious lesion. Multifocal involvement of the anal mucosa may necessitate anectomy as part of an integrated surgical approach.

Karyotypic analysis shows that the vast majority of cases are aneuploid in character. The histogram of a typical lesion demonstrates the abnormal amounts of DNA present in comparison to a normal cell population from the same individual (Fig. 41). Yet, despite this change, lesions have been observed to regress spontaneously over periods of observation lasting from three months to two years. Follow-up biopsies from the sites of previous disease showed normal epithelium with euploid karyotype. Some of these patients have remained disease free for over ten years, and the number of spontaneous regression cases in the literature actually exceeds the number reported to have progressed to invasion.

As far as the natural history of the disease is concerned, it may be said that an analysis of the untreated cases reported shows that the disease is as likely to regress as it is to progress. Thus, in a philosophic sense, it is not at all certain that what we label "carcinoma in situ," by agreement and convention on the basis of its histologic appearance, actually represents the precursor of invasive squamous cell malignancy. The age grouping is wrong, the anatomic distribution of the lesions is wrong, and the natural history does not fit well. And so for selected patients who may be reliably followed, especially those who are pregnant or temporarily immunosuppressed and relatively asymptomatic, an extended period of observation is certainly justified.

With intractable symptoms, advanced age, lack of follow-up capability, or failure to regress, patients become candidates for treatment on an individualized basis, and a number of options are available.

Surgical removal may be as localized or as extensive as necessary in order to remove all involved tissue. The use of careful plastic techniques can assure excellent cosmetic results and maximum preservation of normal function and appearance. For small unifocal lesions this involves only a simple wide local excision. With diffuse, coalescent, multicentric disease, a partial or total vulvectomy with or without anectomy may be required. Regardless of the procedure the recurrence rate is dependent on the histologic quality of the tissue margins. These must be carefully assessed by the pathologist, for if the margins are involved, there is a fifty-fifty chance that the disease will recur. This fact does not mandate immediate additional surgery. It is just as true that half of the patients will have no future trouble despite the involved margin of resection. So it would seem preferable to wait and re-excise whatever lesions actually recur. If the margins are free of disease, there remains a 10 per cent chance of recurrence, since the original oncogenic stimulus may become operative at different times in different sites within the same vulva.

Destructive methods rely heavily on the odds that lesions that grossly look alike will have similar histology and that the initial biopsy is representative of the entire lesion to be destroyed. The security of total histologic evaluation is, therefore, lacking. Destructive methods require a prolonged period of time for completion of the therapy, and the convalescent interval may be lengthy and relatively painful. However, some methods are effective and give acceptable cosmetic results. The carbon dioxide laser has been applied successfully in the treatment of many cases. Topical 5-fluorouracil (5-FU) has been used, but when the published experience is summarized, a 50 per cent response rate is recorded for 5-FU. The final weeks of therapy are often quite uncomfortable and the results are unpredictable. DNCB-induced hypersensitivy has been noted to eradicate the disease in a small number of patients and may be worthwhile when simpler measures cannot be applied. Cryosurgery has little place in this disease. The depth of destruction is unpredictable, recurrence rates are high, patient discomfort may be severe, and scarring may be extensive.

Carcinoma in situ of the vulva is increasing in frequency throughout the world, and the results of experience with various treatment modalities continue to be reported in the literature. Recommendations regarding therapy must, therefore, remain cautious and thoughtful until the complete pathophysiology of this entity has been elucidated.

Lifetime follow-up is necessary no matter what treatment method is used. After completion of therapy, patients should be seen at three- to six-month intervals in order to detect early recurrence. After two years without disease, annual visits suffice and should include a complete evaluation of the breasts and reproductive tract, with cytology and colposcopy of the cervix and vagina. Toluidine blue directed biopsies should be taken from any suspicious vulvar lesions, and patients should be taught to promptly report the development of pruritus, papules, ulcers, or abnormal bleeding.

PAGET'S DISEASE

At St. Bartholomew's Hospital, London, in 1874, the clinician-pathologist Sir James Paget published the first description of the disease that now bears his name. The original cases occurred on the nipple and areola and were associated with an underlying breast cancer. Twenty-seven years later, the first case of the condition affecting the vulva was reported. Isolated case reports and collected series have been published since, and extramammary Paget's disease is now recognized as a distinct clinicopathologic entity with unique, pathognomonic, large, pale cells noted on histologic section of the epithelium and skin adnexa (Fig. 42). The biologic behavior and significance of this disease set it apart from the more common squamous cell carcinomas in situ and warrant its separate consideration. Although it represents new growth within the confines of the epithelial basement membrane, and as such may be classified as a form of intraepithelial neoplasia, it is rarely preinvasive per se. Isolated reports of a truly

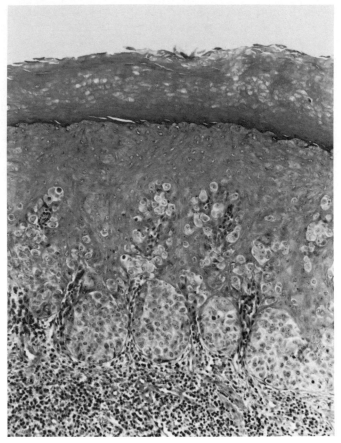

Figure 42. Paget's disease. Nests of large clear cells present at tips of rete pegs and above basal layer. Note hyperkeratosis.

invasive form of Paget's disease have been documented, but this is an unusual variant of an already unusual disorder.

Despite its rarity, Paget's disease of the vulva has absorbed the attention of many clinicians and pathologists. As a result, we know that the usual Paget cell contains a normal euploid complement of chromosomes, manufactures carcinoembryonic antigenlike sweat-gland cells, has cytoplasmic organelles consistent with both squamous and secretory skin cells, and exhibits characteristic staining reactions. Paget cells are classically located just above the replicating basal layer and often occur in clones or nests. They are found in the epithelium, along hair shafts, and in the ducts of the sweat glands. All of these features are explained by Woodruff's theory of histogenesis, in which the Paget cell represents a form of abnormal differentiation of the epidermal stem cell that would otherwise become a normal component of the skin or its adnexa. Long-term experience with Paget's disease substantiates this interpretation. Older theories suggesting that the cells represent migrating sweat gland cancer cells or amelanotic melanoma cells are no longer tenable.

Elegant topographic microscopy studies have shown that the disease process is multifocal with isolated clones of cells arising at various sites. Not all of these foci are clinically evident at any given time so that silent areas of involvement are left unrecognized and account for the high rate of apparent "recurrence."

The disease is largely confined to Caucasians, and the median age at diagnosis is 65. Clinically, it appears as a sharp-bordered, velvety red lesion with white islands of hyperkeratosis. It also may exhibit a bright pink color and have an eczematoid scaly surface. Itching and soreness are the most frequent symptoms, but typically patients delay about two years before seeking help. Unless the lesion is immediately biopsied for diagnosis, it may be misinterpreted as cutaneous candidiasis or severe dermatitis, and physician-related delay occurs in many cases. During this time, the disease process slowly encompasses more of the vulvar tissues and the irritative symptoms increase.

The major significance of Paget's disease in extramammary as well as mammary locations lies in the frequent finding of concomitant invasive carcinomas. Paget's disease of the nipple and breast areola generally signals the presence of an underlying ductal carcinoma of the breast. Similarly, in vulvar Paget's disease, underlying adenocarcinomas of the apocrine sweat glands, adenocarcinomas of the breast, squamous carcinomas of the vulva and cervix, and adenocarcinomas of the gastrointestinal tract have all been noted. Paget's disease should then be viewed as a raised red flag on the mailbox—it means that something may well be inside. The same kind of exlusional work-up proposed for the pretreatment evaluation of carcinoma in situ is therefore indicated, including: barium enema, mammography, and cytologic/colposcopic examination of the uterine cervix and vagina.

Once other malignancies have been either treated or ruled out, the primary therapy should consist in the surgical excision of the entire vulva to a depth inclusive of all adnexal structures and into the subcutaneous fat. Only by multiple sections through the complete surgical specimen have underlying and occult adenocarcinomas of the sweat glands been discovered. These tumors are true carcinomas, not simply sweat glands involved by Paget cells. Most authorities now agree that they are found in less than 20 per cent of the cases. Even when such tumors are present, the overall prognosis is good provided a follow-up radical vulvectomy with bilateral groin node dissection is performed. Shallow "skinning" procedures, which excise only a superficial portion of the vulva, run the risk of leaving behind small foci of adenocarcinoma deep in the adnexa, with a resultant tragic and unnecessary decrease in prognosis. Such suboptimal excisions also contribute to the high rate of local recurrence.

In general, partial excision, radiotherapy, topical chemotherapy, cryocautery, and laser vaporization have no place in the ideal primary treatment of vulvar Paget's disease. But risk/benefit considerations may dictate otherwise in the occasional patient. If for some reason complete surgery cannot be performed, it is still advisable to remove or destroy as much of the visible lesion as possible to prevent continued local spread and to control symptoms.

Recurrent lesions, which appear after total vulvectomy, constitute a different therapeutic problem. Wide initial margins do not completely preclude the possibility of recurrence. Extramammary Paget's disease has even been noted to recur in areas subjected to excision and primary skin graft. But recurrent sites constitute only a local threat. They are often symptomatic and they may enlarge to encompass wider areas. Surgical management by multiple repeated excision has traditionally been used, but extensive scarring may result. For such recurrent cases, laser vaporization or topical chemotherapy using a six-week course of 5-FU should be considered.

Routine follow-up observation is extremely important. Because of the high incidence of recurrence, regular visits should be scheduled every six months for the first year or two after initial excision. Thereafter annual examinations should include breast screening and a stool guaiac determination in addition to cytologic and colposcopic evaluation of the cervix and vagina. Recurrent soreness or itching in the vulvar area should prompt an immediate examination along with biopsy of any suspicious lesions.

BASAL CELL CARCINOMA

Although a relatively common tumor on exposed body surfaces, basal cell carcinoma rarely occurs on the vulva. When these lesions are seen, they, like Paget's disease, are most often found in Caucasian women over the age of 50. The clinical appearance is commonly that of a rolled edge "rodent" ulcer, but red and brown macules and hypertrophic polypoid excrescences have also been described. This wide range of clinical manifestations makes excisional biopsy the only sure method of diagnosis.

Death from basal cell carcinoma is almost unknown and essentially 100 per cent cure rates are reported. Overzealous therapy, however, may result in operative mortality. Wide local excision is all that is necessary. Provided the margins are free of tumor, the prognosis is excellent, although local recurrences are found in approximately 20 per cent of the cases. If the margins are involved, further excision is in order. Occasionally, normal mature squamous cells are noted within the basal cell cords and represent a histologic variant of the basic tumor. When these more mature cells themselves show evidence of anaplasia, then the tumor is termed "mixed basosquamous" and its biologic behavior and indicated therapy may become more like that of invasive squamous cell carcinoma. This differentiation is extremely important and often requires multiple sections, interpreted by an experienced pathologist. As in patients with carcinoma in situ and Paget's disease, there is an increased incidence of antecedent or concomitant malignancy elsewhere in the body in those with basal cell carcinoma. This incidence is noted in some series to be one in five. Pretreatment evaluation then must consist of an exclusional survey to rule out other tumors, and follow-up care should be planned to include frequent searches for other primary malignancies.

VERRUCOUS CARCINOMA

Another unusual tumor that must be separated from the common invasive squamous cancer is that of verrucous carcinoma. It may be thought of as an aggressive condyloma and in the earlier literature was known as the "giant condyloma of Buschke-Löwenstein." The lesion represents a point in the spectrum of disease represented at one end by the squamous papilloma, encompassing virally-induced benign condylomata and their dysplastic variants, through verrucous carcinoma and well-differentiated squamous carcinoma, to anaplastic undifferentiated tumors at the far extreme of neoplasia.

Like basal cell carcinoma, verrucous carcinoma is a locally invasive process that characteristically does not metastasize. The lesions are clinically dramatic. In fact, it is their alarming appearance that generally prompts a sufficiently generous biopsy to allow the pathologist to make an accurate diagnosis. Frequently, small histologic specimens look like nothing more than benign condylomatous tissue. Only when the broad front of deeply advancing epithelium is examined can the diagnosis be confirmed. There is usually no individual cellular atypia but rather an overall abnormal tissue pattern. The masses of unremarkable cells are organized in an abnormal way, encroaching on dermal connective tissue and causing a visible cauliflowerlike lesion.

Complete local excision is the only treatment necessary and more radical surgery is inappropriate. The nodes are not at risk in verrucous carcinoma. Radiotherapy is contraindicated. A number of cases have been documented in which the use of radiotherapy has transformed these more or less benign growths into aggressive, anaplastic tumors that rapidly metastasize and result in the patient's death.

INVASIVE SQUAMOUS CELL CARCINOMA

Invasive squamous cell carcinoma of the vulva accounts for 5 per cent of all female genital cancers. With a practice confined to gynecology and obstetrics, one might expect to encounter a single case about every five years. Vulvar cancer is not a clinically subtle lesion. As a rule, a grossly obvious abnormality is present and careful questioning often reveals that it has been present for some time. The disease is predominantly one of older women, with the peak incidence occurring in the seventh decade. While some series have noted a history of antecedent granulomatous infections, vulvar carcinoma is essentially a disease without clear-cut precursors.

Many years ago, women were reluctant to consult a physician regarding minor changes on the genitalia and routine screening was unknown. As a consequence, the patient with vulvar cancer usually presented with established, advanced disease. Attempts to help these patients gave dismal results until innovative and aggressive surgery was recognized as the treatment of choice and was made possible by improved anesthetic techniques.

John L. McKelvey was born in Ontario, Canada, in 1901. He obtained his M.D. degree at Queen's University and took his training in Obstetrics and Gynecology at Montreal, at the Johns Hopkins Hospital, and in Germany at both Kiel and Berlin before returning to Baltimore. As professor and head of the department in Peiping, China, from 1934 until 1938, he was asked to treat many advanced cases of vulvar carcinoma, "dreadful lesions" in his own words. It was there that he worked out his en bloc approach of radical vulvectomy and bilateral groin dissection. He did not expose the retroperitoneal space and did not excise the pelvic nodes.

Many of his techniques were performed using only local anesthesia until he returned to the United States as Professor and Head of the Department of Obstetrics and Gynecology at the University of Minnesota, a post he held until his retirement in 1967. His many papers and discussions did much to focus attention on vulvar cancer and the excellent results that could be achieved using a standardized surgical approach.

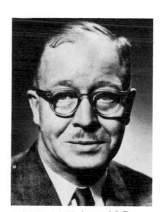

John L. McKelvey, M.D.

Led by trail-blazing surgeons such as John McKelvey in this country and Stanley Way in England, gynecologists have traditionally approached invasive vulvar carcinoma with radical vulvectomy and en bloc bilateral dissection of the lymph node groups. Their combined results upheld the superiority of radical surgery as the primary approach to this disease. The survival rates at all stages were significantly better than those obtained when other forms of therapy or lesser surgery had been employed.

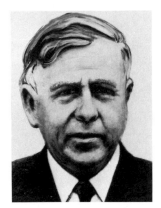

Stanley Way, F.R.C.O.G.

Born and raised in Portsmouth, England, Stanley Way completed his medical and gynecological training at Middlesex Hospital in London. Like McKelvey, he too had to confront the problem of advanced vulvar cancer. One of his mentors challenged him to "do something about it." And so, as consultant at the Royal Victoria Infirmary in Newcastle and later at the Queen Elizabeth Hospital in Gateshead, he independently designed an en bloc procedure that included routine extraperitoneal deep pelvic node dissection. Optimistic and determined, he often fought alone against a medical establishment that refused to see the advantages of a standardized approach. Over the years he kept careful records, examined and re-examined the pathological specimens, and was able to identify a new histologic variant, the "giant cell" squamous tumor. He modified his techniques to allow primary skin closure and included transplant of the sartorius muscle. His patients were kept on prolonged bed rest and were not anticoagulated. Yet, with vigorous physiotherapy, his rate of pulmonary emboli is the lowest of any series.

As a cancer surgeon consultant he had little experience with benign vulvar dystrophies or even carcinoma in situ. Patients were largely referred to him for surgery after a diagnosis of invasion had been made. But in the operating theatre he had no peer, and his legendary dexterity inspired a generation of graduate fellows, including the author, who were privileged to work with him for a time.

In 1982, he published in book form a summary of his lifetime experience, with 642 cases, under the title Malignant Diseases of the Vulva. *It is unlikely that any single surgeon will again be able to discuss a personal series of that magnitude.*

But patient attitudes have changed over time and today's woman is no longer hesitant to call her physician's attention to any vulvar abnormality. The annual check-up has become an established health habit that has provided the opportunity to identify early asymptomatic lesions. As a result, invasive squamous cell carcinoma of the vulva is now recognized in younger women who present with early lesions. This change has prompted a re-examination of the surgical protocols that have been applied so successfully in the past.

MICROINVASIVE CARCINOMA

If it were possible to identify that early tumor whose characteristics marked it as one without risk of node development, therapy could be confined to the vulva itself. Time in the hospital, long-term and short-term morbidity, and the cost of care could all be decreased. We know that the biology of the cervix differs greatly from that of the vulva. The existence of a continuum of dysplasia characterized in the cervix as CIN I–III does not apply to vulvar atypias nor to in situ carcinoma. The age group and other epidemiologic factors are not parallel. Still, the temptation is great to extrapolate cervical concepts to vulvar neoplasia. One of these concepts is that of "microinvasion." Those involved with cervical pathology now feel they are able to recognize that early lesion whose incidence of node involvement is so low that treatment of the nodes can be safely ignored. But much more data is needed before the same can be defined for vulvar carcinoma.

Those invasive squamous carcinomas of the vulva that invade less than 1.5 mm when measured from the basement membrane of the adjacent most superficial dermal papilla have a total tumor volume of less than one cubic centimeter and a very low incidence of nodal metastases. Mature differentiation, lack of confluency, and absence of vascular space involvement are good secondary prognostic factors. But until sufficient data has been collected to justify an official definition, patients with small invasive tumors, regardless of depth, should probably be treated as having stage I disease.

While depth of invasion is highly significant, the quality of the measurement varies from series to series, so that the data are not comparable. From the growing tip of the tumor, measurements are made to differing points: the immediate overlying surface, the nearest intact surface, the tip of the deepest rete peg, the depth of the deepest skin appendage, or the basement membrane of the adjacent most superficial dermal papilla. The last of these points would seem to be the most constant (Fig. 43). But until there is universal agreement on the manner of measurement, the comparison of statistics will remain hazardous.

Yet even today, most patients with vulvar carcinoma present with lesions more advanced than any definition of microinvasion would encompass, and groin node involvement is a very real possibility. In order to assess the prognosis and provide for a comparative evaluation of treatment methods, a universal system of staging is essential. In 1970, a staging system for invasive squamous cell carcinoma of the vulva, incorporating the TNM (Tumor–Node–Metastases) classification, was adopted by the International Federation of Obstetrics and Gynecology (FIGO). This system is outlined in Table 3. Patients are separated into one of four stages utilizing size and location of the lesion, clinical status of groin lymph node groups, and presence or absence of clinically demonstrable metas-

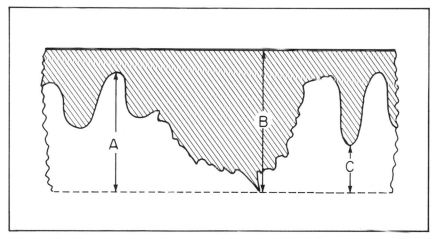

Figure 43. Depth of invasion should be measured from *A*, the top of the most superficial dermal papilla, rather than *B*, the inconstant surface, or *C*, the deepest ridge. (From Wilkinson, et al.: Microinvasive carcinoma of the vulva. Int. J. Gynecol. Pathol. 1:29, 1982.)

Table 3. FIGO Classification and Staging for Invasive Carcinoma of the Vulva

Stage I	All lesions confined to the vulva with a maximum diameter of 2 cm. or less and no suspicious groin nodes.	T_1	N_0	M_0
		T_1	N_1	M_0
Stage II	All lesions confined to the vulva with a diameter greater than 2 cm. and no suspicious groin nodes.	T_2	N_0	M_0
		T_2	N_1	M_0
Stage III	Lesions extending beyond the vulva but without grossly positive groin nodes.	T_3	N_0	M_0
		T_3	N_1	M_0
		T_3	N_2	M_0
	Lesions of any size confined to the vulva and having suspicious nodes.	T_1	N_2	M_0
		T_2	N_2	M_0
Stage IV	Lesions with grossly positive groin nodes regardless of extent of primary.	T_1	N_3	M_0
		T_2	N_3	M_0
		T_3	N_3	M_0
		T_4	N_3	M_0
	Lesions involving mucosa of rectum, bladder, urethra, or involving bone.	T_4	N_0	M_0
		T_4	N_1	M_0
		T_4	N_2	M_0
	All cases with pelvic or distant metastases.	M_1A		
		M_1B		

tases. Other postoperative staging systems outlined in the first edition of this book were applied retrospectively in two large series. While possibly helpful in terms of future therapeutic design, they did not prove to be clinically useful and have not been pursued.

It is now known that whenever the deep pelvic lymph node groups (iliac, obturator, and hypogastric) are involved by metastatic tumor, so also are the groin nodes. Similarly, the deep pelvic nodes are not found to be involved when the groin nodes are clear. In other words, the tumor follows the lymphatic pathways, metastasizing first to the primary drainage site—the groin—and only secondarily involving the deeper pelvic lymphatics.

For this reason, the classical practice of performing an extraperitoneal pelvic lymphadenectomy as part of the initial surgery has been abandoned by most oncologic surgeons. The usual approach is now that of radical vulvectomy and bilateral groin dissection. If careful histologic evaluation of the excised specimen reveals tumor metastases in the groin nodes, the possibility of deep pelvic node involvement then exists. These deep nodes may then be explored at a second surgical procedure or treated with radiotherapy. The prognosis is progressively diminished as the extent of node involvement increases. This disease most often occurs in elderly patients who may succumb within five years of diagnosis from completely unrelated causes. Consideration of such deaths in the survival statistics gives an unrealistic picture of the hazard posed by the treated disease alone. Like all of us, the patient has already faced and accepted the inevitability of death and the natural risks of aging. What she really wants to know is how her vulvar disease will affect that longevity.

Looking only at deaths due to the vulvar cancer, if the groin nodes are negative, the five-year survival should exceed 90 per cent; the presence of groin metastases alone reduces this figure to less than 70 per cent. When dissection or biopsy shows involvement of the deep pelvic nodes, less than 20 per cent can expect to remain tumor free. New techniques of radiotherapy may improve these statistics somewhat.

Groin node involvement thus represents a crucial factor influencing further therapy and indicating the prognosis. Clinical palpation may be misleading. Yet evaluation of node involvement must be as accurate as possible. Painstaking histologic study after removal constitutes the best means of assessment, but even here errors may occur and false-negative reports especially may have devastating consequences. Xerography of the surgical specimen is one technique that may aid the pathologist by providing a "road map" showing the number and location of lymph nodes embedded in the fatty tissue. Every node can thus be identified and removed. Formerly, these nodes were simply bisected, but this procedure may miss small foci of tumor. The probabilities of finding micrometastases are greatly improved if all nodes are quartered rather than bisected. Alternate tissue faces should then be embedded for microtome sectioning. This method of critical assessment could reduce the incidence of false-negative reports.

If the excised groin nodes are found to be completely free of tumor, the patient is considered to have been fully treated. Some centers may still make an exception to this procedure if the clitoris is involved, but direct lymphatic connections from the clitoris to the deep pelvic nodes are clinically nonexistent and central lesions can be treated without pelvic exploration. Such midline tumors do require bilateral groin dissection, however, since there are a number of connections crossing from side to side within the superficial lymphatic system.

Finally, if advanced lesions involving bladder or rectum are thought to be resectable, anterior or posterior pelvic exenteration may be included as part of the primary surgical approach.

Radiotherapy has found a new place in the tratment of vulvar carcinoma. A direct attack on the vulvar lesion is still inadvisable. Whether teletherapy or implants are used, the vulva does not tolerate radiation well and a nonhealing slough is the usual result. The vulva itself then must still be approached surgically. But adjunctive radiation techniques now allow for adequate exposure in order to sterilize microemboli of tumor that may be present in the groin nodes and the pelvic nodes as well. The incidence of long-term complications, especially leg edema, can be reduced and even the skin can be spared any visible reaction.

Systemic chemotherapy has been rarely used for the palliation of recurrent or disseminated disease. Objective regressions have been recorded using such single agents as bleomycin and doxorubicin (Adriamycin); but the numbers are small and the response durations usually short.

The average patient with invasive squamous cancer of the vula is an older woman with many of the medical complications characteristic of this age group. Although these patients represent a challenge of medical and surgical management, successful treatment of their disease can be accomplished with negligible mortality, acceptable morbidity, and gratifying long-term survival without tumor. The valid and accurate message to the patient then should always be one of increasing hope.

103

OTHER MALIGNANCIES

Malignant melanoma; adenocarcinomas of the sweat glands, Bartholin glands, and ectopic breasts; sarcomas of the connective tissue; and endodermal sinus tumors have all been reported to occur on the vulva. Each of these entities requires specialized primary therapy. Depending on the clinical stage and histologic type, many of these unusual tumors can be successfully managed with current techniques available to the trained oncologist. All, however, carry a much graver prognosis if they have been mismanaged initially or if well-meaning but misguided attempts at treatment have resulted in a delay of primary therapy.

Malignant melanoma of the vulva accounts for less than 5 per cent of all melanomas and less than 10 per cent of all vulvar malignancies. While it is extremely rare before puberty, it may occur at any age thereafter. In a recently reported series, almost half of the patients noted a pre-existing tumor or enlarging mole. The staging system used for squamous cell carcinoma of the vulva is not suitable for application to malignant melanoma. Instead, melanomas are graded according to the depth or level of skin involvement (Table 4). The prognosis is excellent tor level I and II lesions, fair for those in level III, and poor when levels IV and V are involved. Vulvar melanomas are either of the superficial spreading or nodular variety. The former are more common and have a better long-term outlook. Radical vulvectomy and bilateral groin dissection are usually recommended as the treatment of choice, but many series contain cases of long-term survival after only wide local excision. These are most certainly the cases of very early tumor, with level I or II involvement, and demonstrate again the fact that early discovery of superficial lesions is the best key to improved salvage. A knee-jerk response of radical surgery may not be justifiable for small superficial lesions, and there is room for individualization.

The occurrence of apocrine adenocarcinomas in conjunction with Paget's disease of the vulva has already been discussed. Adenocarcinoma may also arise within the Bartholin glands. Most of these lesions occur in women over 40, a time when the likelihood of inflammatory involvement of these structures is decreasing. Therefore, never assume that a Bartholin enlargement in patients over 40 represents a simple cyst or abscess. Marsupialization, incision and drainage, or sitz bath observation cannot yield histologic information. For these patients, at least a biopsy of the deep tissue should be performed. If adenocarcinoma is present, radical vulvectomy and node dissection can then be carried out. Lying on the "milk line," the labia are occasionally the site of accessory breast tissue.

Table 4. Levels of Cutaneous Involvement Corresponding to Prognosis in Melanoma

Level I	Intraepithelial—above the basal lamina
Level II	Extension into papillary layer of dermis
Level III	Filling dermal papillae—accumulating at junction of papillary and reticular layers
Level IV	Invading bundles of collagen in reticular dermis
Level V	Invading subcutaneous fat

At least three cases of breast carcinoma arising primarily in such ectopic structures have been reported. The vulva was the site of breast cancer metastasis in three other cases and has been known to harbor other metastatic tumors as well.

Sarcomas of the vulva are extremely rare, comprising less than 2 per cent of most series of vulvar cancers. They may occur at any age and, in general, have a poor prognosis. Leiomyosarcomas, fibrosarcomas, neurofibrosarcomas, liposarcomas, rhabdomyosarcomas, angiosarcomas, and epithelioid sarcomas have all been described. Patients who have survived are those with relatively small tumors who have been treated with adequate surgery.

Because these tumors are rare, the clinician's index of suspicion is generally low. Hoofbeats usually mean horses, not zebras. And yet, if the poor survival figures for melanoma, adenocarcinoma, and sarcoma are ever to improve, we must begin to discover them much earlier in their course. Only by keeping in mind the possibility of their existence, along with liberal use of the biopsy, can this goal be accomplished. Simple removal of all isolated pigmented lesions, solitary tumors, and biopsy of enlargements of the Bartholin gland in women over 40 would greatly decrease the mortality from these unusual malignancies.

FURTHER READING

CARCINOMA IN SITU

Friedrich, E.G., Wilkinson, E.J., and Fu, Y.S.: Carcinoma in situ of the vulva: a continuing challenge. Am. J. Obstet. Gynecol. 136:830–838, 1980.
   A personal series of 50 cases with DNA histograms and clinicopathologic analysis. Five cases of spontaneous regression are documented.
Knight, R.D.: Bowen's disease of the vulva. Am. J. Obstet. Gynecol. 46:414–424, 1943.
   The source article that reviewed the previous world's literature and began the American investigation.
Seski, J.C., Reinhalter, E.R., and Silva, J.: Abnormalities of lymphocyte transformations in women with intraepithelial carcinoma of the vulva. Obstet. Gynecol. 52:332–336, 1978.
   A landmark paper presenting evidence that the occurrence and course of carcinoma in situ of the vulva may be related to a defect in cellular immunity.
Stein, D.S.: Transmissible venereal neoplasia. Am. J. Obstet. Gynecol. 137:864–865, 1980.
   A case report that documents genital carcinoma in situ occurring concomitantly in sexual partners.
Wade, T.R., Kopf, A.W., and Ackerman, A.B.: Bowenoid papulosis of the genitalia. Arch. Dermatol. 115:306–308, 1979.
   A landmark paper describing the disease in women by the authors who first described it in men.
Wilkinson, E.J., Friedrich, E.G., and Fu, Y.S.: Multicentric nature of vulvar carcinoma in situ. Obstet. Gynecol. 58:69–74, 1981.
   Do widespread confluent lesions evolve from the coalescence of many individual clones? According to this study, the answer is yes most of the time.

PAGET'S DISEASE

Creasman, W.T., Gallagher, H.S., and Rutledge, F.: Paget's disease of the vulva. Gynecol. Oncol. 3:133–148, 1975.
   A good discussion of the M.D. Anderson experience with 15 cases. Well written and illustrated.
Gunn, R.A., and Gallager, S.: Vulvar Paget's disease: a topographic study. Cancer 46:590–594, 1980.
   A major study of serially sectioned specimens proving the multifocal nature of the disease and identifying the cause of "most recurrences."
Hart, W.R., and Millman, J.B.: Progression of intraepithelial Paget's disease of the vulva to invasive carcinoma. Cancer 40:2333–2337, 1977.
   Summarizes the available literature and presents convincing evidence for the occurrence of this rare phenomenon.

BASAL CELL CARCINOMA

Breen, J.L., Neubecker, R.D., Greenwald, E., and Gregori, C.A.: Basal cell carcinoma of the vulva. Obstet. Gynecol. 46:122–129, 1975.
A classic that analyzes 17 new cases and reviews the literature.

VERRUCOUS CARCINOMA

Japaze, H., van Dinh, T., and Woodruff, J.D.: Verrucous carcinoma of the vulva: study of 24 cases. Obstet. Gynecol. 60:462–466, 1982.
This superb report fully covers the clinical presentation, pathologic features, treatment, and results in a large series.

INVASIVE CARCINOMA

Deppe, G., Cohen, C.J., and Bruckner, H.W.: Chemotherapy of squamous cell carcinoma of the vulva. Gynecol. Oncol. 7:345–348, 1979.
An excellent summary of the available data on this topic.
Iversen, T.: Squamous cell carcinoma of the vulva. Acta Obstet. Gynecol. Scand. 60:211–214, 1981.
The final proof showing that pelvic lymphadenectomy does not influence the prognosis regardless of stage and only adds needless morbidity.
Iversen, T., Abeler, V., and Aalders, J.: Individualized treatment of stage I carcinoma of the vulva. Obstet. Gynecol. 57:85–89, 1981.
A retrospective look at the Norwegian experience suggesting ipsilateral node dissection for selected cases with unilateral lesions.
Lundwall, F.: Cancer of the vulva—a clinical review. Acta Radiol. (Stockholm) Suppl. 208:1–326, 1961.
A masterpiece of review and organization that completely covers the subject prior to 1960.
McKelvey, J.L., and Adcock, L.L.: Cancer of the vulva. Obstet. Gynecol. 26:455–466, 1965.
A review of a great surgeon's experience from 1938 to 1965 using a standardized approach.
Sengupta, B.S.: Vulvar carcinoma in premenopausal Jamaican women. Int. J. Gynaecol. Obstet. 17:526–530, 1980.
An important look at what may be a new variant of this disease, preceded by LGV, granuloma inguinale, or warts and occurring in a very young age group.
Way, S.: Malignant Disease of the Vulva. Churchill-Livingston, Edinburgh, 1982.
A complete summary of a personal experience with 642 cases seen between 1939 and 1975.

MICROINVASIVE CARCINOMA

Barnes, A.E., Crissman, J.D., Schellhas, H.F., and Azoury, R.S.: Microinvasive carcinoma of the vulva: a clinicopathologic evaluation. Obstet. Gynecol. 56:234–238, 1980.
At Cincinnati the patients could be separated into two categories. Those with overlying atypia, shallow depth of invasion, and no confluency were successfully managed with conservative surgery.
Kneale, B.L.G., Elliott, P.M., and McDonald, I.A.: Microinvasive carcinoma of the vulva: clinical features and management. Chapter 24. In: Gynaecologic Oncology (M.A. Coppleson, ed.). Churchill-Livingstone, Edinburgh, 1981.
A principal reference that collates the literature and sets the problem in perspective.
Wilkinson, E.J., Rico, M.J., and Pierson, K.K.: Microinvasive carcinoma of the vulva. Int. J. Gynecol. Pathol. 1:29–39. 1982.
A landmark paper reviewing all criteria and proposing the standard of measurement to be taken from the dermoepidermal junction at the tip of the adjacent dermal papilla. Measured in this way, tumors of less than 1.5 mm depth have less than 1 ml of volume and no nodal metastases.

OTHER MALIGNANCIES

Chung, A.F., Woodruff, J.M., and Lewis, J.L.: Malignant melanoma of the vulva: a report of 44 cases. Obstet. Gynecol. 45:638–646, 1975.
An important contribution that adapted Clark's classic levels to the vulvar skin and found no patient with a level II lesion or less dying of melanoma, but their recommendation for inflexible treatment seems unwarranted now.
Davos, I., and Abell, M.R.: Soft tissue sarcomas of the vulva. Gynecol. Obstet. 4:70–86, 1976.
Reviews the broad range of sarcomatous tumor types found on the vulva and illustrates these in a clinicopathologic study of 15 cases.

Dehner, L.P.: Metastatic and secondary tumors of the vulva. Obstet. Gynecol. 42:47–57, 1973.
   A landmark paper that reviewed this unusual subject for the first time.
Leuchter, R.S., Hacker, N.F., Voet, R.L., et al.: Primary carcinoma of the Bartholin gland. Obstet. Gynecol. 60:361–368, 1982.
   A large series of 14 cases is reported with outstanding clinical and pathologic detail and an excellent review of the literature.
Mader, M.H., and Friedrich, E.G.: Vulvar metastasis of breast carcinoma. J. Reprod. Med. 27:169–171, 1982.
   Distinguishes those cases of true metastasis from those arising primarily in accessory tissue.

6

RED LESIONS

CANDIDA

REACTIVE VULVITIS

SEBORRHEIC DERMATITIS

PSORIASIS

PAGET'S DISEASE

SQUAMOUS CELL CARCINOMA

TINEA CRURIS

PITYRIASIS VERSICOLOR

VESTIBULAR ADENITIS

ERYTHRASMA

FOLLICULITIS

RED LESIONS

The flesh tone color of normal skin is due in part to the redness of blood cells coursing through the superficial capillaries, muted by the overlying cell layers of epidermis. Abnormal erythema results from an increased visibility of the capillary bed. This in turn is dependent on the dilatation, engorgement, total number, and concentration of the capillaries as well as the thickness of the epidermal layers interposed between the vessels and the surface. Vasodilatation is part of the local immune and inflammatory response and accounts for the redness of lesions of disorders such as candidal infections, allergic responses, seborrheic dermatitis, folliculitis, and vestibular adenitis.

In carcinoma, a tumor angiogenesis factor brings about an increase in the total number of surface capillaries. In fact, without this factor and its subsequent effects, the growth capacity of any invasive tumor would be severely limited. Neovascularization, then, is present in all clinically overt invasive squamous cell carcinomas. Carcinomas in situ, as well as psoriasis, Paget's disease, and acute reactive vulvitis, are red because of a decreased number of cell layers between the surface and the vascular dermal papillae. With upward proliferation of the papillae, only a few cells of the granular zone and stratum corneum intervene above the dilated and twisted capillary loops in the papillary apex. This is the histologic picture in the erythroplastic variety of carcinoma in situ. It also prevails in psoriasis, where it accounts for the characteristic Auspitz's sign (fine capillary bleeding points on the surface of a lesion after blunt scraping). In Paget's disease, normal epidermal cells are gradually replaced by the larger and more transparent Paget's cells. The total thickness of the epidermis may remain constant, but the number of cells and the opacity of their cytoplasm has decreased. With acute reactive changes, ulceration may actually occur as layers of epithelium undergo desquamation, revealing patches of the vascular dermis.

Red lesions are usually symptomatic. The woman with carcinoma in situ may be unaware of her condition, but as a rule, the patient with a red lesion presents at the physician's office with definite specific complaints. Many of the red lesions cause itching; some result in soreness or pain; because of the fragility of surface capillaries, some present with gross bleeding. A diffuse erythema of the vulva signals a benign process, but localized red lesions are suspicious for neoplasia. Contact dermatitis develops as a result of sensitization of the vulvar and perineal skin to a specific agent. It may be possible to identify the offender by means of patch tests, but the following substances are especially suspect: detergents, bleaches, fabric softeners, perfumes, presoaks, chlorine, vinyl shields, propellants, preservatives, and even saliva and semen. Cutaneous candidiasis, seborrheic dermatitis, and psoriasis are long-term problems that may require extended management over a lengthy period of time. Patients with these disorders can become bitter and discouraged by what they perceive to be a failure of modern therapy. The psychologic as well as physical comfort of these women must be patiently considered by the clinician who would be truly effective in their care.

Candida

Candida infection of the vulva and intertriginous areas of the groin and buttocks is a common disease. This infection may be found in a primary cutaneous form, but usually a concomitant candidal vaginitis is coexistent and the vulvar involvement is secondary. Diabetics are particularly prone to the development of the disorder, and cutaneous candida may be the first sign of occult diabetes. Fully two-thirds of the women with cutaneous vulvar candidiasis are known diabetics or will be found to be such after investigation. Therefore, blood glucose tests are indicated in order to rule out the presence of metabolic disease. The high sugar content of diabetic urine bathing the vulvar tissues is thought to be one of the factors responsible for the development of such infections.

The erythema is intense and the deep red color is frequently overlaid with a fine, gray sheen. In moist intertriginous locations, this gray film may appear thick and white. The presence of satellite pustules on the fringe of the lesion helps to distinguish candida from erythrasma and tinea cruris. Wet smears, using KOH, are easily done with scrapings from the surface of the affected skin.

Keratinized cells do not lyse as quickly as do vaginal squames. If the smear is warmed with a match, the reaction is accelerated. When further confirmation is desired, an office culture for fungus can be done using Nickerson's media or dermatophyte test medium (DTM). Diabetics in poor control may develop a persistent shiny erythema of the vulvar skin ("diabetic vulvitis") after the candidal infection has been completely treated. Even after diabetic control is established, patients on oral agents may continue to complain of burning and soreness. Switching to insulin results in dramatic relief for some of these patients. Diabetics frequently suffer from peripheral neuropathies, and when these affect the pudendal nerves, vulvar symptoms may persist despite a healthy-appearing skin. Oral phenytoin (Dilantin) is sometimes successful in alleviating this problem.

Consider: The presence of candidal vaginitis suggests the diagnosis, but primary skin involvement must be differentiated from tinea cruris, erythrasma, and seborrheic dermatitis. Acute reactive vulvitis, if severe and ulcerative, may present a similar picture but rarely will this involve the genitocrural folds and buttocks. Paget's disease of the vulva may also resemble candida, but usually affects a smaller surface area and is asymmetric. The margins of Paget's involvement are sharp, but those of candida characteristically exhibit satellite inflammatory pustules.

Treatment. Treatment and control of candidal vaginitis are paramount. The cutaneous lesions should then be painted each week with 1 per cent aqueous gentian violet for two or three weeks or until the condition is resolved. Oral nystatin tablets taken three times daily will decrease the candidal colonization of the gastrointestinal tract—the major source of reinfection. Mild corticosteroid creams are helpful in between applications of gentian violet. Clotrimazole creams and lotions are also highly effective. Once the acute phase is controlled, topical boric acid in lanolin (Borofax) can be used to provide a protective fungistatic "raincoat" and prevent urine contact. Oral tranquilizers (Atarax, Vistaril, Benadryl) help to control anxiety and pruritus. One hundred per cent cotton underwear should be worn next to the skin and should be changed frequently. Rinsing the vulva with saline or tap water after voiding is a good practice. When severe candidal vulvovaginitis is a recurrent problem, oral contraceptives should be discontinued. If this is done, however, alternative methods of contraception should be suggested, since the avoidance of pregnancy may be mandatory in such cases.

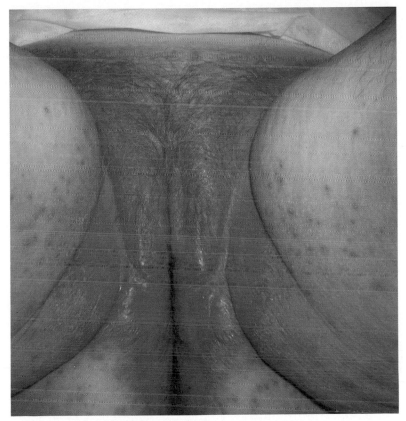

Candidal vulvitis with satellite pustules.

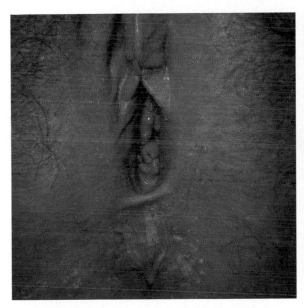

Diffuse erythema with gray sheen of candida.

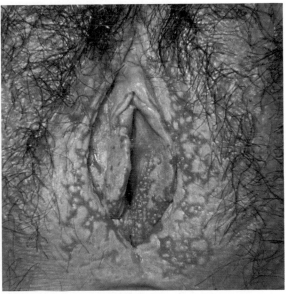

Thick film of candida gives pseudoulcerative appearance.

111

Reactive Vulvitis

A wide variety of physical and chemical stimuli can cause acute reactive changes in the vulvar skin. The mechanical trauma of scratching and rubbing; contact with synthetic fabrics, detergents and presoaks, perfumed oils, fabric dyes, hygiene sprays, or condom lubricants; and misuse of home remedies or prescribed medications such as podophyllin, gentian violet, or 5-FU are but some of the more common causes of this disorder.

A good history is of the utmost importance in such cases. Pruritus is the usual presenting symptom—when did it start? Was there contact with poison ivy or other plants? Did the onset coincide with or shortly follow any change in clothing or washing habits? Some artificial fabrics release formaldehyde vapor. Have new laundry products been tried? Oral-genital foreplay can be extremely irritating to the mucosa of the introitus and this same region may become secondarily inflamed by the discharge emanating from a concomitant vaginitis. Topical applications of potentially caustic compounds may have been used to relieve a mild pruritus, only to result in a more severe one because of contact irritation.

A wide range of clinical manifestations may be seen in this disorder and the distribution of the lesions often provides a clue to their possible cause. If only localized areas of the introitus are involved, coital trauma, vaginal discharge, perfumed suppositories or douches, or condom lubricants should be suspected. The labia minora are usually spared from exposure to contact irritants unless the agent was a component of a deliberate topical application. Diffuse reaction in the "saddle area" sometimes follows unaccustomed bicycle or horseback riding. Fabric irritants often imprint the skin with a diffuse outline of the guilty article of clothing.

Consider: Any diffuse erythema can represent acute reactive vulvitis. Candida, tinea, erythrasma, and hyperplastic dystrophy may look the same.

Treatment. Identification and interdiction of the irritant is the key to successful therapy. An axiom of dermatology states that the more severe the skin reaction, the more gentle must be the initial treatment. For exudative, weeping lesions, dilute astringents (1:40 Burow's solution in a wet compress) are soothing. These may be applied for 30 minutes, three or four times a day, and should be followed by gentle drying with cool air (hair dryer). Topical application of a corticosteroid preparation will decrease the inflammation. In lotion form these preparations are expensive, but such gentle vehicles may be necessary in the initial phases of therapy. Thereafter, creams may be used and should be gently applied two or three times a day. Topical anesthetics should be avoided. The propellants used in anesthetic sprays are irritating and the drugs themselves may cause sensitization. Oral analgesics are a better choice, and antihistaminic tranquilizers (Atarax, Vistaril, Benadryl) will potentiate their effect. Only 100 per cent cotton underwear, separately washed in a pure mild soap solution and thoroughly rinsed, should be allowed.

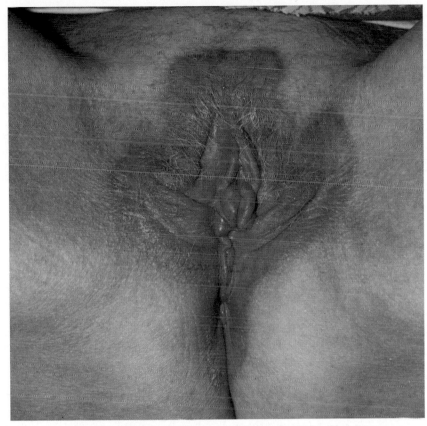

Reactive vulvitis from detergent. (Courtesy Dr. J. W. Glasser.)

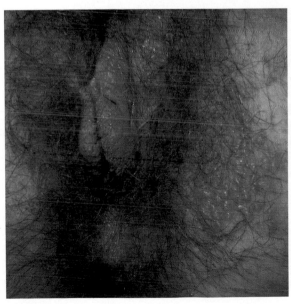

Poison ivy reaction.

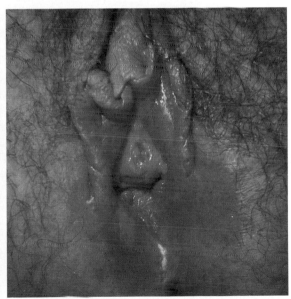

Inner vulva reacting to discharge.

113

Seborrheic Dermatitis

Seborrheic dermatitis is a term applied to a chronic skin eruption occurring in an area of high sebaceous gland activity but not necessarily related to the sebaceous cells themselves. Recurrent attacks are precipitated by fatigue, infection, and emotional stress, and most patients can recall the occurrence of similar rashes in the past. Although the eruption may take many forms, it is generally red and may be covered with a fine scale that is sometimes greasy. Past or present lesions on the scalp, behind the ears, on the sternum, or between the scapulae help to corroborate the diagnosis. There may be no symptoms, but vulvar involvement is usually pruritic and intense scratching may result in secondary bacterial infection.

Excessive sweating may itself be irritating. Women with sedentary occupations will benefit from using a ventilating cushion of wicker or fiber as well as loose clothing to maximize air circulation between the thighs. Absorbent powders are also helpful.

The labia minora are usually not involved and this feature helps to distinguish this disorder from fungal and bacterial infections. Seborrheic dermatitis usually causes symmetric lesions. Although chronic and recurrent, seborrheic dermatitis can be predictably improved with proper therapy. Since the cause is unknown, there is no "cure" as such. Patients do respond, however, to careful "management," a major part of which must be directed at the psychologic factors underlying the recurrent attacks. If a good rapport is established with the clinician, patients are often able to vocalize a great deal of hidden anxiety.

Consider: Atypical isolated foci of vulvar involvement may mimic a chronic epithelial dystrophy. Histologically and conceptually, these two lesions overlap. Separation is academic, however, since the treatment for both is virtually identical.

Treatment. In severe exudative cases, wet dressings of 1:40 Burow's solution are helpful. Pruritus, if present, must be relieved. A mixture of 7 parts Valisone cream to 3 parts Eurax applied twice daily often results in dramatic alleviation of the symptoms and a temporary disappearance of the rash. Some lesions tend to become resistant to whatever is initially prescribed. Changing to a different corticosteroid preparation may again produce good effect. The substitution of lotion or foam vehicles for cream is sometimes beneficial. Synthetic fabrics should be avoided. If scratching complicates the problem, the patient should wear white cotton gloves to sleep. Symptoms are often aggravated at night and insomnia is not uncommon. Oral Atarax or Vistaril given on retiring are both soporific and antipruritic. Understanding that the lesion will probably recur, and knowing that she has a sympathetic clinician to consult if and when it does, may help more than anything to decrease the severity of the patient's condition.

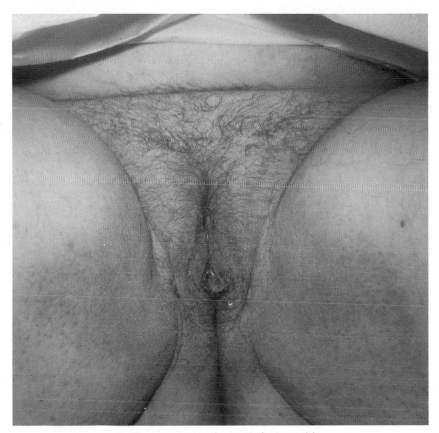

Diffuse erythema of seborrheic dermatitis.

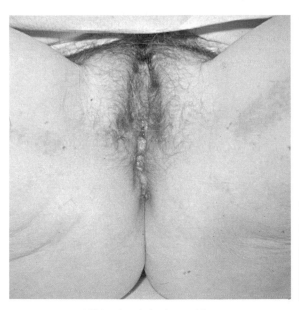

Mild seborrheic dermatitis.

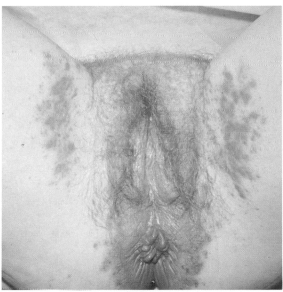

Severe seborrheic dermatitis.

115

Psoriasis

This relatively common skin disease affects over two million women in the United States and is caused by an inherited tendency to altered epidermal growth rate. While psoriatic plaques may be found on the vulva, they are rarely confined to that location. Careful inspection of the total skin surface usually reveals other sites of involvement. Rubbing or scratching may cause the formation of new lesions (the Koebner phenomenon). The uncomplicated lesion has a sharply limited border and a dull red surface covered with a fine, silvery scale. This scale may be absent in moist vulvar patches. If the scales are scratched off, fine punctate bleeding points may be noted (Auspitz's sign). Biopsy material from a psoriatic plaque will often show the intraepidermal abscesses of Munro as well as areas of superficial parakeratosis. Retention of topical toluidine blue stain should therefore be expected.

Consider: Central clearing of the lesion may render the gross appearance similar to that of tinea infection or nummular (coinlike) eczema, but the silvery scales, the involvement of other sites, and the response to scraping aid in the diagnosis.

Treatment.   Trauma and stress should be avoided. Suppression of the rapid epithelial cell turnover is the goal of therapy. Fluorinated corticosteroid preparations (Lidex, Valisone, Halog) may be applied topically twice daily on an intermittent basis. A longer-lasting effect is achieved if plastic film wrap is placed over the treated vulva to act as an occlusive dressing, but rarely is this necessary. Intralesional injection of triamcinolone suspensions in a concentration of no more than 2 to 4 mg/ml will often produce rapid involution of isolated lesions. Coal tar preparations are poorly tolerated by intertriginous areas such as the vulva.

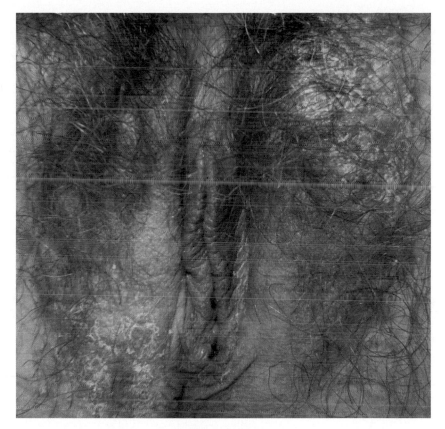

Patches of psoriasis.

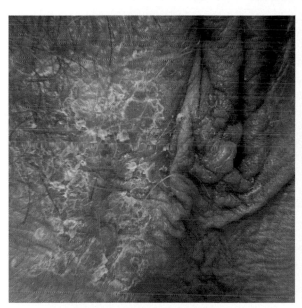

Psoriatic scaling is typical.

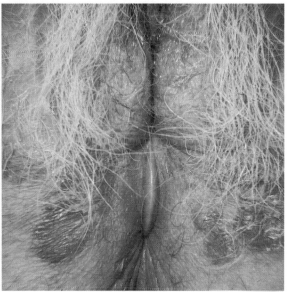

Psoriasis.

117

Paget's Disease

Paget's disease of the vulva, like Paget's disease of the nipple, represents an unusual form of differentiation of the primitive stem cell of the epidermis. These stem cells normally form squamous keratinocytes, hair shaft cells, apocrine cells, eccrine cells, and sebaceous cells. Paget's cells may then be found, singly or in nests, within the skin adnexae as well as the epidermis proper and are usually first noted just above the basal layer. The Paget's cells alone are rarely malignant. Their existence, however, is an ominous sign that frequently signals the presence of anaplasia elsewhere. In the breast, Paget's disease of the nipple is the hallmark of an underlying adenocarcinoma. Paget's disease of the vulva may also develop before, concomitantly with, or after carcinoma of the breast, and it must be remembered that both structures are in the "milk line."

Most patients are white and postmenopausal. Localized to the vulva, this disease results in an erythematous lesion interlaced with islands of hyperkeratosis that give a white speckled appearance to the surface. The margins of the lesion appear grossly well defined, but histologic involvement may extend for great distances beneath the normal-appearing skin. These occult foci are probably responsible for the high recurrence rate characteristic of the disease. Itching and soreness are the primary complaints and usually the condition will have been present for many months prior to the diagnosis.

Consider: It is frequently confused with a cutaneous candidal infection, but the raised white areas in candida are usually not as thick. Candida is diffuse and symmetric, while Paget's disease tends to be localized. Candida responds rather quickly to therapy, whereas Paget's disease is slowly progressive. An acute reactive vulvitis can mimic Paget's disease, but again, the course of irritant vulvitis is one of rapid onset and quick response to therapy. The red areas of Paget's disease will avidly retain toluidine blue dye, which is not usually the case in reactive vulvitis. Occasionally, Paget's disease may appear eczematoid (pink and scaly), resembling a chronic reactive vulvitis or hyperplastic dystrophy. Such cases can only be properly differentiated by biopsy, since the histologic features are pathognomonic. The long delay time noted in most cases of vulvar Paget's disease therefore reflects a lack of suspicion and infrequent use of biopsy procedures.

Treatment. A diagnostic survey should be performed to rule out concomitant carcinomas. A total vulvectomy with wide margins and a careful histologic search for underlying adenocarcinoma is the recommended initial therapy. A full discussion of the management of vulvar Paget's disease, both primary and recurrent, is presented in Chapter Five.

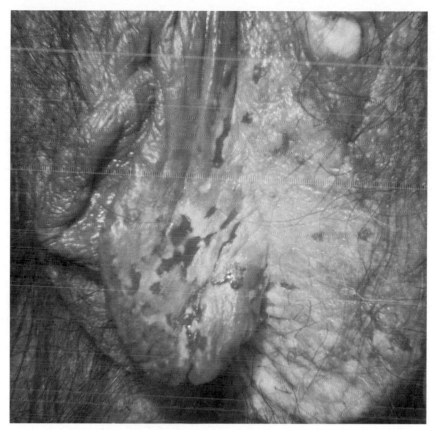

Paget's disease—unilateral.

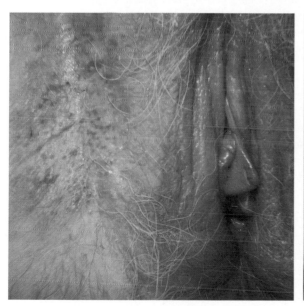

Paget's disease—single visible focus.

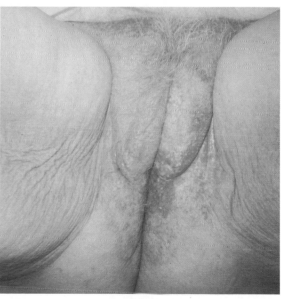

Extensive Paget's disease.

119

Squamous Cell Carcinoma

Invasive. The growth of any solid tumor beyond a diameter of one or two millimeters depends on the development of an angiogenesis factor that results in the elaboration of new capillaries. As these vessels proliferate in surface lesions, a red color is imparted to the tumor mass. Such red lesions almost always take up toluidine blue dye. Raised, red lesions with sharply defined margins should arouse immediate suspicion, and biopsy is indicated. Invasive squamous cell carcinomas are most commonly seen after age 50 and on the anterior portions of the labia majora, but they are by no means confined to this age group or location. Granuloma inguinale and giant condylomata, on the other hand, are usually seen during the reproductive years and more often begin posteriorly on the nonkeratinized surface of the introitus. A generous biopsy under local anesthesia is the only secure diagnostic procedure.

In Situ. The red variety of vulvar carcinoma in situ was formerly called erythroplasia of Queyrat. The red color is due to the prominence of the dermal papillae, which reach upward close to the cutaneous surface. The vessels located at the apices of these papillae may have a punctate or mosaic appearance when viewed under high (colposcopic) magnification. The lesions may be flat or raised and usually retain toluidine blue dye. Pruritus may be present, and contact bleeding may occur, but most patients are completely asymptomatic. These lesions are easily overlooked or regarded as localized examples of acute reactive vulvitis. The diagnosis then, depends on keen powers of observation, a high index of suspicion, and liberal use of the sampling biopsy technique.

Consider: Granuloma inguinale and giant condylomata can produce exuberant beefy red lesions that closely resemble invasive carcinoma, and many small reddish tumors may look like carcinoma in situ.

Treatment. The management of both in situ and invasive squamous cell carcinoma of the vulva is discussed at length in Chapter Five.

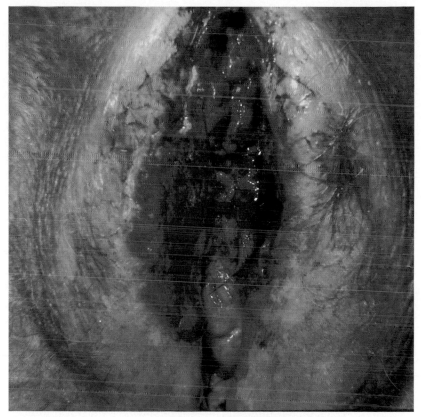

Invasive squamous cell carcinoma.

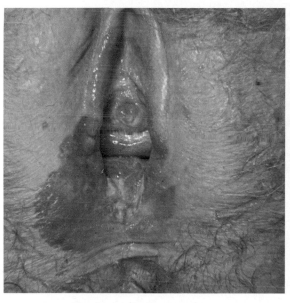

Carcinoma in situ—macular.

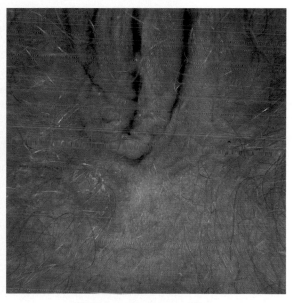

Carcinoma in situ—papular.

121

Tinea Cruris

Superficial infection of the groin and upper thighs by dermatophytic fungi results in a red, usually symmetric lesion with sharp margins and raised advancing edges. Involvement of the perineum, perianal area, and gluteal cleft is not as common in women as it is in men but accompanies a similar infection of the feet in both sexes. Therefore, looking between the toe webs for tinea pedis (athlete's foot) may give a clue to the diagnosis. Itching is often present and the infection is aggravated by obesity, sweat, friction, and heat. Exact identification of the causative fungal species is not clinically important, although most infections are caused by *Trichophyton rubrum*. The KOH wet smear will usually identify a *Candida albicans* infection. Use of the in-office DTM culture of scrapings from the active border of the lesion will further characterize a dermatophyte infection by the color change from yellow to red. Candida organisms rarely produce this color change. Tinea cruris lesions do not fluoresce under Wood's light, whereas erythrasma produces a distinctive orange to coral-red fluorescence.

Consider: The disease must be differentiated from candida and erythrasma, both of which may have a similar gross appearance.

Treatment. Hydrocortisone cream, applied twice daily, will relieve the itching and decrease the inflammatory response. Topical clotrimazole and miconazole creams or lotions are specific for tinea infections and also effective for cutaneous candida.

Pityriasis Versicolor

A common fungal infection of skin elsewhere on the body, pityriasis versicolor is unusual in the vulvar area. It is asymptomatic and especially liable to occur in patients on systemic corticosteroid therapy. The red/brown/yellow patches may fluoresce a gold color under Wood's light, but diagnosis is usually made by the clinical appearance of the lesion. Scrapings from a ringworm plaque will produce a color change on DTM culture, whereas those from a versicolor lesion will not do so. The disease is thought to be caused by transformation from the spore phase to the mycelial phase of the organism *Pityrosporum orbiculare*.

Consider: Ringworm and nummular eczema may resemble versicolor, but these lesions have a more raised edge, whereas those of versicolor are generally flat.

Treatment. Clotrimazole cream or one of the selenium sulfide shampoos used as a soap may be applied. Both are effective when applied twice a day for two or three weeks. Hypopigmentation may persist for some time after treatment.

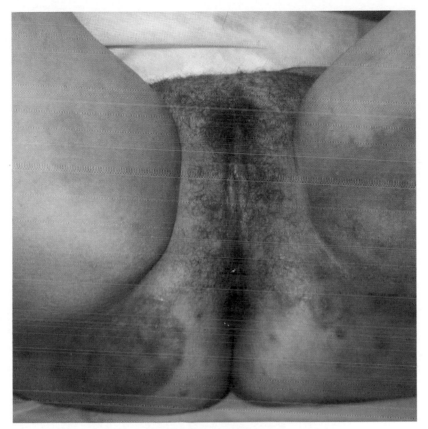

Tinea cruris.

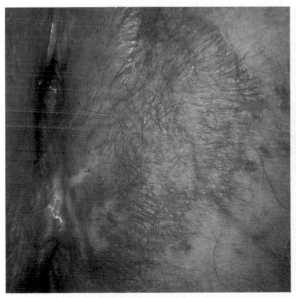

Sharp centrifugal border of tinea.

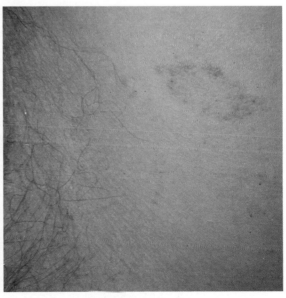

Pityriasis versicolor.

123

Vestibular Adenitis

Every student of anatomy is familiar with the paired major vestibular glands of Bartholin, but few are aware that there are minor vestibular glands as well. Since the vestibule derives embryologically from the endoderm of the hindgut, it is not surprising that mucus-secreting epithelium could be present. In fact, the entire vestibule from hymenal ring to the minora may contain any number of these structures, and they have been histologically demonstrable in over half of normal women in an autopsy study.

The minor vestibular glands are simple tubules with secretory columnar acini at their bases whose cytoplasm stains positive for mucus (Fig. 44). Their openings onto the surface are difficult to see even with a colposcope, although edema or past trauma and infection can render their ostia obvious. What function these glands serve is not known, but presumably they contribute to coital lubrication.

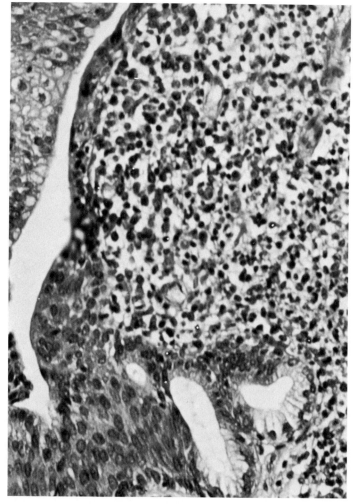

Figure 44. Inflamed minor vestibular gland with mucous acini at lower right; duct along left side supported by inflamed stroma, rich in plasma cells.

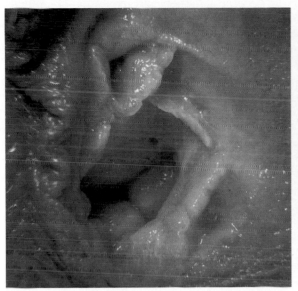

Red gland openings—left vestibule.

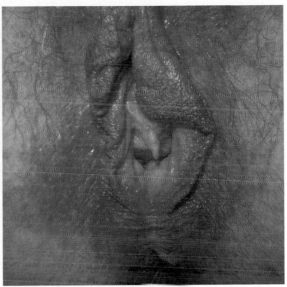

Red fourchette in vestibular adenitis.

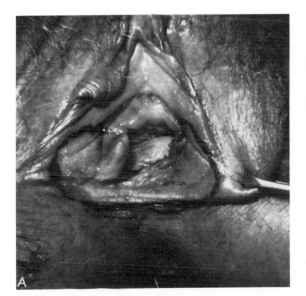

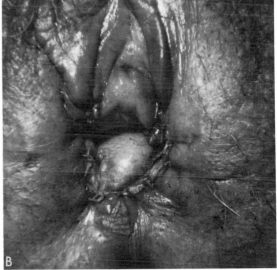

Figure 45. A, Vestibule containing inflamed glands outlined with marking pen for excision. *B,* Vagina undermined and advanced to form new introitus. Perineum left intact.

It is possible for these glands to become inflamed and symptomatic. When this occurs the involved area is slightly erythematous and if one looks closely, the tiny gland openings may be seen. Histologic section of such glands shows a chronic inflammatory infiltrate with many plasma cells.

Consider: The visible change caused by adenitis is easily overlooked. Though not a common entity, vestibular adenitis should be considered in the differential diagnosis of women who present with vulvar burning pain of unknown etiology or with dyspareunia.

Treatment. The bacteriology of such inflammations has not been studied. However, some patients have experienced relief after massaging the area with vitamin creams or estrogen creams. If this proves ineffective, the laser may be used. It is a simple matter to lase the entire gland-bearing area to a depth of 1 to 2 mm. When all else fails, the involved vestibular tissue is excised. The vaginal edge is then undermined and brought downward to cover the defect. This supplants the vestibular skin with estrogen-responsive vaginal epithelium and forms a reliable and comfortable coital platform (Fig. 45).

Erythrasma

This is an unusual disorder, but in the groin area it may mimic tinea and candidal infections by producing a symmetric erythematous lesion. Erythrasma is usually asymptomatic and the margins are not elevated. The causative organism is *Corynebacterium minutissimum.* This aerobic species may be present as part of the normal skin flora, but in diabetes and other chronic disease states of low resistance, the organism may become pathogenic. The orange to coral-red fluorescence of the lesion under the black light of the Wood's lamp is diagnostic. Such fluorescence is thought to be due to the presence of a porphyrin produced by the organism. The bacteria are difficult to culture on most media and give no reaction on DTM.

Consider: Candida and tinea may look much the same.

Treatment. Washing with antibacterial soaps is helpful as is topical clotrimazole. Oral erythromycin (500 mg twice daily for 5 to 10 days) is curative in most cases.

Folliculitis

The genitalia are second only to the feet in the density of their overall bacterial populations. Staphylococcal and streptococcal species predominate. Chronic disease states with lowered resistance, poor hygiene, localized trauma (scratching) resulting in mechanical breaks in the skin surface, or long-term occlusion (beneath a wet garment such as a bathing suit) may all encourage overgrowth of the skin flora. Infection around the hair follicles may result, with small red papules developing at the follicular sites. Tiny pustules at the center of these lesions are pierced by the hair shaft. The relationship of the papule and its pustular center to the hair follicle can be appreciated only on close inspection, and this feature differentiates the condition from Fox-Fordyce disease, in which nonerythematous, flesh-tone papules of similar size are noted.

126

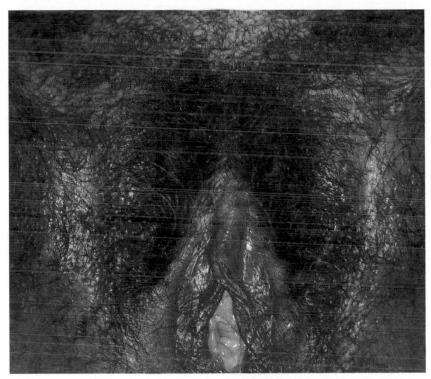

Erythrasma.

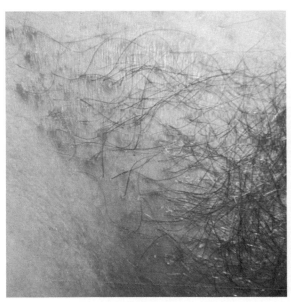

Pubic folliculitis.

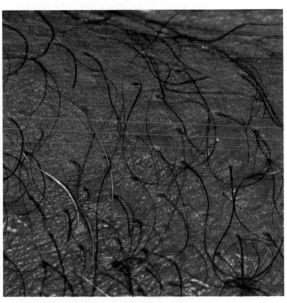

Folliculitis papules with central hair shafts.

127

Consider: Molluscum contagiosum also results in small, umbilicated papules, but they are not inflamed, lack central pus formation, and bear no relation to the hair shaft. Scabies is an uncommon disease in the vulvar area, but presents as a more diffuse red maculopapular rash.

Treatment. Folliculitis is treated first by cleansing with germicidal soap prior to the application of gentamycin or Neosporin ointment. Cases not responding within a week merit systemic antibiotic therapy, and penicillin or erythromycin are the drugs of choice.

FURTHER READING

REACTIVE VULVITIS

Chang, T.W.: Familial allergic seminal vulvovaginitis. Am. J. Obstet. Gynecol. 126:442–444, 1976.
The symptomatic allergic reaction to semen, manifestated as erythema and swelling, was genetically mediated in these cases.
Davis, B.A.: Salivary vulvitis. Obstet. Gynecol. 37:238–240, 1971.
An unusual cause for acute reactive vulvitis, worth considering in perplexing cases.
Mathias, C.G.T., and Maibach, H.I.: Cutaneous irritation: factors influencing the response to irritants. Clin. Toxicol. 13:333–346, 1978.
A thorough discussion by dermatologic authorities on the response to cutaneous irritants.

SEBORRHEIC DERMATITIS

Derbes, V.J.: Seborrheic dermatitis. Cutis 4:553–558, 1968.
An excellent review of this entity, with a complete discussion and further references.
Medansky, R.S., and Handler, R.M.: Dermatopsychosomatics: classification, physiology, and therapeutic approaches. J. Am. Acad. Dermatol. 5:125–136, 1981.
An excellent discussion of the dermatologic manifestations of anxiety and depression and the therapeutic role possible for antidepressant drugs, behavioral counseling, and doctor/patient rapport.

PAGET'S DISEASE

Breen, J.L., Smith, C.I., and Gregori, C.A.: Extramammary Paget's disease. Clin. Obstet. Gynecol. 21:1107–1115, 1978.
A careful group of clinicians looks at the relevant aspects of a large personal series of this unusual disease.

PITYRIASIS VERSICOLOR

Catterall, M.D.: Tinea versicolor—a reappraisal. Int. J. Dermatol. 19:84–85, 1980.
A short discussion that ascribes the cause of this condition to the yeast Pityrosporum orbiculare.

ERYTHRASMA

Montes, L.F., Dobson, H., Dodge, B.G., and Knowles, W.R.: Erythrasma and diabetes mellitus. Arch. Derm. 99:674–680, 1969.
Excellent color photographs of erythrasma including its Wood's light appearance, along with a good correlative discussion.

GENERAL

Korting, G.W.: Practical Dermatology of the Genital Region. W. B. Saunders Company, Philadelphia, 1981.
A good source of additional discussion and clinical photographs of dermatologic conditions with excellent presentations of the same lesions as they appear in the male.
Lynch, P.J., and Epstein, S.: Burckhardt's Atlas and Manual of Dermatology and Venereology. 3rd ed. The Williams & Wilkins Company, Baltimore, 1977.
An excellent text illustrating many of the red lesions and dermatologic conditions discussed in this chapter.

7

WHITE LESIONS

LICHEN SCLEROSUS
HYPERPLASTIC DYSTROPHY
MIXED DYSTROPHY
CARCINOMA IN SITU
VITILIGO
PARTIAL ALBINISM
LEUKODERMA
INTERTRIGO
RADIATION REACTION

WHITE LESIONS

White lesions of the vulva were traditionally treated as a group, with the misguided perception that they were premalignant. Three factors, operating independently or in concert, account for their white appearance: keratin, depigmentation, and relative avascularity. When keratin is wet, it becomes opaque and appears white or gray. The thicker the keratin layer, the more this is true; the sole of the foot after lengthy water immersion is the prime example of this phenomenon. For the same reason, any skin lesion that is hyperkeratotic appears white if located in an area of constant moisture such as the vulva. Depigmentation occurs when the basal layer melanocytes are lost or destroyed, or when because of chemical malfunction, they are unable to manufacture melanin pigment. Skin appears pale whenever superficial blood vessels are constricted, when the interposing distance between them and the surface is increased, or when they are numerically decreased by a sclerotic process.

All three of these "white producing" mechanisms are active in the vulvar dystrophies. In vitiligo, the melanocytes actually disappear from localized aras of skin; in leukoderma, newly formed skin has not yet acquired a melanocytic population; and in albinism, the otherwise normal melanocytes are prevented from forming melanin by an enzymatic defect. In the past, ionizing radiation was given for pelvic tumors with equipment that produced obliterative and fibrotic changes in the dermal vasculature and resulted in atrophy and loss of melanocytes. The net result was a pale, white appearance with depilation.

The white lesions of the vulva are not premalignant and they do not deserve the sinister reputation accorded them in the past. Much of the confusion regarding their behavior resulted from a lack of uniform terminology, and the patient's welfare was lost in the semantic shuffle. When a patient presents with a vulvar lesion that is white, gray, or simply pale in which there is a change in skin surface architecture and to which a specific cause cannot be ascribed, the clinician must ask, "Do I watch this lesion, do I put medication on it, or do I cut it off?" The answer is that the lesion should be biopsied for diagnosis. Based on its histologic features, the disease can then usually be assigned to one of the categories listed in this chapter and be given appropriate therapy.

DYSTROPHY

The vulvar dystrophies as a group constitute the most common entity in all of vulvar disease. So numerous are the patients who suffer from these disorders that if there were no other entities that afflicted the vulva, the dystrophies alone would justify special interest in this area. Because of the intense pruritus that often accompanies dystrophy, some patients may actually become disabled shut-ins for fear of scratching in public. Apprehension over the possibility of cancer and guilt because of a supposed lack of hygiene adds to the patient's misery. For these reasons, the correct diagnosis and effective treatment of a patient with dystrophy can be one of the most rewarding experiences in the field of vulvar disease.

Clinics around the world report that lichen sclerosus is by far the most common single entity and accounts for over 70 per cent of most series. The hyperplasias are actually unrelated to lichen sclerosus, although they may occur concomitantly and constitute a mixed dystrophy. But until a new nomenclature is devised, the hyperplastic conditions will continue to be protected under the term dystrophy lest they again be mistaken for some premalignant condition and become the targets of surgery. For in the past, when the histologic examination of radical vulvectomy specimens became possible, white areas of skin with disordered epithelial architecture were sometimes found adjacent to the carcinomatous growth. Early observers concluded that the white change preceded the cancer and led to its development. The same logic could have been used in the reverse interpretation: that the presence of carcinoma caused the surrounding white change. But, in fact, there is no good evidence to substantiate either theory. White changes are common; cancer is rare. Occasionally both are found to coexist on the same vulva, but such coincidence does not imply a causal relationship. Prospective studies and a review of the world's literature over 25 years have shown conclusively that the likelihood of carcinoma developing within a pre-existing area of benign white change is less than 5 per cent. Nevertheless, the erroneous concept that "leukoplakia" of the vulva is premalignant continues to be reproduced in textbooks, and needless vulvectomies are still performed in the name of prophylaxis.

In order to correct this widespread misconception and neutralize the bias associated with the older inaccurate terminology, the International Society for the Study of Vulvar Disease promoted a new nomenclature recommending that dystrophy be used as a general heading to denote the many disorders of epithelial growth and nutrition that may result in a white surface change on the vulva (Table 5). Based on clinical and histologic characteristics, the vulvar dystrophies may be subclassified into three groups: lichen sclerosus, hyperplastic, and mixed. Within the latter two groups epithelial atypia is sometimes noted, but the incidence of this is not great. Only in unusual cases in which the degree of atypicality approaches that of carcinoma in situ is there any suspicion of a premalignant tendency. It must be emphasized that this statistical improbability of cancer arising from dystrophy is based on cases in which biopsy has been performed to rule out already existent neoplasia. Without liberal use of the vulvar biopsy, the accurate diagnosis and proper treatment of vulvar dystrophy is impossible. In addition to the initial diagnostic biopsy, follow-up biopsies should be obtained, especially in those cases marked by an incomplete therapeutic response.

Table 5. Classification of Vulvar Dystrophies Adopted by the International Society for the Study of Vulvar Disease

	CLINICAL	HISTOLOGIC
Lichen sclerosus	Pruritic, thin, parchment, "atrophic," introital stenosis.	Thin, loss of rete, homogenization inflammatory infiltrate.
Hyperplastic°	Pruritic, thick, gray or white plaques, skin or mucosa.	Acanthosis, hyperkeratosis, inflammatory infiltrate.
Mixed°	Areas compatible with both forms may be present at the same time.	

°Atypia may accompany hyperplastic dystrophy and is graded mild, moderate, or severe.

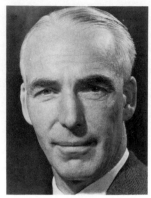

Sir T.N.A. Jeffcoate, M.D.

Dystrophy *is a term that denotes a disturbance of nutrition and was suggested for vulvar white lesions by T.N.A. Jeffcoate, M.D., who had established himself as one of the foremost gynecologic authorities in England. Educated at the University of Liverpool, he remained in that city for most of his postgraduate work, eventually becoming Professor of Obstetrics and Gynecology at the University of Liverpool until his retirement. Along the way, he became a member of the American Association of Obstetricians and Gynecologists and served as President of the Royal College of Obstetricians and Gynecologists. His book the* Principles of Gynecology *ran to four editions and became a classic text.*

In 1942, he diagnosed his first case of carcinoma in situ of the vulva, and subsequently reported it as a first in Britain, for the condition was rare in those days. In 1961, he delivered the Emily Blake Memorial Lecture at Newcastle upon Tyne, which was later published in the British Medical Journal *under the title "Premalignant conditions of the vulva with particular reference to chronic epithelial dystrophies." It was this paper that challenged the time-honored concepts of premalignant leukoplakia and proposed that most white lesions were benign disorders that did not lead to cancer. Summarizing the literature, demonstrating the histology, and detailing his own cases followed over time, he concluded that in the "majority of cases of chronic epithelial dystrophy there is no special risk of malignant change and vulvectomy is not justified. . . ."*

Within the present nomenclature the dystrophies are defined by their histologic appearance. In lichen sclerosus, the criteria include variable degrees of thinning of the squamous epithelium with progressive loss of the epithelial folds

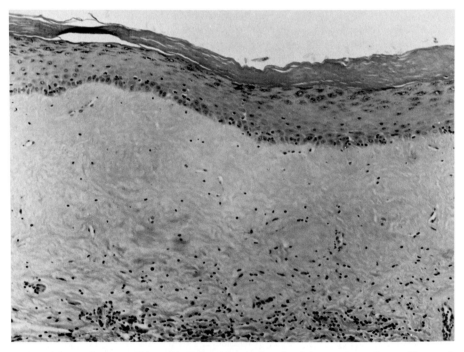

Figure 46. Lichen sclerosus. Thin epithelium with paucity of cell layers; loss of rete ridges, subepithelial homogeneous zone and deep inflammatory infiltrate.

(rete ridges). Vacuoles may be noted in the basal layer of cells. The dermis just beneath the squamous epithelium has a characteristic acellular, homogeneous appearance, and chronic inflammatory cells are found deep to the homogeneous zone. Hyperkeratosis or parakeratosis may be present, but often the keratin layer is normal (Fig. 46). Biopsies from hyperplastic dystrophy exhibit acanthosis with elongation and blunting of the epithelial folds. Chronic inflammation within the dermis will vary from mild to severe, and hyperkeratosis is usually present (Fig. 47). A mixed condition exists when both forms of dystrophy are noted on the same vulva simultaneously. In areas of hyperplasia, atypia may occur. Atypical features include the presence of individually keratinized cells, corps ronds, abnormal nuclei, ectopic mitoses, and discrepancies in the nuclear/cytoplasmic ratio. An increased density of the cell population is sometimes noted, as are alterations in the overall architecture of the epithelium. Some degree of atypia is found in approximately 5 per cent of all dystrophies, and most of these are mild or moderate and amenable to medical therapy.

In the future, this histologic classification may be expanded by the International Society Committee on Nomenclature to separately identify a number of dermatologic entities (e.g., lichen planus, lichen simplex chronicus, interface dermatitis, etc.) currently encompassed within the category of hyperplastic dystrophy.

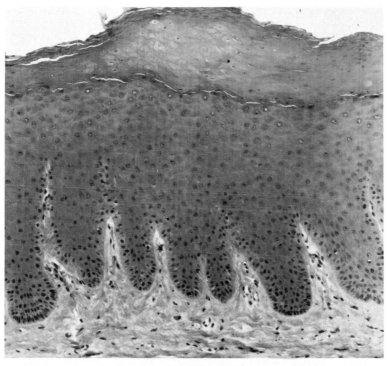

Figure 47. Hyperplastic dystrophy. Thickened epithelium with deep, broad rete ridges and hyperkeratosis.

Lichen Sclerosus

The lichen sclerosus variety of vulvar dystrophy is the most common of all the white lesions. Formerly known with a suffix as lichen sclerosus et atrophicus (LS & A), it has also been called atrophic leukoplakia, kraurosis vulvae, senile atrophy, and atrophic vulvitis. In the male, it may affect the glans penis and is known as "balanitis xerotica obliterans." It was first described as an entity in 1887 by the French dermatologist Hallopeau, who named it in the botanical tradition of the time.

The disease may occur at any age and has been reported in young children, in whom it causes special therapeutic problems. At puberty, the disease will sometimes resolve spontaneously. But women in the reproductive age group may also be affected, so it is not related to simple estrogen lack. Marked remissions are sometimes noted by these patients during pregnancy, with postpartum re-exacerbation. In addition to the vulva, patches of similar skin change may sometimes be found on the neck, trunk, and extremities. But by far the most common presentation is on the vulva and perineum of the postmenopausal woman.

Although not present at the onset, pruritus eventually accompanies the lesion in almost all cases, and may prompt vigorous scratching with subsequent ulceration and the formation of ecchymoses. The vulvar architecture is progressively destroyed as the labia minora undergo adhesion to the adjacent majora prior to their eventual dissolution. Edema, scarring, and agglutination of the prepuce and frenulum gradually bury the glans of the clitoris in an amorphous mass of pale tissue. These structural alterations are clinical hallmarks of lichen sclerosus. Without regular coitus or dilatation, the diameter of the vaginal opening may shrink and result in a true kraurosis, or contraction of the introitus. Untreated cases, irritated by years of grattage, can develop reactive hyperplastic change which may be accompanied by atypia. From such foci, carcinoma may develop. But lichen sclerosus by itself does not eventuate in cancer, and patients should be firmly reassured on this point.

The cause of lichen sclerosus remains unknown and the disease has not attracted the research attention it deserves. We do know that the siblings and offspring of affected individuals, who possess certain HLA antigens in common, may manifest the disease. There is an increased incidence of pernicious anemia, achlorhydria, and autoimmune disorders found in some series of patients with lichen sclerosus. Biochemically, a two- to threefold decrease in elastin has been noted in affected skin, and immunofluorescent studies show an increased deposition of fibrin in the homogeneous upper dermis. Patients with lichen sclerosus have been found to have decreased serum levels of dihydrotestosterone compared to age-matched controls without the disease.

More information is gained from a study of case histories that shows this usually diffuse condition sometimes sharply limited to a single facet of one labium minus. In a landmark case reported from Argentina, lichen sclerosus developed within myocutaneous grafts transplanted from the thigh for vulvar reconstruction. This occurrence would seem to eliminate local blood supply or local dermal factors as causative. While the search for an etiology slowly proceeds, women continue to present with the disease and are dependent on the physician's skill for recognition, management, and long-term observation.

The surface epithelium is pale. Varying degrees of hyperkeratosis may be

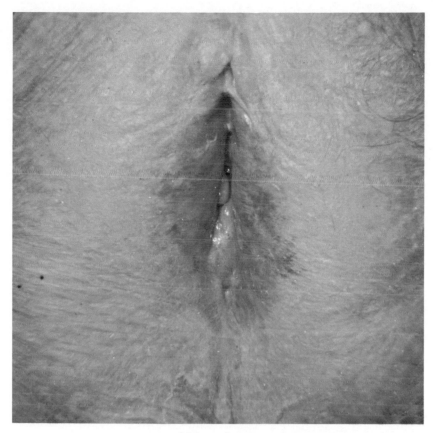

Lichen sclerosus.

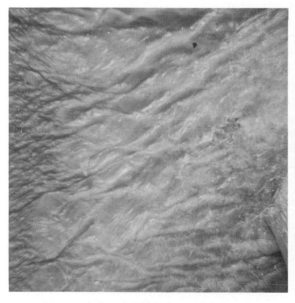

Characteristic wrinkling of superficial layers.

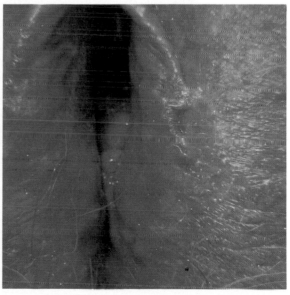

Early adhesion of minora.

135

present, but more usually the surface is shiny and crinkled, not unlike wrinkled parchment or tissue paper. These changes are usually symmetric, diffusely involving the entire vulva and perineum, and producing shapes similar to a "figure 8," a "butterfly," a "lotus flower," or a "keyhole." Although poetic, such patterns have no individual significance.

In early cases, the initial adhesions are noted between the minora and underlying majora and around the prepuce and frenulum. Unchecked, this process eventually obliterates the minoral and periclitoral structures. Fissures and small thickened areas may be noted and it is not possible to rule out foci of hyperplasia, atypia, or carcinoma in situ on the basis of gross appearance alone. Toluidine-blue directed punch biopsies must initially be performed, sampling representative areas of involvement. If these show only the classic histologic features of lichen sclerosus, the nature of the disorder should be explained and definitive therapy begun.

Consider: Few lesions resemble lichen sclerosus, but many may coexist with it. Vitiligo exhibits no surface change but when present with lichen sclerosus makes the area of involvement seem larger. Foci of atypicality or cancer should always be sought, especially at the time of initial evaluation.

Treatment. Many schemes of therapy have been advocated for lichen sclerosus but none has worked as well in the postmenopausal patient as the topical application of 2 per cent testosterone propionate in Vaseline. The use of this drug is fully discussed in Chapter Three. If testosterone therapy is discontinued, the lichen sclerosus will usually recur. Lifetime maintenance therapy using testosterone ointment once or twice a week is therefore recommended to achieve "permanent" control of this disorder. Occasionally, cases are found to be resistant to this approach. Some patients report aggravation of their symptoms when they ingest "acid" foods like tomatoes, citrus fruits, or pickles; simple antacids are extremely helpful for this group. Paradoxically, if achlorhydria is present and properly treated, the dystrophy may improve.

In children and in some older women in whom testosterone side effects prove intolerable, topical progesterone creams have been helpful. The drug probably acts through local conversion to the androgen, but it is amazingly well tolerated and free of masculinizing effects.

The disease recurs in over half of those treated with total vulvectomy and in most of those postmenopausal women treated with deep laser vaporization, so surgery is not the answer. Some young women of reproductive age have remained disease free for as long as three years after laser treatment, and investigation of this mode of therapy is being continued. When all else fails, alcohol injection may produce relief from the symptom of itching, but seems ineffective if a painful or burning sensation is present.

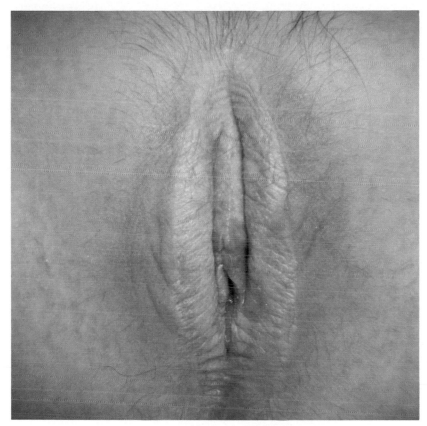

Childhood lichen sclerosus.

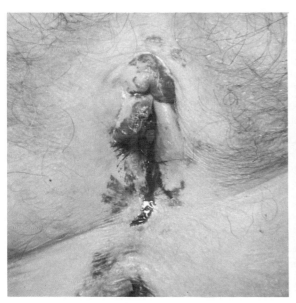

Friable lichen sclerosus with ecchymoses.

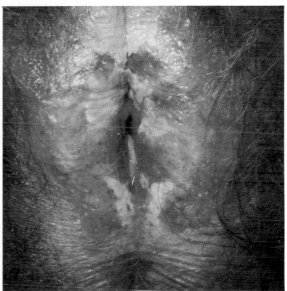

Severe untreated lichen sclerosus.

137

Hyperplastic Dystrophy

The hyperplastic dystrophies are characterized by a thickened, white keratinized surface (hyperkeratosis), along with enlargement of the epidermal rete pegs (acanthosis), and a dermal inflammatory infiltrate. These are all nonspecific dermatopathologic features that may be found in neurodermatitis, lichen simplex chronicus, hypertrophic vulvitis, chronic reactive vulvitis, eczema, etc. There is little point in the delicate differentiation of these entities. They are alike in their gross appearances, have identical histologic features, and show similar therapeutic responses. Accordingly, they are conveniently considered as a single group.

The age of these patients varies widely throughout the reproductive and postmenopausal years. Isolated areas of involvement are seen more frequently than with lichen sclerosus, and the dystrophic remodeling of the labia minora and clitoris is usually absent. In black women, the appearance of hyperplastic dystrophy may be dramatic, and it is often confused with vitiligo. The rapid turnover of the keratinocytes does not permit them to acquire their usual amounts of melanin pigment. The basally situated melanocytes are so far from the surface that their contribution to skin color is negated by the dense, opaque, superficial keratin. Over a period of time, the pigment usually returns to these areas, once the fundamental problem of dystrophy has been reversed.

Pruritus is the cardinal presenting symptom, and the degree of surface alteration depends, in part, on the amount of previous scratching. Surface appearance cannot be used as an indicator of histology, however. Foci of atypia may lie within the hyperplastic areas, and the total significance of any lesion depends upon the amount and severity of the atypical change. For this reason, toluidine-blue directed biopsies are necessary, both to secure the diagnosis of hyperplasia and to rule out atypicality.

Consider: Carcinoma in situ, Paget's disease, lichen sclerosus, and mixed dystrophies may all give a similar clinical appearance.

Treatment. The relief of itching must be the first aim of any therapy. If anxiety and nervous agitation are evident, oral tranquilizers may be used and are especially helpful at bedtime. Topical corticosteroids are the mainstay of therapy for hyperplastic dystrophies. The potent fluorinated compounds, in cream or ointment vehicles, applied twice daily will bring about an impressive regression of the lesion within four to eight weeks. If Eurax is combined with the steroid, a powerful antipruritic effect is achieved. A combination of 7 parts Valisone and 3 parts Eurax in a cream base applied twice daily seems particularly effective. Unlike lichen sclerosus, once the condition has completely regressed, recurrence is uncommon, providing any aggravating irritant is identified and removed from the patient's environment. Laundry products and underwear fabrics are particularly likely offenders. Should hyperplasia develop again at a later date, it must be treated as a new lesion. Diagnostic biopsies must be obtained and therapy reinstituted. Total vulvectomy is unnecessary and often futile, since the dystrophic process frequently recurs at the surgical site. When severe pruritus is unresponsive to long-term topical therapy, alcohol injection should be considered.

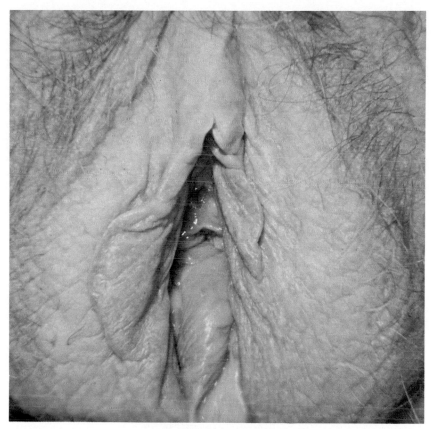

Hyperplastic dystrophy.

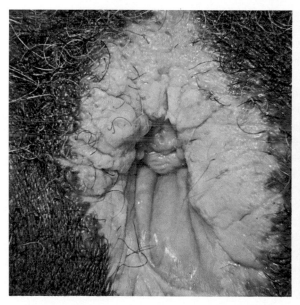

Hyperplastic dystrophy, recurrent postvulvectomy.

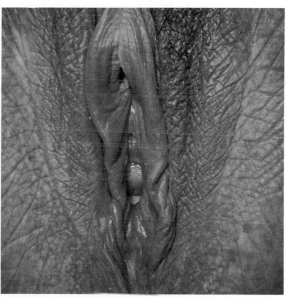

Hyperplastic dystrophy—"cross-hatch" pattern.

139

Mixed Dystrophy

Both lichen sclerosus and hyperplastic dystrophy may be found on the same vulva and constitute the condition known as mixed dystrophy. If all vulvar dystrophies are taken together, a mixed variety is present in about 15 percent of the cases. There may be no clear delineation visible on the surface between the areas of thick and thin epithelium. Occasionally, a wrinkled parchment appearance will signify an area of lichen sclerosus and a heaped-up white plaque will betray an underlying hyperplasia. But only numerous punch biopsies, preferably directed by prior staining with toluidine blue, can establish the complete diagnosis.

Mixed dystrophies have a slightly higher incidence of atypia than do the hyperplastic lesions alone. The reason for this is not clear, but histologic sampling of all representative areas becomes even more important when a mixed situation occurs. Although these conditions may show a gratifying response to treatment, the patients should continue to be followed throughout their lives. Little is known of the incidence of recurrence, regression, or progression of vulvar atypias. Severe atypia is probably best managed as if it were carcinoma in situ. Mild and moderate changes, however, seem to regress when the basic dystrophy is treated, and follow-up biopsies usually show a normal-appearing epithelium.

Atrophic vaginitis frequently accompanies vulvar dystrophy in elderly patients. For a long time, the vulvar changes were thought to be part of the involutional process resulting from estrogen deprivation. Estrogen-containing creams were therefore advocated for both conditions. The vaginal mucosa would predictably improve and vulvar itching would be diminished, but the underlying dystrophic process would continue its inexorable course, sometimes resulting in near total occlusion of the vaginal outlet. When present, atrophic vaginitis should be specifically treated, but estrogen-containing creams have no place in the therapy of vulvar dystrophy itself.

Consider: Lichen sclerosus with hyperkeratotic plaques, or superimposed candidal infection, and carcinoma in situ may give a similar appearance.

Treatment. The treatment of mixed dystrophy may be accomplished in one of two ways. The entire vulva may be treated with corticosteroids first, as if it were uniformly hyperplastic. This will usually require about six weeks. Once the hyperplastic areas have receded to normal, testosterone therapy is instituted to reverse the zone of lichen sclerosus. A much slower but in the long run equally effective method consists of using corticosteroid and testosterone preparations on alternate days. Over a period of one or two years, the testosterone effect will predominate and the lichen sclerotic areas will improve. This latter approach has the advantage of preventing the macerations and ulcers that occasionally accompany the vigorous use of testosterone alone. The clitoral enlargement and libido surge, sometimes seen with unopposed testosterone, are also minimized. The overall response is much slower, however, so that when atypia is present, the more rapid method is preferred.

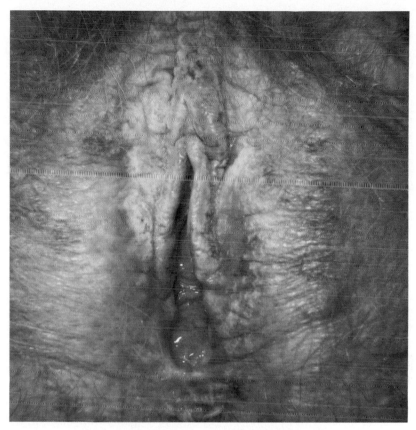

Mixed dystrophy—foci of hyperplasia with lichen sclerosus.

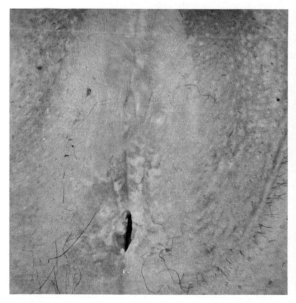

Mixed dystrophy with true kraurotic vaginal stenosis.

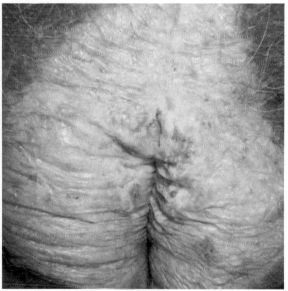

Mixed dystrophy—hyperplasia at introitus.

141

Carcinoma in Situ

The lesions of carcinoma in situ may be brown, red, gray, white, or any combination of these colors. Their particular shade depends on the histologic construction of the individual lesion. Cases in which a white change is predominant usually exhibit a heavy layer of superficial hyperkeratosis or parakeratosis (presence of nuclear material within a keratinized stratum). This latter feature can be grossly demonstrated by the retention of toluidine blue dye and is one of the characteristic hallmarks of the disease. When the decolorizing 1 per cent acetic acid is applied, it may serve to make the lesion more obviously white and raised. By dehydrating densely packed cells, acetic acid renders them more opaque, just as it does when used in cervical colposcopy.

The precursors of carcinoma in situ, if there are any, have yet to be identified. But it is logical to assume that at least some severely atypical hyperplastic lesions may progress to the full-thickness change necessary for the diagnosis of in situ cancer. Just what percentage of atypias behave in this manner is unknown. For this reason, it is best to manage dystrophic lesions with foci of severe atypia as if they were indeed in situ carcinoma. In like manner, it is possible to find foci of dystrophy associated with carcinoma in situ, but this is not usually the case. The lesions may appear superficially identical, but carcinoma in situ has a median age incidence between 30 and 40, while that of dystrophy is somewhat higher. Both lesions are usually pruritic. When a neoplastic process arises in a pigmented epidermis, a dark appearance may result as long as the normally functioning melanocytes continue to produce pigment. By the same token, a white change occurring in previously pigmented skin as a result of neoplasia may indicate destruction of the basal melanocytes and serve as a signal of early stromal invasion. For this reason, multiple biopsies should be taken to sample as much of the lesion as possible and a blade is sometimes better suited to this purpose than is the Keyes cutaneous punch.

Consider: Carcinoma in situ may be either discrete or diffuse, but as a rule, the lesions are more localized than those of dystrophy and their appearance is more variegated. Some areas of carcinoma in situ resemble Paget's disease, and the similarities of surface appearance make biopsy the only secure method of diagnosis.

Treatment.   The management of carcinoma in situ must be individualized. Much depends on the age of the patient, extent of the lesion, and quality of follow-up observation. The white hyperkeratotic lesions are least likely to respond to topical chemotherapy, which then becomes an even less attractive treatment alternative. The available methods of therapy are fully discussed in Chapter Five.

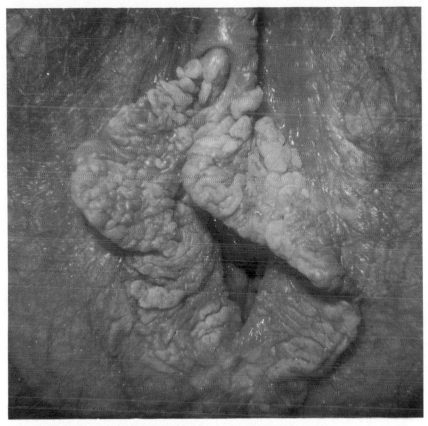

Extensive carcinoma in situ resembling condylomata.

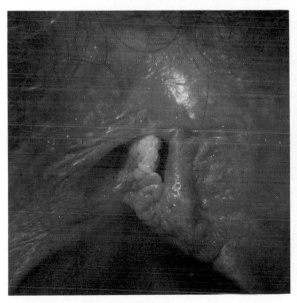

Clitoral carcinoma in situ.

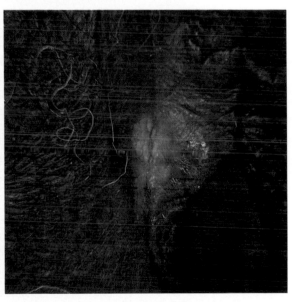

Carcinoma in situ.

143

Depigmentation Disorders

The depigmentation disorders of the vulva include *vitiligo,* which commonly affects the genitalia; *partial albinism* (piebaldism), which rarely does so; and *leukoderma* (postinflammatory depigmentation), which is a common sequel to any destructive process.

Vitiligo is an inherited disorder related to a dominant gene with variable penetrance, in which the epidermal melanocytes are progressively lost, possibly related to an autoimmune mechanism or to toxic by-products of prostaglandin metabolism. Within a given area, those melanocytes associated with pigmented hairs are among the last to be affected, so often black hairs will paradoxically be growing from an amelanotic patch of skin. Any area of the body may be involved in addition to the genitalia. The borders of the lesion are often scalloped with milky white convexities invading the normal dark concavities. The edge is usually well defined and may even be hyperpigmented. Under a Wood's light, the affected areas appear bright white—totally devoid of pigment. Patients with vitiligo may give a positive family history of the disease and begin to notice the condition early in life. Uveitis, lymphoma, thyroid disease, and Addison's disease are found more frequently in affected individuals. Late onset vitiligo has been associated with a higher incidence of diabetes mellitus and pernicious anemia. Chronic exposure to phenols appears to cause similar lesions.

Partial albinsim (piebaldism) is a dominant multigenic trait. It is characterized by the presence (generally from infancy onwards) of patches of nonpigmented skin and hair commonly on the forearms and forehead. In this disorder, the melanocytes are present, but a local enzymatic deficiency prevents the normal formation of melanin pigment. Hairs in the affected areas are therefore white. Such patches may occur on the labia and are usually unilateral and striking. But despite their appearance, they are of no clinical significance and require no treatment.

Leukoderma is a descriptive term for the lack of pigment seen in scarred areas resulting from trauma or ulceration. It may be permanent or temporary. Herpes infections often show this as a transient reaction during the later stages of healing, and the scars of syphilitic ulcers may give a similar appearance. In time, normal melanocytes will usually populate the new skin from the periphery. Leukoderma differs from vitiligo and albinism in that the skin surface in the white area is often thin, there is a history of previous inflammation, a familial history is lacking, and other body areas are not affected.

Consider: It is possible for any of these entities to simulate one another, but since none are amenable to therapy, only vitiligo is of clinical consequence. The history, normal skin surface, and presence of lesions elsewhere should assist in its identification.

Treatment. There is no specific therapy for these three disorders as they affect the vulva. Once associated diseases have been excluded, the problem is a cosmetic one, generally covered by ordinary clothing. Lesions elsewhere on the body, however, should be evaluated for therapy by a dermatologist.

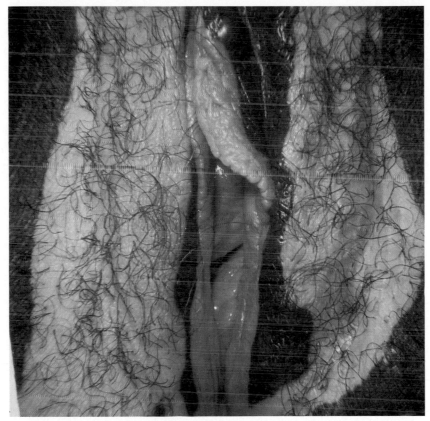

Vitiligo.

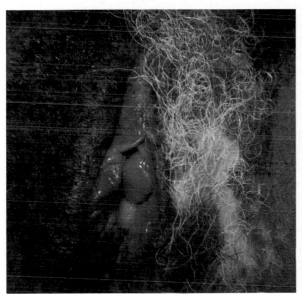

Partial albinism.

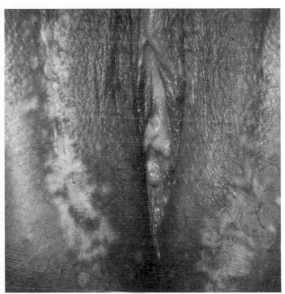

Postherpetic leukoderma.

145

Intertrigo

Literally translated, intertrigo means "between the three corners" and refers to a nonspecific inflammatory condition usually found in the genitocrural folds and beneath the abdominal panniculus. Because of the constant moisture present on the opposing skin surfaces, the superficial keratin is white. Squamous debris, adnexal gland secretion, superficial fungi (usually candida), and bacteria (often *E. coli*) contribute to the accumulation of matter that may have a white, yellow, or gray color and overlies a dull, red, somewhat shiny skin fold. The borders are not sharp and distinct as in tinea cruris, and the satellite pustules characteristic of superficial candida are usually lacking.

Consider: Either candida or tinea may be present and are easily investigated with a wet smear or fungus culture.

Treatment. Anything that can be done to minimize the aggravating factors of obesity and moisture will help. Wet packs (1:40 Burow's solution) aid in achieving dryness if acute maceration and breakdown are present. Correction of urinary incontinence, use of absorbent cotton undergarments, better air circulation, and simple talcum powder as a skin lubricant are all beneficial. If fungi are documented, 1 per cent gentian violet paint is curative.

Radiation Reaction

The advent of supervoltage equipment has given the radiotherapist the ability to deliver tumorcidal doses of pelvic radiation with a negligible effect on the overlying skin. This was not always the case, however, and many patients still bear the cutaneous scars of old orthovoltage therapy. That they are still alive and free of tumor is a tribute to the success of radiation therapy and to the skill of the physicians who employed it. But when the external fields overlapped onto the mons or vulvar areas, a recognizable change in the skin was produced.

Such areas are generally devoid of active hair follicles. The melanocytes have been damaged or destroyed, and an obliterative endarteritis has produced a devascularization of the sclerotic dermis. Superficial venules may have become telangiectatic. The net result is a diffusely bald, pale vulva. A history of prior radiation helps to differentiate this lesion from dystrophy.

Consider: Carcinoma in situ may present in a similar fashion and may even be more likely to arise in previously radiated skin. Toluidine-blue directed biopsy is therefore indicated in order to rule out the possibility of an in situ carcinoma.

Treatment. There is no therapy available that can repair the damage caused by ionizing radiation. Such lesions should be observed at regular intervals, however, lest a carcinomatous change arise within the damaged epithelium.

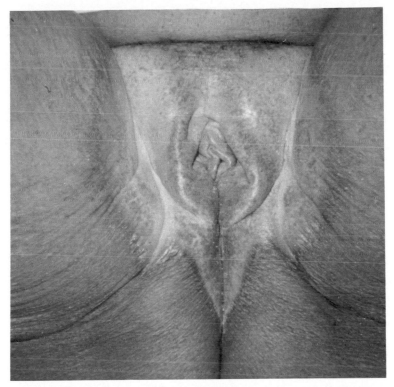

Intertrigo.

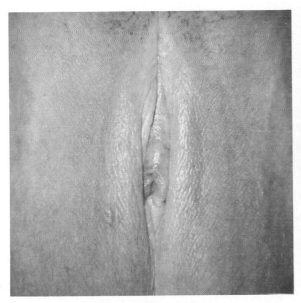

Chronic radiation reaction.

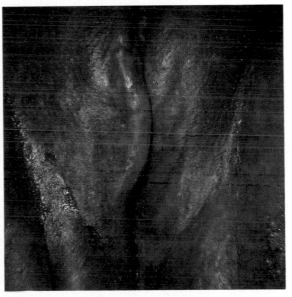

Acute radiation epithelitis.

147

FURTHER READING

DYSTROPHY

Bushkell, L.L., Friedrich, E.G., and Jordan, R.E.: An appraisal of routine direct immunofluorescence in vulvar disorders. Acta Dermatovener. 61:157–161, 1981.
The reactions in vulvar pemphigus and pemphigoid were characteristic. Surprising was the finding of upper dermal fibrin in 12 of 24 cases of lichen sclerosus.

DiPaola, G.R., Rueda-Leverone, N.G., and Belardi, M.G.: Lichen sclerosus of the vulva recurrent after myocutaneous graft. J. Reprod. Med. 27:666–668, 1982.
A landmark occurrence, this report will greatly influence future thought on the etiology of this disease.

Flynt, J., and Gallup, D.G.: Childhood lichen sclerosus. Obstet. Gynecol. 53:79S–81S, 1979.
An excellent review of the disease in premenarchial girls and the special problems they can present.

Harrington, C.I., and Dunsmore, I.R.: An investigation into the incidence of auto-immune disorders in patients with lichen sclerosus and atrophicus. Brit. J. Dermatol. 104:563–566, 1981.
Fifty patients with lichen sclerosus showed more tissue antibodies and autoimmune disorders than did age-matched controls.

Hart, W.R., Norris, H.H., and Helwig, E.B.: Relation of lichen sclerosus et atrophicus of the vulva to development of carcinoma. Obstet. Gynecol. 45:369–377, 1974.
A landmark paper from the Armed Forces Institute of Pathology experience with over 100 cases, showing only one carcinoma developing in association with lichen sclerosus and this was from an isolated area of hyperplasia.

International Society for the Study of Vulvar Disease: New nomenclature for vulvar disease. Obstet. Gynecol. 47:122–124, 1976.
A definite end to the semantic confusion, this publication set the terminology for the following decade.

Jasionowski, E.A., and Jasionowski, P.A.: Further observations on the effect of topical progesterone on vulvar disease. Am. J. Obstet. Gynecol. 134:565–568, 1979.
Progesterone cream is useful as a second-line approach in the treatment of some dystrophies and may be safely used in children.

Jeffcoate, T.N.A., and Woodcock, A.S.: Premalignant conditions of the vulva with particular reference to chronic epithelial dystrophies. Brit. Med. J. 2:127–134, 1961.
A landmark of historical significance that marked the "beginning of benignity."

Jeffcoate, T.N.A.: Chronic vulval dystrophies. Am. J. Obstet. Gynecol. 95:61–73, 1966.
Excellent summary of personal experience from this thoughtful observer.

Kaufman, R.H., and Gardner, H.L.: Vulvar dystrophies. Clin. Obstet. Gynecol. 21:1081–1106, 1978.
An excellent summary of the problem and of the literature.

Murphy, F.R., Lipa, M., and Haberman, H.F.: Familial vulvar dystrophy of lichen sclerosus type. Arch. Dermatol. 118:329–331, 1982.
Identifies three sisters who developed lichen sclerosus in a family with pernicious anemia.

Sanchez, N.P., and Mihm, R.C.: Reactive and neoplastic epithelial alterations of the vulva. J. Am. Acad. Dermatol. 6:378–388, 1982.
A classification of the vulvar dystrophies from the dermatopathologist's viewpoint.

Zelle, K.: Treatment of vulvar dystrophies with topical testosterone propionate. Am. J. Obstet. Gynecol. 109:570–573, 1971.
Careful investigation into the response and side effects to be expected from androgen therapy.

CARCINOMA IN SITU

Caglar, H., Tamer, S., and Hreshchyshyn, M.M.: Vulvar intraepithelial neoplasia. Obstet. Gynecol. 60:346–349, 1982.
A study of 50 patients that nicely details the clinical and therapeutic aspects of the disease.

Rastkar, G., Okagaki, T., Twiggs, L.B., and Clark, B.A.: Early invasive and in situ warty carcinoma of the vulva: clinical, histologic and electron microscopic study with particular reference to viral association. Am. J. Obstet. Gynecol. 143:814–820, 1982.
Despite their size, the lesions are benign, but their incidence is increasing and viral particles can be demonstrated in the lesion.

VITILIGO

Nordlund, J.J., and Lerner, A.B.: Vitiligo. It is important. Arch. Dermatol. 118:5–7, 1982.
All you need to know about this disorder with the statement of a new hypothesis relating its occurrence to prostaglandin metabolism.

8

DARK LESIONS

LENTIGO

CARCINOMA IN SITU

NEVI

REACTIVE HYPERPIGMENTATION

SEBORRHEIC KERATOSES

MELANOMA

HISTIOCYTOMA

PUBIC LICE

DARK LESIONS

Derived from the neural crest, melanocytes are specialized cells found in the basal layer of the epidermis. They possess the enzymatic equipment necessary to convert the amino acid *tyrosine* to the pigment *melanin*. This substance is packaged within the cell into organelles called melanosomes, the size and character of which are racially determined. Like nerve cells, melanocytes have dendritic processes that intercalate between the other epidermal cells. Via these dendrites they "eject" melanosomes into the cytoplasm of the cutaneous squamous cells. Leftover melanosomal material is taken up by dermal macrophages, which, when filled with melanin, are known as melanophores. So melanin pigment is found in all the skin layers in a form, amount, and concentration that is, in part, genetically determined.

The concentration of melanocytes also varies depending on anatomic location. The genitalia characteristically have a high number of melanocytes per square millimeter of skin surface. Hence, genital skin is generally darker than that covering the rest of the body. Within this background, any localized stimulus to an increase in the number of melanocytes or an increase in the production rate of melanin will result in an increased depth of color, which may be perceived as a dark lesion.

The relative frequency of the various entities that may present in this manner can be gained from a study that looked at biopsies from 100 consecutive patients with dark lesions (Table 6). Lentigo, a freckle-like concentration of melanocytes, was the most common member of the group. Unexpectedly carcinoma in situ was next at about the same frequency as that of nevi or moles. After mild to moderate trauma, especially inflammation, an increased amount of melanin is found in the dermal melanophores as well as the epidermis. The reactive hyperpigmentation is diffuse and more or less symmetric. Seborrheic keratoses become more common with advancing age and are very common elsewhere on the body. But on the vulva, as isolated lesions, they mimic melanomas, nevi, and other dark lesions. Melanoma is a rare tumor and accounts for an extremely small, albeit dangerous percentage of vulvar dark lesions. Basal cell carcinoma is also rare but can present as a freckle-like lesion.

Table 6. The Histologic Diagnosis in 100 Consecutive Dark Lesions

LESION	NUMBER OF PATIENTS
Lentigo	36
Carcinoma in situ	22
Nevi	21
Junctional (7)	
Compound (8)	
Intradermal (6)	
Reactive hyperpigmentation	10
Seborrheic keratoses	5
Hemosiderin deposit	3
Melanoma	2
Basal cell carcinoma	1

Finally, there are dark lesions that owe their color to old blood pigments rather than to melanin. Organizing hematomas and hemosiderin-containing histiocytomas are two examples. The transparent pubic louse would be practically invisible were it not for the ingested blood present in the alimentary tract.

Taken altogether, then, dark lesions comprise about 10 per cent of all vulvar diseases. Most lack pathognomonic clinical features and a secure diagnosis is possible only after biopsy. Junctional nevi are usually flat macules; but then, so are lentigines, the benign freckle-like concentrations of normal melanocytes. Melanomas are usually elevated with an irregular surface, but so are the benign and more common intradermal nevi and seborrheic keratoses. Nor can depth of color be used as a guideline. Melanomas, for example, may vary from deep black to flesh colored (amelanotic melanomas).

It does little good to suggest that intradermal nevi are benign and should be left untreated, while melanomas must be excised and seborrheic keratoses should be curetted. The three lesions may look exactly alike, and without histologic confirmation, both diagnosis and treatment remain in doubt. Melanomas account for less than 2 per cent of all vulvar dark lesions, but their prognosis is extremely grave and much depends on early diagnosis. For safety then, all dark lesions of the vulva should be biopsied. Most are small and circumscribed, so that excisional biopsy is easily accomplished. When larger lesions are encountered, do not be apprehensive about incisional biopsy. Much has been said about the potential dangers of incising a true melanoma, but a number of studies have shown that incisional biopsy of a melanoma has no effect whatsoever on the prognosis of the lesion, providing the biopsy is correctly interpreted and followed promptly by surgical therapy. Pregnancy may cause transient changes in depth of pigmentation. As a general rule, however, any change in color, size, or texture, as well as bleeding or ulceration occurring in a vulvar dark lesion, should be regarded as suspicious and the lesion should be immediately excised.

Lentigo

Lentigo is the most common vulvar dark lesion and usually first appears on the vulva in early to mid-adult life. Frequently multiple (lentigines), these lesions are flat, circumscribed macules of varying size (1 to 10 mm). They appear on both skin and mucous membrane and may be found anywhere from the hymenal ring outward. They are asymptomatic, light brown in color, and closely resemble freckles. True freckles, however, are localized areas of sensitive melanocytes stimulated to excess pigment production by the tanning rays of the sun. As such, they do not occur on the vulva. Similar in both clinical and histologic appearance, lentigo occurs on nonexposed areas of skin and mucous membrane, and bears no relation to sunlight. Histologically, lentigines are areas of skin within which the melanocytic population present in the basal layer produces an excessive amount of melanin. Prominence of the rete ridges is a variable feature. But lentigo is not a completely casual diagnosis. Some dermatopathologists recognize atypical melanocytes above the basal layer in some of these lesions. Thus, what may appear to be a harmless area of lentigo may, in fact, represent a level I melanoma of the rare lentigo maligna type. This is one more reason to excise all dark lesions regardless of their clinical appearance. Only careful histologic study can confirm the diagnosis.

Consider: The appearance of lentigines grossly mimics that of junctional nevi, superficial melanomas, small pigmented basal cell carcinomas, and foci of carcinoma in situ.

Treatment. Excisional biopsy is both diagnostic and curative. For extensive lentigo, once the diagnosis is firmly established, no further treatment is necessary.

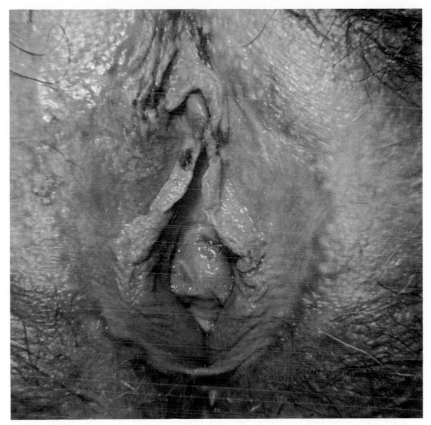

Lentigo.

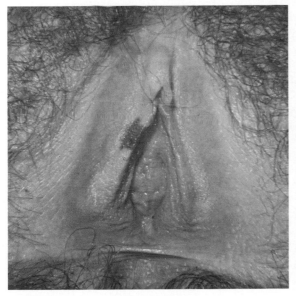

Unifocal lentigo.

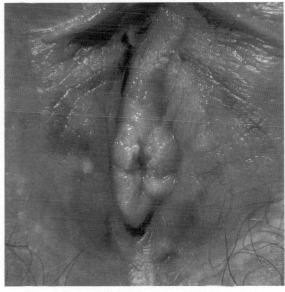

Vestibular melanosis (lentigo).

153

Carcinoma In Situ

The proliferation of abnormal squamous cells in areas of carcinoma in situ stimulates the production of melanin in some cases. In an effort to provide the same amount of pigment to each new squamous keratinocyte, the melanogenic process is accelerated within each local melanocyte. Some of the atypical squames may lose their ability to contain the pigment manufactured by the melanocytes. They become "incontinent" of this pigment, which is then carried upward in the epidermis in the form of individual granules of melanin located between the surfaces of adjacent squamous cells. Some of the pigment "leaks" out into the dermis and is incorporated by the histiocytic macrophages, which then become melanophores. These large cells full of pigment are often located near the tips of the dermal papillae, close to the skin surface. Along with the epidermal pigment granules, these melanophores account for the dark color of the atypical areas. Continued production of pigment depends on normally functioning melanocytes and an intact basal layer. Invasion of the dermis by squamous carcinoma would destroy these cells. Dark-colored areas of carcinoma in situ are therefore less likely to harbor foci of microinvasion.

About one third of all vulvar carcinomas in situ appear hyperpigmented; this feature constitutes one of the major hallmarks of the disease and should always prompt a diagnostic biopsy. The individual areas are often multiple and may be confluent. The lesion is almost always raised or papular, and the surface may be smooth and nevoid or rough and warty.

Consider: Isolated lesions closely resemble nevi, seborrheic keratoses, melanomas, and lentigines. Confluent and multiple examples mimic dark condylomata, syphilids, and reactive hyperpigmentation. Only biopsy is reliable for diagnosis. Unifocal lesions can be totally excised. Confluent areas require incisional biopsy, removing a portion of one or two separate areas. This will permit an accurate diagnosis and will not affect the subsequent prognosis of the disease.

Treatment. *VD alert.* This disease is frequently found in younger women and is often associated with condylomata acuminata, trichomonas, herpes, gonorrhea, and syphilis. In addition, there is a high incidence of concomitant or antecedant carcinoma in situ of the cervix. Cytology and colposcopy are mandatory as is careful inspection of the anal canal, which harbors foci of occult disease in over 20 per cent of the cases. Individualized therapy is warranted for carcinoma in situ and is fully discussed in Chapter Five.

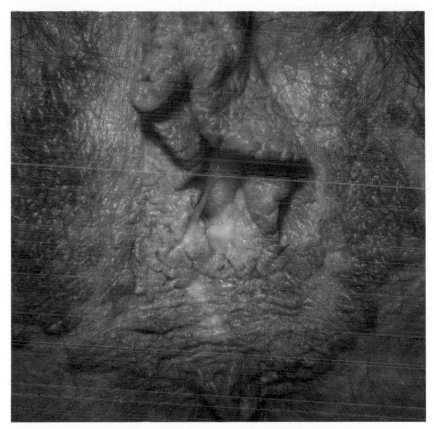

Coalescent carcinoma in situ.

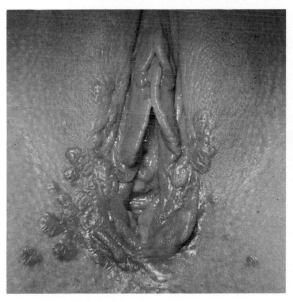

Multicentric carcinoma in situ.

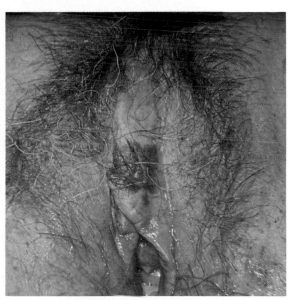

Unifocal carcinoma in situ.

155

Nevi
(*Moles*)

Localized clusters of neural crest cells in an undifferentiated form, present from birth, are called nevi. As juvenile nevi they exhibit a high degree of activity at the junctional (basal) layer of the epithelium, are invisible, and usually go unrecognized until after puberty, when pigmentation occurs. If biopsied at this early stage, they are called junctional nevi. These are young lesions and usually appear as round flat macules closely resembling lentigines. As the nevus matures, the cells begin to occupy the dermis as well as the epithelium, and when present both above and below the basement membrane they are known as compound nevi. Eventually, the nevus cells are completely confined within the dermis and no junctional activity is noted. These are intradermal nevi. As the nevus evolves over time from junctional to intradermal, there is a corresponding decrease in the tendency to melanoma transformation and an increased height of surface contour. Very few nevi eventuate in melanomas, but approximately 30 per cent of all melanomas arise in pre-existing nevi.

There is a wide variation in the depth of color found in these lesions. Some nevi are flesh colored or light tan and almost "amelanotic." Most, however, are dark enough to be distinguished from the surrounding skin. Nevi are completely asymptomatic. Rarely is the patient aware of their presence unless it has been called to her attention during a previous examination. Her estimate of the historical course of the lesion is therefore uncertain.

Consider: Depending on their stage of development, nevi may resemble melanomas, carcinomas in situ, basal cell carcinomas, seborrheic keratoses, histiocytomas, and lentigines. The raised intradermal nevus may also resemble an acrochordon, hidradenoma, granular cell myoblastoma, pyogenic granuloma, or accessory breast tissue. Only histologic assessment can be considered diagnostically reliable. Sudden growth, ulceration, bleeding, or the development of satellite lesions are ominous signs that warrant immediate attention.

Treatment. Excisional biopsy is both diagnostic and curative. In order to encompass all the nevus cells, the dissection should be three-dimensional and include the underlying dermal tissue as well. Nevi should not be treated by destructive techniques that prevent histologic evaluation.

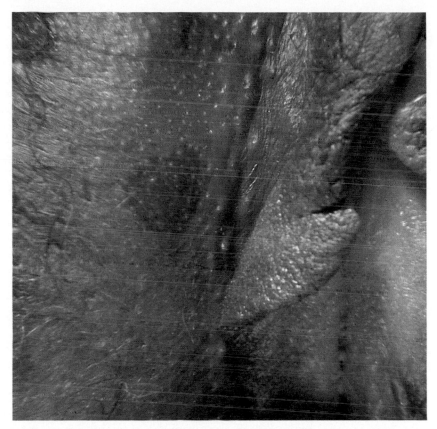

Junctional nevus—flat.

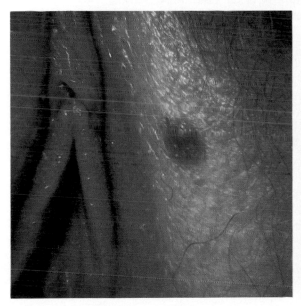

Compound nevus—slightly raised.

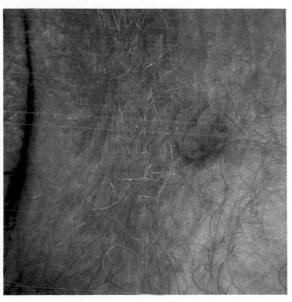

Intradermal nevus—polypoid.

157

Reactive Hyperpigmentation

In response to chronic inflammation, persistent low-grade irritation, or mild to moderate injury, pigmented skin can react with a compensatory hyperpigmentation. Such change may be seen in a diffuse form in obese women who suffer from constant chafing, and in diabetics with chronic cutaneous fungal infections. A more localized process is noted on the periphery of healing ulcerative diseases, in some mature condylomata, and paradoxically in vitiligo. As a rule, reactive hyperpigmentation shows no surface change under magnification. It is a totally flat lesion without an elevated component.

Consider: Lentigo may be extensive and symmetric and is also completely flat. Focal areas of reactive change are unusual but would resemble junctional nevi.

Treatment. No one treatment is required provided the diagnosis is secure. Histologic confirmation is desirable.

Seborrheic Keratoses

Seborrheic keratoses are the most common tumors of the body skin occurring in the postmenopausal age group. Although they are frequently seen on the scrotum, they are relatively unusual on the vulva. They account for a correspondingly small percentage of vulvar dark lesions. Sebaceous glands play no part in the formation of these excrescences; the term "seborrheic" refers instead to their frequently greasy appearance. These flat-topped papular lesions are raised above the level of the surrounding skin and often appear as if they could simply be "picked off" or bluntly shaved from the skin surface, as indeed they may be with a dermal curette. Inspection of other skin areas often reveals additional similar lesions, and their presence may suggest the clinical diagnosis of the vulvar lesion.

Histologically the papule is made up of proliferating basal cells that are growing upward in a controlled fashion and are generously interlaced with melanocytes. Cystic spaces filled with keratin are a common feature. The sudden appearance of large numbers of seborrheic keratoses is ominous and may signal the development of an unrelated internal malignancy. Seborrheic keratoses themselves are asymptomatic and believed to have no appreciable malignant potential, although isolated cases in which carcinoma has developed have been reported.

Consider: The clinical features of seborrheic keratoses may mimic those of melanomas, compound or intradermal nevi, or carcinomas in situ. Therefore, while their gross appearance may be adequate for diagnosis in some cases, they are sufficiently rare on the vulva to warrant excisional biopsy in order to rule out more serious disease.

Treatment. Excisional biopsy for diagnostic purposes is also curative. If scraped off with a dermal curette, the specimen should be sent for histologic confirmation.

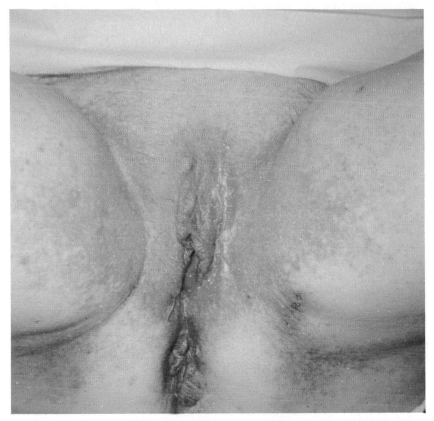

Postinflammatory hyperpigmentation.

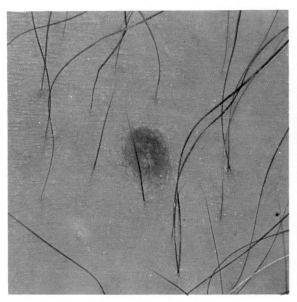

Seborrheic keratosis.

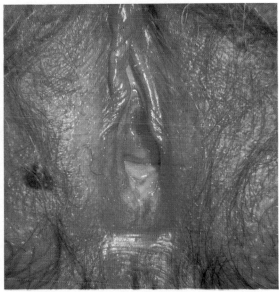

Seborrheic keratosis.

Melanomas

Current usage applies the term "melanoma" only to malignant lesions. Melanomas are rare tumors, but they account for approximately 10 per cent of all vulvar cancers. The vulva constitutes only 1 per cent of the total skin surface, yet approximately 5 per cent of all melanomas in females arise in this organ. There are three basic varieties of this tumor. The first is called lentigo maligna melanoma and is a flat freckle or lentigo-like lesion that frequently has a speckled appearance. It may be quite extensive, but tends to remain superficial and is extremely rare on the vulva. The second type is the superficial spreading variety. This is by far the most common type found on the vulva. Because of its superficiality, it retains a fairly good prognosis if discovered early in its course even though its surface measurements may be well beyond 2 or 3 cm in diameter. The third variety is the nodular melanoma, a raised tumor with an irregular surface, which carries an ominous prognosis. Though relatively small in diameter, it often involves the deeper levels and is frequently as deep as it is wide. The degree of pigmentation is variable and "amelanotic" varieties are reported, but most lesions are darker than the surrounding skin.

Vulvar melanomas may occur at any age but are most frequent after age 50 and almost always found in Caucasians. Unfortunately many patients present with a palpable "lump" even though an asymptomatic dark lesion may have been present for some time. It has now been convincingly demonstrated that the prognosis is directly related to the depth or level of cutaneous invasion rather than to the size of the tumor. The patient with an early superficial lesion has an excellent chance of survival. It is for this very reason that all vulvar dark lesions should be biopsied. Excisional biopsy with deep margins should be done whenever feasible, but cutting into such a lesion and removing only a portion for diagnosis does not alter the prognosis if prompt definitive surgery is performed within a short time.

Consider: Depending on the type of tumor, melanomas may be flat or raised and therefore they may resemble almost any of the other dark lesions. The surface features of melanomas, nevi, lentigines, seborrheic keratoses, carcinomas in situ, and histiocytomas are often identical.

Treatment. Optimium therapy is dependent on depth of the tumor invasion. According to many authorities, needless node dissection can be safely avoided if the lesion is of the superficial spreading variety and has not invaded below 0.76 mm from an intact surface. Similarly, an overly wide margin of resection does nothing to improve the already excellent prognosis in such cases. Deeper lesions correspondingly justify more extensive dissection. These options are more fully discussed in Chapter Five.

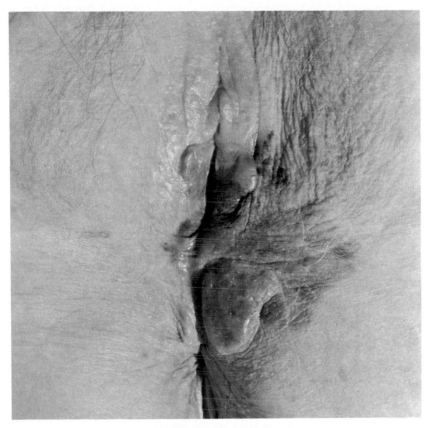

Superficial spreading melanoma. (Courtesy Dr. F. J. Fleury.)

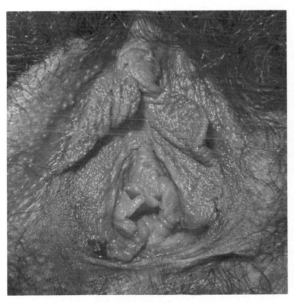

Early melanoma.

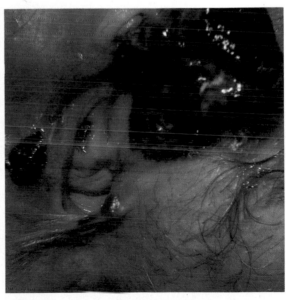

Nodular melanoma with satellites. (Courtesy Dr. J. D. Woodruff.)

Histiocytomas

Formerly known as sclerosing hemangiomas or dermatofibromas, these connective tissue tumors are now felt to be composed of histiocytes, multipotential cells that are capable of functioning as fibroblasts and producing collagen. More vascular variants of this tumor are rich in capillaries and contain numerous histiocytes that have phagocytosed hemosiderin as well as lipid. This accounts for the pale brown color of these tumors, which are considered to be benign, although some have been noted to recur locally years after wide excision. They are asymptomatic and their appearance may mimic that of melanomas, compound or intradermal nevi, and papular syphilids.

Treatment. Excisional biopsy is both diagnostic and curative.

Pubic Lice

The pubic louse is an obligate parasite whose specific host is man. Unlike the less fastidious body lice, pubic lice are usually confined to the hair-bearing regions of the genitalia and are only occasionally found in axillary or eyelash hair. While sexual contact is a frequent mode of transmission from one individual to another, bed linen, upholstery, and personal clothing can also serve as sources of infestation. The pale gray nymph and adult forms are almost transparent. They would be all but invisible against the skin were it not for the hemosiderin pigments present in their digestive tract. Under high-power magnification, this blood-filled alimentary canal will be seen to have a horseshoe or wishbone shape. To the unaided eye, the louse appears as a tiny (1mm) rusty spot on the skin surface closely related to the base of the hair shaft. There may also be tiny specks of "ground pepper" visible on the nearby skin. These represent excreta of the louse. The nits (louse eggs) are olive-shaped, pale gray excrescences that are cemented to the hair shafts and have the appearance of "dandruff." The louse is a very slow moving creature that prefers to establish itself in a single location where it remains attached to the skin, grasping the hair shafts and feeding intermittently on blood from the skin capillaries. A female extrudes about two nits per day, cementing these to the hair shafts throughout her one-month life span (Fig. 48).

Pruritus of the mons is the most common complaint, although the upper labia majora may be involved as well. Most patients will have already identified the organisms and will present promptly for treatment. When a colposcope is available, the appearance of the nits and lice under high magnification is diagnostic. A hand lens will serve the same purpose. Alternatively, one of the rusty spots may be teased from the skin surface under a drop of mineral oil, placed on a slide, and examined with a microscope.

Consider: Severe pruritus in the absence of vaginitis or obvious vulvar lesion is also a hallmark of Fox-Fordyce disease, which should be considered in the differential diagnosis.

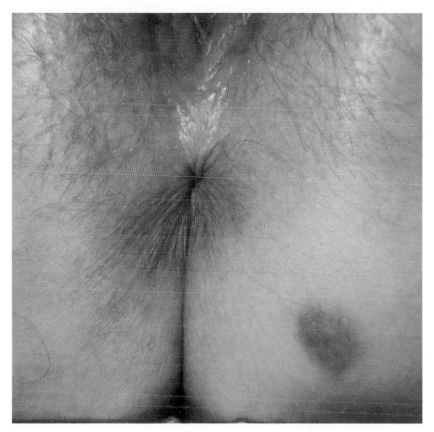

Histiocytoma.

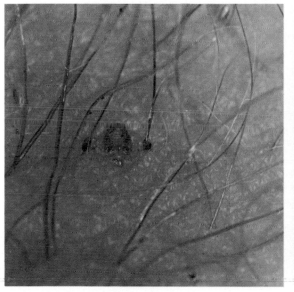

Pubic louse in situ.

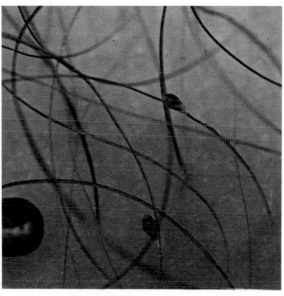

Louse nits. Probe tip gives size comparison.

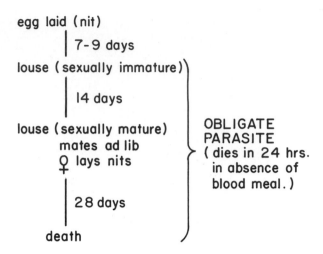

egg laid (nit)

| 7-9 days

louse (sexually immature)

| 14 days

louse (sexually mature)
mates ad lib
♀ lays nits

| 28 days

death

OBLIGATE
PARASITE
(dies in 24 hrs.
in absence of
blood meal.)

clothing contaminated with nits and not laundered will be self-sterilizing *if not worn for 10-14 days* giving time for all the nits to hatch & the immature lice to die without blood meal.

Figure 48. Life cycle of Phthirus pubis.

Treatment. VD alert. As many as one third of women with pubic lice will be found to harbor another sexually transmitted disease. One per cent lindane, the gamma isomer of benzene hexachloride (Kwell), is available on prescription in cream, lotion, and shampoo forms. It is effective with only one or two applications, provided repeat contamination is avoided. The cream or lotion is applied and left on for 12 to 24 hours. The shampoo is lathered into the affected area for four minutes and then thoroughly rinsed. A fine comb is used to remove the nit shells that remain. An over-the-counter product with a pyrethrin base (RID) is also available. It is applied to the affected area, left on for 10 minutes, then thoroughly washed away. Both forms of treatment may be repeated if necessary, but prolonged exposure may be toxic to the central nervous system. No data exists to support the safety or danger of either drug when used during pregnancy. All clothing and bed linen should be freshly laundered as part of the treatment regimen.

FURTHER READING

MELANOMA

Silvers, D.N., and Halperin, A.J.: Cutaneous and vulvar melanoma: an update. Clin. Obstet. Gynecol. 21:1117–1133, 1978.
   Excellent capsule review of melanin physiology and the classification and staging of cutaneous melanoma in general and vulvar melanomas in particular.
Chung, A.F., Woodruff, J.M., and Lewis, J.L.: Malignant melanoma of the vulva. Obstet. Gynecol. 45:638–646, 1975.
   A series of 44 cases that are well presented and illustrate the epidemiology of the disease.

Epstein, E., Bragg, K., and Linden, G.: Biopsy and prognosis of malignant melanoma. JAMA 208:1369–1371, 1969.
An important paper that showed that survival rates in melanoma patients with and without pretreatment incisional biopsy were not different.
Breslow, A., and Macht, S.D.: Optimal size of resection margin for thin cutaneous melanoma. Surg. Gynecol. Obstet. 145:691–692, 1977.
Another important study that established that the width of margins of resection were insignificant when the depth of invasion was less than 0.76 mm.

OTHER DARK LESIONS

Jones, I.S.C.: Assessment of vulval pigmentation. N.Z. Med. J. 89:348–350, 1979.
A unique autopsy study of postmenopausal women that details the pathology of pigmentation in various locations.
Felman, Y.M., Phil, M., and Nikitas, J.A.: Pediculosis pubis. Cutis 25:482–559, 1980.
An up-to-date summary of the problem that nicely covers all its aspects.

9

ULCERS

HERPES SIMPLEX
SYPHILIS
BEHÇET'S DISEASE
CROHN'S DISEASE
PEMPHIGUS
PEMPHIGOID
HIDRADENITIS SUPPURATIVA
INVASIVE CARCINOMA
BASAL CELL CARCINOMA
GRANULOMA INGUINALE
PYODERMA
TUBERCULOSIS
VACCINIA

ULCERS

An ulcer is a defect in the integrity of the skin due to localized destruction of the epidermis. Most ulcerative lesions are the result of primary infectious processes, but secondary infection may develop in cases where self-induced (factitious ulcer) or accidental (abrasion) trauma has occurred. Since the majority of vulvar ulcerations are associated with communicable agents, the physician should take special care with these patients to reduce the possibility of inadvertent transmission within the office setting.

Herpes became a household word after the "epidemic" that occurred in the 1970s and 1980s. Large numbers of people remain infected with latent virus capable of causing recurrent disease in themselves and primary infection in others. Lack of a real cure has set the disease and its victims apart. But those who have contracted syphilis or granuloma inguinale are equally unfortunate—even though treatment is available—if their ulcers are unrecognized and lead to chronic sequelae. The classic hard chancre of syphilis is rare on the vulva, and most syphilitic lesions, both primary and secondary, will be soft. As such, they mimic closely the other ulcerative conditions. It is a good rule, then, to obtain serologic tests for syphilis in all patients with vulvar ulcers. Not only does this serve to identify the syphilitic lesion, but it is also indicated as part of the *VD alert* work-up that should be performed in cases of primary herpes and other sexually transmitted diseases. Fixed Pap smears from the ulcer surface may also be of great help. Herpes, carcinoma, and syphilis may all be identified by this technique.

Some ulcerative conditions are not contagious. Behçet's disease, for example, is one of uncertain etiology. Bacterial opportunists can often be cultured from Behçet's ulcers, but they do not represent causative organisms. Instead, the etiology is more related to the type of process responsible for ulcerative colitis or Crohn's disease. Autoimmune phenomena definitely play a role in these conditions, as they do in pemphigus and pemphigoid. So there is a considerable overlap among all of these entities, each of which may present as a vulvar ulceration.

Neoplasms of the vulva may at times present as ulcerations, and invasive carcinomas commonly exhibit this feature. The basal cell carcinoma, granular cell myoblastoma, and hidradenoma are unusual vulvar tumors rarely considered in the differential diagnosis of ulcerative lesions. Yet all three of these entities may ulcerate and resemble syphilitic chancres in their clinical appearance. They must therefore be considered in differential diagnosis, especially when there is little change in the lesion from week to week. Such ulcers, as well as those in which a diagnosis cannot be otherwise confirmed, should be biopsied.

Tuberculosis of the vulva is most unusual, but when present takes the form of an ulcer. Among other rare causes of vulvar ulcerations are discoid lupus, necrotizing spider bites, human bites, and accidental vaccine infection which may be transmitted from a recently vaccinated spouse or child. Chancroid of the vulva has become so unusual in the United States that few physicians have ever seen or treated a verified case. In many reports, the diagnosis was one of exclusion and *Hemophilus ducreyi* was never actually cultured from the lesion. The literature on chancroid deals largely with its occurrence in male armed forces personnel stationed overseas, and even in those cases, the diagnosis was often problematic. Reports in the female are increasingly rare. Within the United States,

167

therefore, a soft painful chancre-like ulcer of the vulva is in all likelihood due to herpes unless proven otherwise, and chancroid has become a diagnosis of exclusion at the very bottom of the differential list.

Herpes Simplex

Herpes is now recognized as the most common cause of vulvar ulcers. Herpes simplex virus (HSV) is an enveloped DNA-containing virus that is species specific for man. It occurs in two varieties, type I and type II, which are antigenically and structurally distinct. The type II herpes virus (HSV-2) is usually transmitted sexually and accounts for most cases of genital infection, although either type may occur at any site. The disease is so common and may be so variable in clinical presentation that, like syphilis, it should be considered in the differential of all vulvar ulcers and ruled out by smear or culture.

HSV-2 infections are associated with the development of cervical cancer and, in the pregnant woman, may cause spontaneous abortion, neonatal morbidity, and infant mortality. Once contracted, the disease may become recurrent with successive attacks occurring in the absence of repeated exposure. The virus resides in a latent form in the pelvic nerve ganglia and within autonomic nerves along the uterosacral ligaments. While the process of reactivation is not completely understood, it frequently occurs after events associated with a rise in local or systemic prostaglandins. Prostaglandins have also been shown to enhance the cell-to-cell spread of herpes in vitro, so that antiprostaglandins may prove to be of future therapeutic benefit. The incubation period is variable, but symptoms usually arise from 48 hours to 7 days after initial infection. Partial protection may be provided and the risk of recurrence decreased by circulating antibodies developed during the convalescent phase of prior herpes infections. Thus, previous type I infections (oronasal "cold sores") may attenuate the severity of an initial HSV-2 infection. A suppression of cell-mediated immunity due to pregnancy, leukemia, or chemotherapy may have the opposite effect and increase the probability of recurrence and exaggerate its severity.

Active replication of the virus results in localized tissue destruction and the formation of vesicles that are often asymptomatic on the vulva. If this is the patient's first experience with HSV, a prodromal illness characterized by malaise, fever, and inguinal lymphadenopathy may occur. The vesicles then enlarge and rupture, exposing shallow ulcerations that are usually multiple, frequently coalescent, and exquisitely painful. It is at this stage that the patient seeks relief. If the ulcers are within the urethra or located such that they contact the urine stream, she may be unable to void and urinary retention may result. The frequency of urethral mucosal involvement precludes the use of transurethral indwelling catheters, and such patients are ideal candidates for temporary suprapubic cystotomy. The cervix and vagina are involved in over 50 per cent of cases with vulvar ulcers. Due to the relative lack of free nerve endings within these structures, lesions in these locations are generally asymptomatic. Even after the overt clinical episode, unpredictable asymptomatic shedding may occur from the cervix and vagina. Inspection and cultural or cytologic evaluation of these organs is therefore indicated.

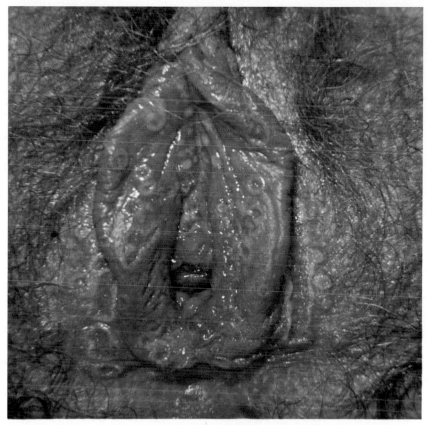

Severe herpetic vulvitis.

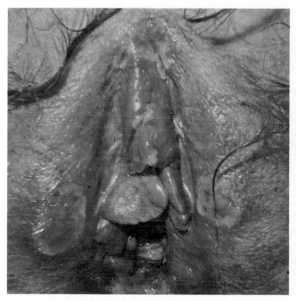

Atypical large herpetic ulcers.

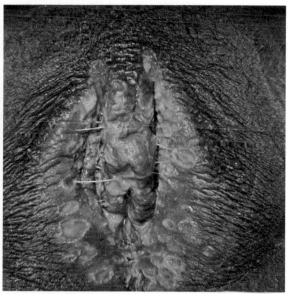

Severe herpes with secondary infection.

Depending upon the severity of the infection and the immune status of the patient, the ulcers persist for one to three weeks and heal spontaneously. Secondary bacterial infection will prolong the healing phase. Although usually mild and localized, recurrent infections are painful and exasperating. Coital activity is suspended, and some patients are unable to perform their daily tasks.

Herpes often occurs in association with other sexually transmitted infections, and its dramatic symptoms may effectively mask the concomitant presence of syphilis or gonorrhea. Serologic tests for syphilis and a cervical culture for gonorrhea should therefore be performed on every patient with primary herpes. Frequently, it is not possible to insert a speculum for cervical culture until later on during the healing phase, but this step should be performed eventually.

Multiple, shallow, exquisitely painful lesions that are coalescent with serpiginous red borders and pale yellow centers are typical. Extensive involvement with secondary labial edema and tender inguinal lymphadenopathy indicates the probability of primary infection. More localized and less symptomatic lesions tend to occur in recurrent cases with previous exposure to the virus. Cytologic imprint smears of the ulcers for Pap staining or antibody identification, viral cultures, and serologic tests are all capable of providing confirmation of the diagnosis. Viral isolation by culture and the cytologic smear are most accurate during the first three days of the infection. If seen later with established ulcers, negative results do not rule out herpes and additional confirmation must be sought during the present or following episodes. Such confirmation is extremely important, and serologic tests may be helpful in the later stages of an infection. The diagnosis of herpes carries many grave connotations and should always be based on proven fact.

Consider: Single or large lesions are atypical and mimic secondary syphilis, Behçet's disease, and invasive carcinoma.

Treatment. VD Alert. The management of HSV-2 infections is directed at relief of pain, inactivation of virus, inhibition of secondary infection, prevention of recurrence, and destruction of the potentially oncogenic viral genome. Antibiotic vaginal creams have no effect on the clinical course of the disease and should be avoided. Symptomatic relief can be obtained with oral analgesics, topical anesthetics, cold wet compresses of 1:40 Burow's solution, and artificial seawater sitz baths. Inactivation of the surface virus can be accomplished with the topical application of 10 per cent povidone-iodine or thymol solutions. Both of these afford some relief of pain after the initial application, inhibit secondary infection, and promote drying, thereby accelerating the healing phase. Acyclovir and its related analogues, cytotoxic drugs activated by the thymidine kinase present in herpes-infected cells, have been found useful in the immunosuppressed patient and may decrease the period of symptoms and shedding in other HSV infections. They have not, however, reduced the incidence of latency or recurrence. Smallpox, BCG, and HSV vaccines and other attempts to stimulate a protective immune system have not been proven helpful. Laser vaporization of the ulcers does not prevent recurrence and the laser ulcers may take longer to heal than the herpes itself. Photodynamic dye therapy has also been shown to be unsuccessful. When developed, the ideal drug will treat the latent virus as well as the surface disease.

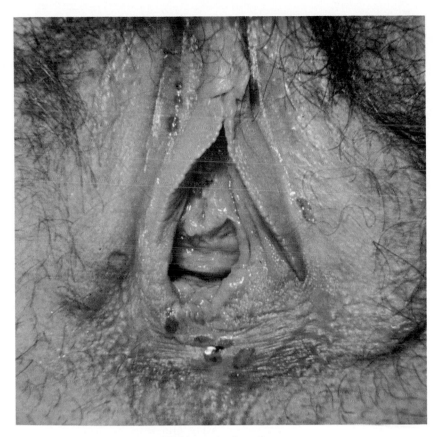

Mild herpetic ulcerations.

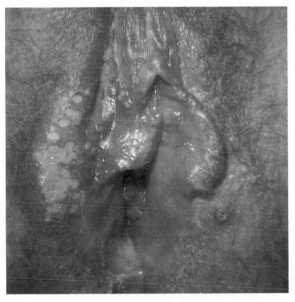

Localized recurrent herpes.

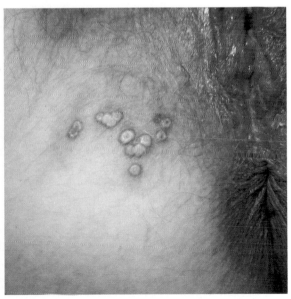

Herpes vesicles.

171

Syphilis

Syphilis continues to represent a major venereal disease problem within urban centers of the United States. The ratio of reported gonorrhea to syphilis is approximately 40:1. Vulvar ulcerations are seen in both primary and secondary stages. The primary chancre is classically single, hard, and painless, but such typical lesions are less frequent than are the atypical ones in which multiple ulcers are seen or where secondary bacterial infection has resulted in a somewhat soft and painful lesion. Almost all vulvar ulcerations, then, should be suspect for syphilis.

The primary chancre appears on an average of three weeks after inoculation and heals spontaneously within one to six weeks. Dark-field examination has almost been replaced by the RPR circle card test, which can be done in the office on the patient's blood. This and the other serologic tests will be positive in over 70 per cent of these cases when first seen by the physician. If negative, such tests should be repeated at weekly intervals for four weeks. Inguinal lymphadenopathy develops three to four days after the chancre and is at first unilateral. The nodes are firm, discrete, and nontender without erythema or suppuration. When acute lymphadenitis with bubo formation occurs, lymphogranuloma venereum (LGV) should be considered and investigated with skin tests and serologic studies.

Secondary syphilis appears from three to six weeks after the development of the chancre and is a systemic disease with a variety of manifestations. The presence of maculopapular lesions elsewhere on the body, especially on the palms and soles, strongly suggests the diagnosis. On the vulva, the ulcerations of secondary syphilis usually present as soft papules or mucous patches that may be coalescent. These lesions are erosive and teem with spirochetes, and the serologic tests are consistently positive at this stage. After therapy, the lesions resolve over a period of two to four weeks. The FTA–ABS test will remain reactive but the VDRL and RPR tests should become negative within a period of one or two years.

Consider: Differentiation from herpes may be quite difficult, but syphilitic lesions are generally larger, more raised, and less tender than herpetic ones. Herpes should always be ruled out, however, with appropriate smears or cultures. When repeated tests for both diseases are persistently negative in the absence of treatment or when the lesions appear stationary after three weeks of observation, biopsy should be done, since basal cell carcinoma and granular cell myoblastoma and other neoplasias may mimic the chancre in gross appearance.

Treatment. VD Alert. Once the diagnosis of syphilis is established, the intramuscular injection of 4.8 million units of benzathine penicillin G is given in two doses of 2.4 million units each, one week apart, and is curative in the primary and secondary stages. Alternatively, the Centers for Disease Control (CDC) recommends a single injection of 2.4 million units of benzathine penicillin if syphilis has been present for less than one year and 2.4 million units weekly for three weeks if present longer than a year. Nonpregnant patients allergic to penicillin should be treated with oral tetracycline, 500 mg four times daily for 15 days. Pregnant allergic patients may be given oral erythromycin, 500 mg four times daily for 20 days.

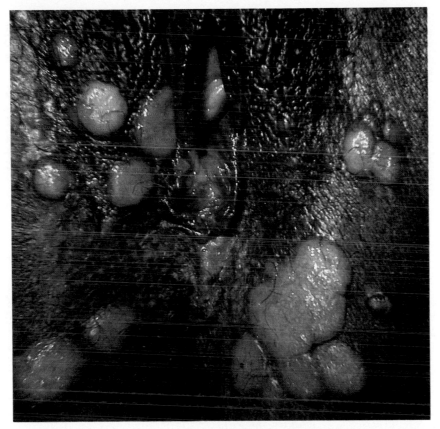

Condylomata lata.

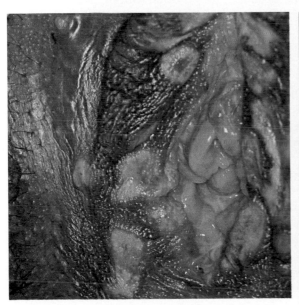

Secondary syphilitic ulcers.

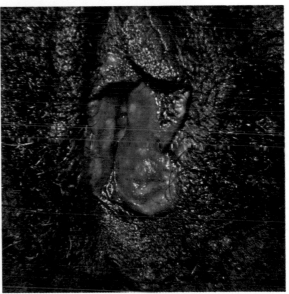

Secondary syphilitic ulcers.

Behçet's Disease

The concurrence of relapsing oral and genital ulcerations associated with ocular inflammation was first described as an entity by the Turkish dermatologist Behçet in 1937. These three major criteria are often associated with the minor criteria of arthritis, thrombophlebitis, acneform skin eruptions, ulcerative colitis, and a variety of neurologic aberrations. The complete disease complex is generally seen in males, and neurologic involvement carries an ominous prognosis. Women more frequently exhibit a modified picture lacking eye involvement. The exact etiology of Behçet's disease remains obscure, but an autoimmune basis has been postulated and there is a high incidence of certain histocompatible antigens, especially HLA–B5, noted in some series.

The oral lesions may occur on lips, tongue, gums, palate, or buccal mucosa and generally have the appearance of common aphthous ulcers. At times they may interfere with eating, but as a rule they cause little distress. The genital lesions are usually more striking and may be highly destructive, resulting in fenestration and scarring with progressive loss of vulvar tissue. Even when small, the lesions are notable for their depth and many are relatively tender. Viral/bacterial smears and cultures will be negative as will the dark-field examination. Serologic tests for syphilis are nonreactive. Even biopsy material is non-specific, showing only chronic inflammation and vasculitis. Immunofluorescent stains on fresh tissue will show a diagnostic pattern in pemphigus, however, and help to rule out this lesion which may look much the same. There is considerable overlap between Behçet's and Crohn's diseases, and both may be present simultaneously. An ESR in excess of 100 argues for Crohn's disease, and radiographic studies of the bowel should be performed whenever there is doubt. The course of the disease is lengthy, and diagnostic studies may need to be repeated over the years as new features become apparent. As in other autoimmune diseases, new data is constantly being developed and new diagnostic and therapeutic measures will become available.

Consider: Both herpes and untreated syphilis may be recurrent and along with pemphigus may cause lesions in the mouth as well as the genitalia. The diagnosis is therefore one of exclusion. Crohn's disease, pemphigoid, and Stevens-Johnson syndrome (erythema multiforme) should also be considered. But unless these diagnoses can be confirmed, the presence of recurring bouts of oral aphthae associated with deeply destructive genital ulcers should be considered to represent Behçet's disease. The presence of any of the minor criteria makes the diagnosis more secure.

Treatment. Avoid the temptation to perform cosmetic surgery. Such well-intentioned whittling often leads to an acute exacerbation of the disease, and the last state becomes worse than the first. Remarkable remissions have been noted after the institution of estrogen-dominant oral contraceptives (Enovid E). Both immunologic and hormonal explanations for this effect have been offered, and when at all possible, it should at least be tried. Intralesional injections of triamcinolone acetonide (10 mg/ml), raising a wheal beneath the entire lesion, may be helpful in some cases. Chlorambucil is recommended for patients with ocular and neurologic involvement.

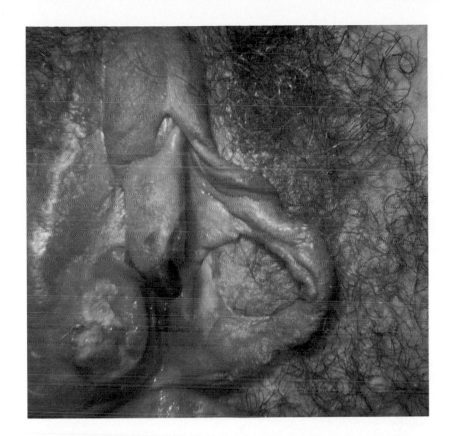

Behçet's disease—genital.

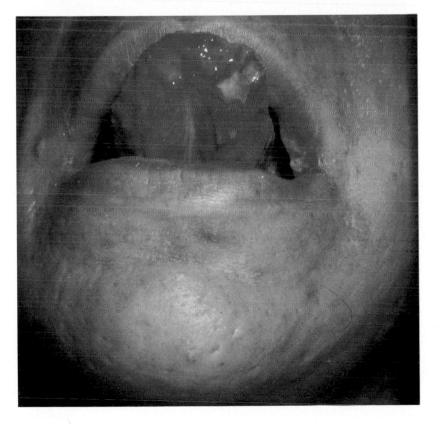

Behçet's disease—oral.

Crohn's Disease

Primarily a disorder of the gastrointestinal tract, Crohn's disease (regional enteritis and ulcerative colitis) may cause primary and secondary cutaneous ulcerations of the vulva and perineum. In fact, these are the presenting complaints in about 25 per cent of cases. Like Behçet's disease, this disease first becomes apparent in early adult life and, like Behçet's disease and pemphigus, may be associated with oral ulceration.

The vulvar manifestations of Crohn's disease may precede the bowel lesions by many years. One of Crohn's original cases had developed linear ulcers of the labia long before her intestinal symptoms began. These "knife-cut" ulcers are characteristic and unlike those due to other causes.

Once the bowel disease is established, secondary involvement of the perianal, perineal, and vulvar areas is common. Edema is frequent, as are draining sinuses and nonlinear ulcers. Biopsy material shows granulation tissue with sarcoidlike granulomas often seen along with acute and chronic inflammation. Eosinophilia may be present as well. A history of intestinal involvement documented by endoscopy with biopsy or radiographic studies strongly supports the diagnosis.

Consider: The clinical appearance may mimic that of almost all the other ulcerative conditions: Behçet's disease, pemphigus, tuberculosis, hidradenitis suppurativa, and granuloma inguinale. The concomitant edema and fistula formation seen in advanced cases may also resemble lymphogranuloma venereum and the skin changes overlying osteomyelitis.

Treatment. In general, the activity of the cutaneous disease parallels that of the bowel lesion. Both respond to long-term metronidazole, sulfones, and steroids. The surgical excision of affected bowel and of chronic vulvar lesions is effective and required by some patients in the absence of medical response.

Pemphigus

Pemphigus is a bullous disease of the skin and mucous membranes with an autoimmune etiology. It is a rare disease whose incidence rate corresponds roughly to that of melanoma. Affecting those in middle and old age, it often involves the vulva, which may even be the site of initial presentation. Although not always present at the onset, oral lesions are eventually found in virtually all cases, a feature shared with Behçet's disease.

The epidermal intercellular deposition of IgG, demonstrable with both direct and indirect immunofluorescent studies of fresh biopsy material, is diagnostic and clearly separates the lesion from pemphigoid and from Crohn's or Behçet's disease. This test is available on request in most pathology laboratories and in all dermatopathology centers.

The bullae or blisters rapidly open, especially in the mouth and on the vulva, so that the lesions are usually ulcerative when first seen.

Consider: In the vagina the ulcers are similar to those associated with tampon use. "Desquamative vaginitis" has been described as an entity but may in fact represent pemphigus in some cases. On the vulva, the lesions resemble the other ulcerative diseases but are generally more extensive and severe.

Treatment. Prior to the use of systemic corticosteroids, the disease was often fatal. Now with high-dose oral steroids and immunosuppressants, the prognosis is much improved. Such patients should be treated by a physician skilled in the use of these drugs and familiar with the various protocols, since many deaths from this disease now relate to long-term complications of therapy.

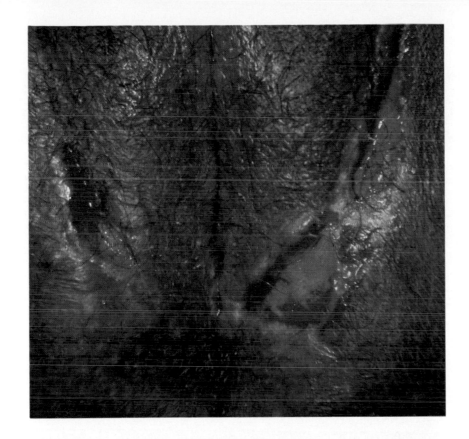

Crohn's disease—"knife-cut" ulcers.

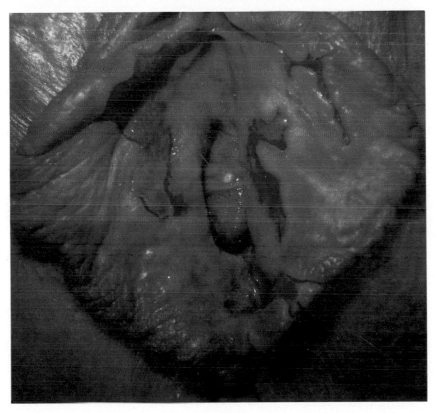

Pemphigus.

Pemphigoid

Another chronic disease of the skin and mucosae that is bullous prior to the formation of ulcers is pemphigoid. Also thought to have an autoimmune basis, this disorder is predominantly one of older patients and usually begins in the seventh decade. Oral lesions may occur but are not characteristic.

As in pemphigus, the large blisters quickly ulcerate on moist surfaces like the vulvar mucosae membranes. One variety, cicatricial pemphigoid, is more common in women and causes scarring when the lesions heal.

Again, biopsy is diagnostic. Immunofluorescent studies of fresh material show pathognomonic deposits of IgG along the basement membrane at the dermoepidermal junction. This location is also the site of subepidermal bullae, which may be seen on ordinary H & E microscopy.

Consider: Dermatitis herpetiformis and erythema multiforme must be included in the differential diagnosis of pemphigoid along with pemphigus and other ulcerative lesions of the vulva, all of which must be considered until the fluorescent biopsy studies are complete.

Treatment. Dapsone, steroids, and immunosuppressants are all helpful, and prompt therapy reduces the chances of irreversible scarring.

Hidradenitis Suppurativa

This is a chronic, recurrent sweat-related disease produced by blockage and subsequent infection of the apocrine glands. The condition is therefore noted most often in the axillae and in the groin and genital areas, and begins after puberty. A wide variety of skin bacteria may be cultured from the chronic, draining sinus tracts, but staphylococcal and streptococcal species predominate. Remissions alternate with exacerbations of tenderness and drainage. Subcutaneous nodules or cords are often palpable and help clinically distinguish the lesion. Although the etiology is not known, deodorants and depilatories have been suggested as contributing to the problem and are best avoided by anyone suffering from the disease.

In its early stages the disorder causes pruritus and burning. Tender skin abscesses form and spontaneously rupture. Repetitive episodes result in deeper involvement, with chronic draining sinuses often anaerobically infected. Hypertrophic scarring is common.

Consider: Early in its course, hidradenitis simulates ulcerating tumors like infected epidermal or pilonidal cysts, pyogenic granulomas, primary abscesses, or basal cell carcinomas. The late vulvar lesions resemble LGV, Crohn's disease, granuloma inguinale, and tuberculosis.

Treatment. Weight loss, oral estrogen (contraceptives) to decrease sweating, and meticulous local hygiene are all helpful in a general way. Specific antibiotics (systemic and topical) given over many months, corticosteroids (both systemic and intralesional), and gentle cleansing scrubs may prevent progression. Surgical excision of localized areas or exteriorization and laying open of all sinus tracts by electrodesiccation offers more permanent relief for advanced disease. Partial vulvectomy with or without skin grafting may be necessary in extreme cases.

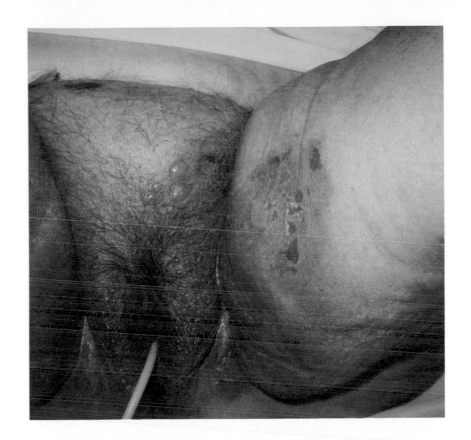

Bullous pemphigoid.

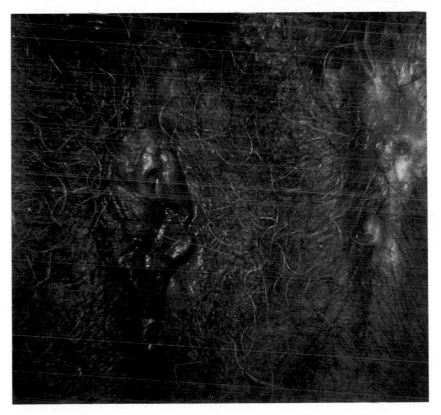

Hidradenitis suppurativa.

179

Invasive Carcinoma

Ulceration is a major finding in approximately one third of all invasive squamous cell carcinomas of the vulva. Bleeding and exudation may accompany the ulcerative process, and when the "sore" fails to heal, the patient finally seeks consultation. Secondary infection may occur and account for the pain that is sometimes noted, but it is remarkable how long many women will tolerate the presence of the disease prior to seeking diagnosis. Squamous carcinomas are usually unifocal. Pain and tenderness are frequently less than what one would expect from looking at the lesion. The edges are generally sharp and often rolled with underlying induration. There is no history of remission and exacerbations. Local therapy may have been tried with no effect. Frequently, the known duration of the lesion can be measured in terms of months, and only biopsy can confirm the diagnosis. Choose a mature site for biopsy that is not necrotic. The edges of the lesion may show only in situ change and be misleading, while the center of the ulcer may contain only inflammatory debris. Sutures must be tied gently, for the tissue is often extremely friable.

Consider: Granuloma inguinale, LGV, giant condyloma, tuberculosis, and syphilis may all coexist with carcinoma and may present with similar clinical findings.

Treatment. Do not suggest the diagnosis unless tissue confirmation has been obtained. The management of established vulvar malignancies is discussed in Chapter Five.

Basal Cell Carcinoma

Approximately one third of all basal cell carcinomas of the vulva present as ulcers. The remainder are dark lesions or small papillomatous tumors. Frequently, the diagnosis is a retrospective one, made after excision of the lesion, and the original clinical appearance is not documented. Although it is a common skin lesion elsewhere on the body, basal cell carcinoma is an unusual finding on the vulva. Most series report a 50:1 ratio of invasive cancers to basal cell tumors, but the same age groups are affected. The sharp "rolled edge" ulcer is classic but not necessarily characteristic.

Consider: A single atypical herpetic ulcer, hidradenitis, syphilis, and pyoderma may look very much like the "rodent ulcer" of basal cell carcinomas.

Treatment. Wide local excision remains the treatment of choice, but there are exceptions, which are fully discussed in Chapter Five.

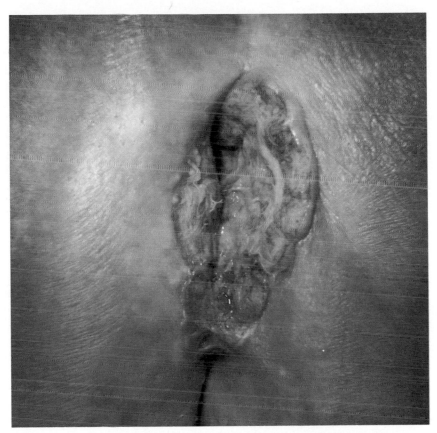

Invasive squamous cell carcinoma—recurrent.

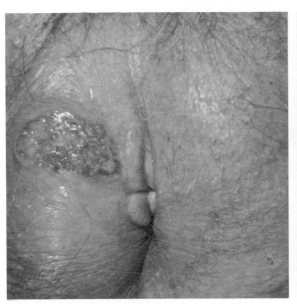

Invasive squamous cell carcinoma.

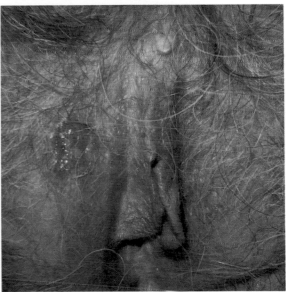

Basal cell carcinoma.

Granuloma Inguinale

Formerly one of the major venereal diseases of the tropics, granuloma inguinale is decreasing in incidence and is very unusual in the United States. The disease is caused by the intracellular *Calymmatobacterium granulomatis* and transmitted by close anogenital contact. Progressive superficial ulceration is an early feature of this disease, though it usually begins as an asymptomatic reddish nodule. The ulcers are characterized by their irregular borders and many have a base of beefy red granulation tissue. True bubo formation does not occur, although the groin lymph nodes may be somewhat swollen. Scarring and lymphedema are present in the later stages. Pseudoepitheliomatous hyperplasia of the adjacent skin is a common biopsy finding and may be misinterpreted as invasive squamous carcinoma. Granulomatous infection may be a precursor to the eventual development of squamous cancer, and in some patients the two diseases coexist. Biopsy material therefore deserves careful study, and these patients require long-term follow-up observation. Smears made from crushed tissue taken from deep biopsies of healthy appearing granulations and stained with Giemsa or Wright's stain are most likely to demonstrate the diagnostic Donovan bodies.

Consider: Lack of true bubo formation differentiates this lesion from lymphogranuloma venereum, and biopsy will distinguish it from squamous cell carcinoma and tuberculosis. Dark-field examinations and serologic tests may be necessary to rule out syphilis. The discrete cords and nodules of hidradenitis are lacking, but the lesions may resemble pyoderma. Only Donovan body demonstration is absolutely diagnostic.

Treatment. VD alert. Oral therapy consists of a tetracycline (500 mg four times daily for three weeks) or ampicillin (500 mg every six hours for two weeks). Intramuscular treatment with gentamycin (40 gm twice daily for two weeks) is also effective.

Pyoderma

Pyogenic bacteria form part of the normal skin flora and when conditions are opportune, they may cause a variety of vulvar problems including acnelike furuncles, primary abscesses, and even necrotizing fasciitis. Pyoderma is a bacterial infection of the skin that is frequently associated with poor hygiene. Children within the same family may have recently developed impetigo. Vicious scratching of the lesions causes infected ulcerations, which heal slowly and may result in scarring. The multiplicity of the ulcers and the similarity of appearance from lesion to lesion help to distinguish this from invasive carcinoma. Involvement of the buttocks and perianal areas may suggest the possibility of hidradenitis. Superficial pus and crust formation are present in both disorders, but draining sinuses are absent in pyoderma and there is no underlying nodule or palpable cord. Bacterial culture of the moist center of the lesion should be performed and antibiotic sensitivities requested. Serologic tests for syphilis are often necessary, and biopsy should be performed if a suspect lesion fails to respond to therapy.

Consider: A relatively acute onset is characteristic of pyoderma, whereas hidradenitis is a much more chronic problem. The irregular shape, multiplicity, and inflammatory aspect of the lesions help to set them apart from syphilitic and neoplastic ulcers.

Treatment. Local cleansing with germicidal soaps will help prevent further spread of the process. For severe cases, both systemic and local antibiotics are used. Erythromycin is a good choice for initial therapy while awaiting the results of sensitivity tests. Vioform cream may be used for local effect.

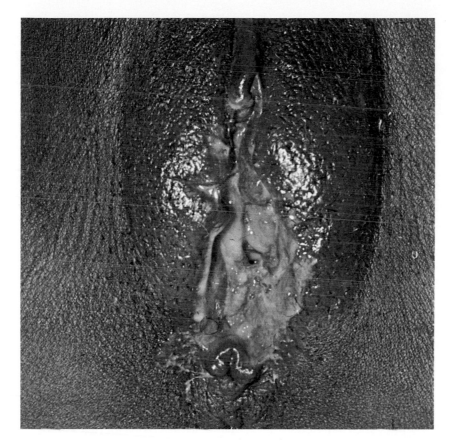

Granuloma inguinale.
(Courtesy Dr. J. StE. Hall.)

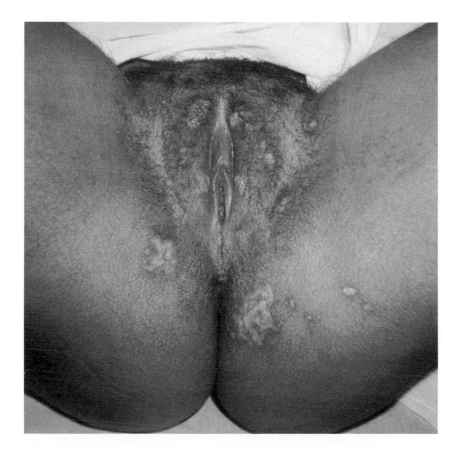

Pyoderma.

183

Tuberculosis

Primary cutaneous tuberculosis of the vulva is extremely rare, and secondary involvement is also uncommon. Sinus tracts may develop from an underlying tuberculous infection of the bony pelvis, lymph nodes, or pelvic viscera. Such lesions are frequently asymptomatic except for their exudative drainage. Radiologic studies usually demonstrate the primary sites of tuberculous involvement. Acid-fast cultures of the drainage material are positive, and the histologic features of caseating granulomas with Langhan's giant cells are present on biopsy. A negative tuberculin skin test makes the diagnosis most unlikely, but a positive test may be related to an old infection. Sometimes the diagnosis is made only when the lesion responds dramatically to specific tuberculocidal drugs.

Consider: Hidradenitis, granuloma inguinale, syphilis, lymphogranuloma venereum, and Crohn's disease may all present in similar fashion and should be considered in the differential diagnosis.

Treatment. The secondary cutaneous lesions respond, as will a primary focus, to long-term systemic therapy with chemotherapeutic agents known for their antituberculous activity (INH, rifampin, ethambutol).

Vaccinia

The fingers may transmit herpes virus to the genitalia from some other infected site or some other individual. In the same manner, vaccinia virus may be transmitted to the vulva from the patient's own recent smallpox vaccination or that of another family member.

Typically, the lesions are painful and appear as umbilicated grouped vesicles that may be widespread. Some may coalesce into large single ulcers with irregular margins. Central dark areas of necrosis characterize the healing phase. The raised, rolled edge of the vesicles and ulcers helps to distinguish them from the more common herpes simplex lesions. Inguinal lymphadenitis is frequently present and bacterial superinfection may occur. Diagnostic confirmation can be made by cytology or viral tissue culture.

Consider: These rare lesions are usually mistaken for herpes simplex lesions, which they resemble. Only careful questioning will uncover the history of recent vaccination.

Treatment: Topical povidone-iodine and Burow's compresses are soothing while the lesions run their course. Permanent scarring is infrequent. Further autoinoculation must be prevented and bacterial infection eliminated.

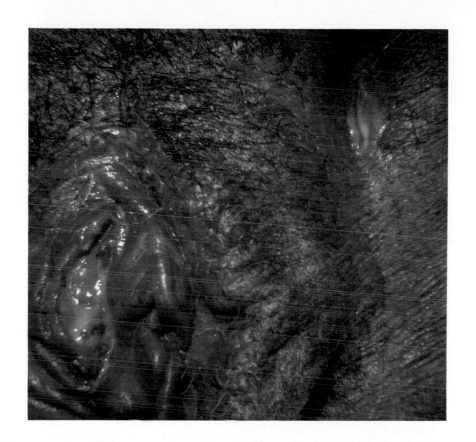

Tuberculosis.

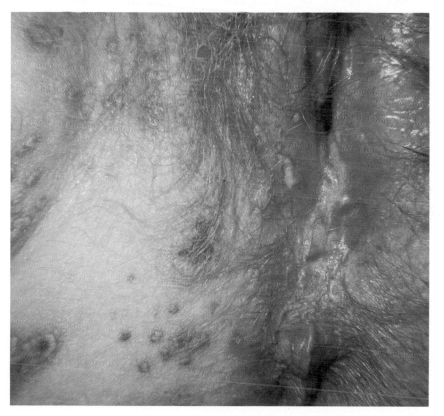

Vaccinia.

FURTHER READING

SEXUALLY TRANSMITTED DISEASES

Felman, Y., ed.: Symposium on sexually transmitted diseases. Dermatologic Clinics 1:1, 1983.
A highly recommended source of review and reference that contains the latest information from various authors, each acknowledged to be the best in the field. Herpes, syphilis, scabies, condylomata acuminata, molluscum contagiosum, and the vaginitides are all discussed in detail.

HERPES

Adam, E., Kaufman, R.H., Mirkovic, R.R., and Melnick, J.L.: Persistence of virus shedding in asymptomatic women after recovery from herpes genitalis. Obstet. Gynecol. 54:171–174, 1979.
The virus was isolated from the cervices of 5 out of 50 women who were asymptomatic and therefore silently shedding the virus.
Fidian, A.P., Halsos, A.M., Kinge, B.R., et al.: Oral acyclovir in the treatment of genital herpes. Am. J. Med. 73(1a):335–337, 1982.
A preliminary report of a multicenter double-blind trial of oral acyclovir in the treatment of initial and recurrent genital herpes showing definite drug effect.
Jarratt, M.: Herpes simplex infection. Arch. Dermatol. *119*:99–103, 1983.
A clear and concise review of all aspects of HSV infection.
Jarratt, M., Smith, R., and Knox, J.M.: Therapy of herpes simplex infection. Int. J. Dermatol. 18:357–361, 1979.
A masterful review of all that has been tried, semi-successful and unsuccessful.
Kawana, T., Kawagoe, K., Takizawa, K., et al.: Clinical and virologic studies on female genital herpes. Obstet. Gynecol. 60:456–461, 1982.
Acute, recurrent, and provoked herpetic infections are discussed and carefully analyzed in this excellent study of 90 women.
Kitchener, H.C., Cordiner, J.W., and Eglin, R.P.: Latency of herpes simplex virus in uterosacral ligaments. Am. J. Obstet. Gynecol. 143:839–840, 1982.
First demonstration of latent virus residing in pelvic tissue distinct from the sacral ganglia.
Reeves, W.C., Corey, L., Adams, H.G., et al.: Risk of recurrence after first episodes of genital herpes. N. Engl. J. Med. 305:315–319, 1981.
A careful study from a leading group of investigators showing the probability of recurrence directly related to the presence and titre of convalescent antibody.

SYPHILIS

Fiumara, N.J.: The treatment of primary and secondary syphilis—serologic response. JAMA 243:2500–2502, 1980.
The leading investigator in the field summarizes the recommended treatment and what can be expected in terms of response.

BEHÇET'S DISEASE

Dodson, M.G., Klegerman, M.E., Kerman, R.H., et al.: Behçet's syndrome with immunologic evaluation. Obstet. Gynecol. 51:621–626, 1978.
A case with complete immunologic investigation is presented combined with clinical evaluation, histology, and a good discussion of differential diagnosis.
O'Duffy, J.D.: Summary of international symposium on Behçet's disease. J. Rheum. 5:229–233, 1978.
A thorough review of this subject that briefly and clearly summarizes all aspects.

CROHN'S DISEASE

Bernstein, L.H., Frank, M.S., Brandt, L.J., and Boley, S.J.: Healing of perineal Crohn's disease with metronidazole. Gastroenterology 79:357–365, 1980.
A comprehensive study of 21 patients, with an excellent discussion of the drug, its side effects, and the striking response to its use.
Burgdorf, W.: Cutaneous manifestations of Crohn's disease. J. Am. Acad. Dermatol. 5:689–695, 1981.
This aspect of regional enteritis that includes the vulvar ulcers is reviewed and expanded to correlate with other manifestations of the disease.
Donaldson, L.B.: Crohn's disease—its gynecologic aspect. Am. J. Obstet. Gynecol. 131:196–202, 1978.

Documents the features that are seemingly unrelated and may present months or years before the main bowel inflammation.

PEMPHIGUS–PEMPHIGOID

Ahmed, A.R., Graham, J., Jordon, R.E., and Provost, T.T.: Pemphigus: current concepts. Ann. Int. Med. 92:396–405, 1980.
An excellent review of this disease covering its various aspects including differential diagnosis and details of therapy.

Rogers, R.S., Seehafer, J.R., and Perry, H.O.: Treatment of cicatricial (benign mucous membrane) pemphigoid with dapsone. J. Am. Acad. Dermatol. 6:215–223, 1982.
Designed as a drug efficacy study, this paper also provides an excellent discussion of the disease and evaluates past and present therapy.

HIDRADENITIS

Gordon, S.W.: Hidradenitis suppurativa: a closer look. J. Nat. Med. Assn. 70:239–343, 1978.
This paper reviews the literature and discusses the disease from all points of view with good tables on the differential diagnosis.

BASAL CELL CARCINOMA

Collins, P.S., Farber, G.A., and Hegre, A.M.: Basal cell carcinoma of the vulva. J. Dermatol. Surg. Oncol. 7:711–714, 1981.
An excellent review of the entity with comprehensive tables and a good summary of the literature.

GRANULOMA INGUINALE

Kuberski, T.: Granuloma inguinale (Donovanosis). Sex. Trans. Dis. 7:29–36, 1980.
An article like this will probably not be written again on this disease for a long time. A fascinating history, good microscopic and clinical pictures, and a thorough bibliography are all added to the general discussion.

OTHERS

Humphrey, D.C.: Localized accidental vaccinia of the vulva. Am. J. Obstet. Gynecol. 86:460–469, 1963.
A classic review of the world literature summarizing 70 cases.

Kanra, G., Sezer, V., Gurses, N., et al.: Accidental vaccinia vulvovaginitis. Cutis 26:267–268, 1980.
Describes a case of vulvar vaccinia transmitted from a recently vaccinated child and successfully treated with cytosine arabinoside.

Magrina, J.F., and Masterson, B.J.: Loxosceles reclusa spider bite: a consideration in the differential diagnosis of chronic nonmalignant ulcers of the vulva. Am. J. Obstet. Gynecol. 140:341–343, 1981.
Just like the title says.

Young, A.W., Tovell, H.M.M., and Sadri, K.: Erosions and ulcers of the vulva. Obstet. Gynecol. 50:35–39, 1977.
This report identifies the conditions presenting as vulvar ulcers seen in an urban clinic over a five-year time span.

10

SMALL TUMORS

CONDYLOMA ACUMINATUM

CARCINOMA IN SITU

MOLLUSCUM CONTAGIOSUM

EPIDERMAL CYST

VESTIBULAR CYST

HEMANGIOMA

HIDRADENOMA

ACCESSORY BREAST TISSUE

ENDOMETRIOSIS

MESONEPHRIC DUCT CYST

PILONIDAL SINUS

NEUROFIBROMA

ACROCHORDON

FOX–FORDYCE DISEASE

SYRINGOMA

SMALL TUMORS

Small tumors of the vulva are those with an average diameter of less than one centimeter. Many of these tumors are inherently restricted in their growth and rarely, if ever, exceed this small size. Others, if undisturbed, might grow to larger dimensions, but because of their symptoms, they cause the patient to present early in the course of the disease. Small tumors may be covered with white keratin, or reveal their red blood circulation. Some reflect a dull blue color, and others are quite variegated and have foci of all these colors in the same lesion. Yet the primary characteristic of these disorders is their three-dimensional growth, and it is this topographic feature that first strikes the attention of the clinician.

Besides the formation of a visible or palpable enlargement, the lesions presented in this chapter have little in common. Some are virally induced, some are embryologic remnants, some are caused by trauma or duct blockage, and still others constitute frank neoplasia. Like their colors, their etiologies differ. But it seems presumptuous to ask a busy clinican, trying to identify an unfamiliar lesion, to seek it out among chapters organized according to etiology. The dysontogenetic cysts, for example, are those in which embryologic anlage have failed to regress. Mucous cysts of the vestibule, mesonephric duct cysts, and some endometriotic cysts all fit into this category. Knowing this helps to understand the lesion, but it has minimal diagnostic value. In a way, we face the same dilemma here as with the group of dark lesions. Benign conditions do not require excision but excision is the only way to tell that they are benign.

Some of the small tumors have such a characteristic appearance that almost every case encountered will look "just like the book." Cherry angiomata are a good example—their features vary little from case to case. Accessory breast tissue, however, may present as a lump of almost any size or any shape, and may look like a hidradenoma, which looks a little like a fibroma, which looks something like a lipoma, etc. Endometriosis is sometimes seen as a classic, blue, cystic mass in the middle of an episiotomy scar. But it can also present as an amorphous lump that may wax and wane with the menstrual cycle. Therefore, many small tumors of the vulva will require a diagnostic (and usually curative) excisional biopsy.

The classification of tumors according to anatomic location aids in the recognition of some entities. If the vulva is thought of as a target, then the concentric rings represent the vagina, vestibule, labia minora, and labia majora. Each of these areas has a unique histologic composition. For this reason, some growths are prone to occur more often in one region than in another. Mucous cysts are practically limited to the vestibule; hidradenomas classically arise between the major and the minor labia. The labia majora, with a full complement of adnexal structures, may be the location of a wide variety of tumors. The list of individual entities is by no means exhaustive, and the diseases are not necessarily confined to the zones indicated. Rather, the diagram simply identifies the most common site of their occurrence (Fig. 49).

A number of other small tumors of the vulva, not illustrated or discussed here, have been the subject of isolated case reports. These include benign mixed tumors, hemangiopericytomas, leiomyomas, and eosinophilic granulomas. The vulva contains such a variety of tissue types that still more small tumors will certainly be found. It is hoped that their discovery and publication will serve to stimulate further interest in the field of vulvar disease.

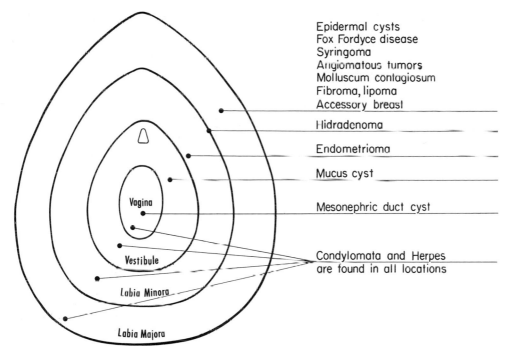

Epidermal cysts
Fox Fordyce disease
Syringoma
Angiomatous tumors
Molluscum contagiosum
Fibroma, lipoma
Accessory breast

Hidradenoma

Endometrioma

Mucus cyst

Mesonephric duct cyst

Condylomata and Herpes
are found in all locations

Vagina

Vestibule

Labia Minora

Labia Majora

Figure 49. Concentric zones of vulva showing common regions of occurrence for small tumors.

Condyloma Acuminatum

By far the most common tumor of the vulva, condyloma acuminatum, if reportable, would qualify as an epidemic disease. Caused by a sexually transmissible, DNA-containing human papovavirus (HPV), the lesions generally appear within three months of exposure, but the incubation period is quite variable. Once present, the growths are unsightly, annoying, often pruritic, and prone to maceration and secondary infection. Most physicians are quite familiar with this entity and with the many frustrations that accompany unsuccessful attempts at therapy. Known to and described by the ancient Greeks, the disease antedates both syphilis and gonorrhea, with which it was often confused. Ancient Romans applied the term "acuminate" (sharply pointed) to the growth, recognizing the fingerlike projections that characterize early lesions. Since then, the disease has been a companion to the human race, but not until recently has its viral etiology and oncogenic potential been fully appreciated.

There are many distinct subtypes of HPV. One that has been associated with genital condylomata is HPV-6. Attempts to identify and grow the virus from suspect tissue failed, and rarely was it visible on electron microscopy. However, a number of virus-specific, cell-staining techniques have shown that it is present in typical vulvar, cervical, and vaginal condylomata as well as in some cases of marked atypia and carcinoma in situ. Condylomata have been observed to undergo malignant transformation through progressive degrees of atypia. This phenomenon was observed especially in cases that had received no treatment over a long period of time and in those that continued to recur despite conventional therapy. Sophisticated genetic probes have shown fragments of the viral

191

genome incorporated into the DNA of verrucous carcinoma and invasive squamous tumors of the vulva.

As with other infections and other forms of neoplasia, the host defense mechanisms play a crucial role in determining the final outcome of the attack. Lesions that dramatically enlarge during pregnancy may completely regress in the puerperium. The condylomata of women who take oral contraceptives are often less responsive to routine attempts at cure. Both of these observations are related to a relative immunosuppression that grants the virus an additional advantage. Lymphocyte transformation studies have shown that recalcitrant condylomata acuminata are but one reflection of an underlying defect in cell-mediated immunity. Autogenous vaccines have helped some patients, but other therapeutic attempts to enhance immune function have so far been unsuccessful. Therefore, this continues to be a promising and important area for future research.

Laryngeal papillomata arising during infancy and early childhood also contain HPV virus. Most of the affected children have been born vaginally by mothers with condylomatous infection. The number of cases is small, but the laryngeal tumors are extremely difficult to treat and cause considerable morbidity. Extensive involvement of the birth canal with condylomata acuminata at the time of delivery may therefore become an indication for cesarean section. The danger of transmission to the newborn should certainly provide an incentive for therapy during pregnancy using laser or electrosurgical techniques.

The natural history of genital warts has been well documented, and the age-incidence curve can be superimposed on that of gonorrhea. Yet cases occur in children without history of sexual contact. Some authorities ascribe these to a merciful lack of memory in the very young and point to the mythical practice of attempting to cure male gonorrhea by touching the penis to the genitals of a young virgin. But that does not help to clarify the truly congenital cases discovered at delivery, in which hematogenous spread from an infected mother seems the only explanation. Even adult patients are sometimes at a loss to explain their own exposure, and it may well be that an asymptomatic carrier state exists whereby the virus is silently transmitted—as is often the case with herpes. This possibility, and the extremely variable incubation period that ranges from a few weeks to many months, often makes identification of the source of infection an impossible task.

Condylomata come in a wide variety of shapes, sizes, and appearances. Young early lesions are pale and have the classic acuminate surface. Their superficial coating of keratin gives them a gray to white aspect. As they grow older, those that arise from pigmented skin tend to become darker, while those from mucosal surfaces appear purple because of their partially visible capillary blood supply. Gross architecture also changes with age. The filiform nature of young lesions gives way to the pedunculated or polypoid growth, and very old lesions may flatten out and spread over wide areas.

Consider: Most condylomata are so characteristic that the diagnosis is obvious. But biopsy is indicated for atypical, isolated, or recurrent lesions, which may represent carcinoma in situ. Verrucous carcinoma cannot be distinguished on the basis of gross appearance alone, but usually these are large lesions that tend to occur in older women who rarely develop condylomata.

A rough, grainy appearance is sometimes noted on the normal introital epithelium of young women that is due to the vestibular papillae, which are discussed in the chapter on special problems. These may be visually confused with extensive early condylomata. Texture alone provides some solution to this diagnostic problem, since early condylomata have a rubbery, almost gritty firmness to them, whereas the variant epithelium is quite soft. Under colposcopic magnification, the condylomata are closely grouped papillae, often with a common base and fairly thick keratin coat. The variant "normal" vestibule, however, shows delicate individual fingerlike projections with a easily visible single capillary loop enclosed by a thin epithelial covering.

Treatment. VD Alert.   Some form of vaginitis is present in almost all cases of condylomata when first seen. Therefore, any direct attack on the lesions themselves must include specific therapy for the coexistent vaginal infection. Other factors contributing to "wetness" of the vulvar and perineal area should be eliminated insofar as possible. Except in very mild cases, oral contraceptives should be discontinued and a barrier or thermal method substituted until the lesions have been totally eradicated. Unless the source of infection can be accurately identified and treated, all sexual partners should wear condoms to prevent both reinfection and transmission.

The treatment of choice for condylomata acuminata, young or old, small or large, is thermal destruction by electrodesiccation and curettage or by laser vaporization. Anesthesia is required, but this method gives the very best results in terms of low recurrence rate and patient acceptance. This method is also the safest and most effective for the management of lesions complicating pregnancy. The routine preoperative "shave and prep" should be forbidden. Instead, clip away excessive hair with a scissors, since shaving may spread the virus and inoculate new areas. Alcohol prep is contraindicated when using electrosurgery or laser because of the danger of fire. A small wire loop is best for large lesions (Fig. 50). Other tips are chosen dependent on lesion site. All visible warts should be destroyed, including those in the vagina and anus.

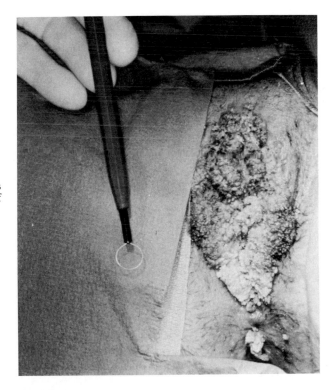

Figure 50. A large Bovie loop is well suited for electrosurgery of large condylomata.

193

Small, early lesions can sometimes be treated with the topical application of 25 per cent podophyllin in compound tincture of benzoin. A little talcum powder dusted on the lesions after treatment prevents the drug from sticking to unaffected areas. Soap and water washing deactivates the drug and must be carried out by the patient within four to six hours. Do not use podophyllin on the cervix or vagina where it cannot be washed off. Do not attempt to treat large or extensive lesions with this drug or to use it in pregnancy, during which systemic absorption, neurotoxicity, and death have been reported. Try another method if no response is observed after two or three applications. Mature lesions are notoriously unresponsive to podophyllin. Since the drug is a mitotic poison like colchicine, it affects rapidly dividing cells but not quiescent ones. The halogenated acetic acids are also topically destructive agents that have been widely used in the past. Commercial preparations (Nevitol) are expensive, but generic trichloracetic acid is reasonably priced for the quantities needed in the office. These compounds denature any protein they contact. The normal surrounding skin must be protected with a mask or with petroleum jelly, or else great care must be taken to apply the chemical only to the wart. The treated lesion will turn white and regress down to the depth treated. Large lesions require multiple treatments. A transient but definite burning sensation is noted at the time of application. Unlike podophyllin, the drug is not washed off or deactivated. For optimum effect, the acid-treated lesion must be kept dry for 12 to 24 hours. Again, powder helps, but in the presence of vaginal discharge and urine, a dry field is often impossible to achieve or maintain.

Topical 5-FU cream 5 per cent (Efudex) applied nightly for one or two weeks may result in dramatic regression without causing irritation to the normal tissue. As expected, it works best on the younger growing lesions, but even if not totally effective, it is often helpful in reducing an extensive lesion to a more manageable size. This same preparation also works well for condylomata of the vagina. After protecting the vulva with a light coating of petroleum jelly, one-half applicator of the 5-FU cream is inserted into the vagina at bedtime for two weeks or until response has been obtained. Of course, this treatment may not be used during pregnancy. Cryosurgery requires an inordinate amount of time and carries a high rate of recurrence. In fact, cold is used to preserve the virus in the experimental situation. In this disease, no program of treatment is 100 per cent effective and fresh crops of lesions may necessitate repetitive therapy.

To help the patient cope with the frustrating phenomenon of recurrence, the "dandelion analogy" can be provided. Everyone is familiar with the little yellow flowers that can spring up in even the most closely tended lawns. Once recognized, they are attacked with chemical poisons, root cutters, and flame throwers. Yet no one is surprised to find that new weeds spring up again within a few weeks of such treatment. The seeds are presumed to be underground and cannot be recognized until they sprout. Only then does direct treatment become possible, and it is very much the same with condylomata acuminata.

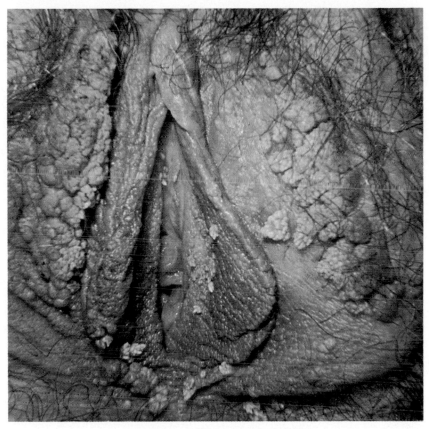

Condylomata acuminata—new and old.

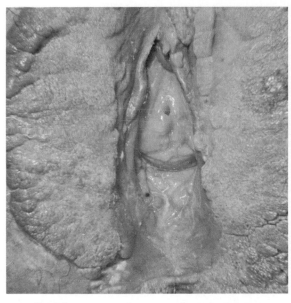

Condylomata acuminata—sessile and confluent.

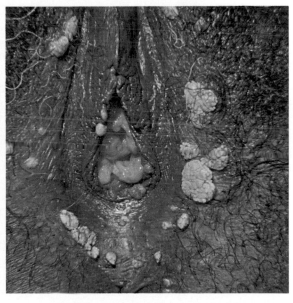

Condylomata acuminata—varicolored.

195

Carcinoma In Situ

Carcinoma in situ has a wider variety of clinical appearances than any other vulvar disorder. At times, it may mimic condyloma acuminatum, presenting as a small nodule of heaped-up hyperkeratosis. When such lesions are isolated and single, it may be easier to distinguish them from the usually multiple condyomata, but multicentric in situ carcinoma occurs so often that this feature is rarely helpful. Both lesions may present in variegated shades of white, brown, or pink. Because of their parakeratosis, both will usually retain toluidine blue dye when topically applied. More and more cases are being noted in which the two lesions are present simultaneously. Since the incidence of both lesions is rising, this concurrence can be expected to increase as well. Biopsy is therefore necessary for an accurate diagnosis, but even this procedure may present problems. If podophyllin has been recently used, a large number of mitotic figures will be seen within a benign condyloma and along with other changes may mislead the pathologist. Such chemical effects last for an unpredictable length of time after treatment, but four to six weeks after exposure should allow sufficient time for their disappearance.

Almost all lesions of vulvar carcinoma in situ are raised. With a colposcope it is possible to appreciate the details of the lesional surface. In situ carcinoma will show a fine-grained irregular surface, almost smooth, whereas condylomata are generally rough and coarsely furrowed.

One presentation of this disease is that of multiple discrete pigmented papules. The term *bowenoid papulosis* has also been used to describe this variation on the theme, but histologically the papules represent carcinoma in situ.

Consider: Carcinoma in situ may closely resemble condylomata acuminata, and when it presents in the form of discrete small papules, it looks very much like molluscum contagiosum. This disease deserves to share with syphilis the epithet of "the great masquerader," since it presents in so many different disguises.

Treatment.   The treatment of this disease must be individualized. Some lesions regress spontaneously; others require extensive surgery. See Chapter Five for a complete discussion of this entity and its therapy.

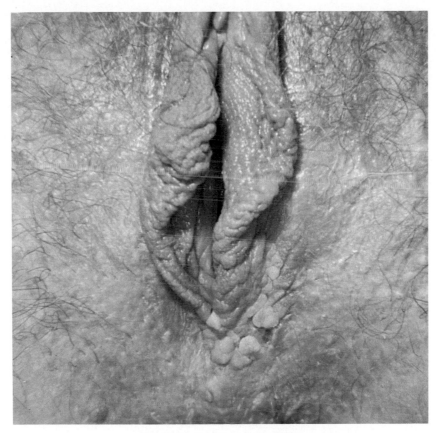

Carcinoma in situ—raised plaques.

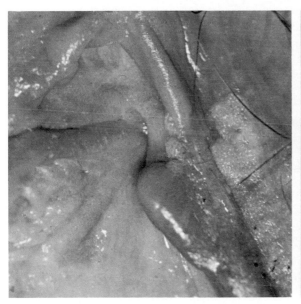

Carcinoma in situ—under magnification.

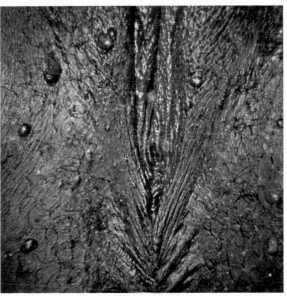

Bowenoid papulosis.

Molluscum Contagiosum

In schoolchildren, molluscum contagiosum is a common viral disease that affects the skin of the trunk, face, and arms. In adults, the lesions are located on the genitalia and are considered sexually transmitted. Intercourse itself probably plays no part in this transmission; close person to person contact is all that is necessary. The virus may also be spread via fomites (contaminated bedclothes) and by autoinoculation from one area to another. These lesions are probably far more common than is realized, since they are asymptomatic and easily overlooked. Also known as "water warts," they present as small, translucent or waxy dome-shaped elevations that may have an umbilicated center. When surrounding erythema is present it gives the papules an appearance similar to that of folliculitis.

The incubation period is from two to seven weeks. The diameter of the smooth papule varies from less than 1 mm to over 5 mm. Giant lesions of up to 1 cm also occur. Molluscum contagiosum is asymptomatic and causes no known morbidity.

Some lesions disappear spontaneously in about six months, but others last for many years. Throughout this time they may be transmitted or autoinoculated. The causative DNA poxvirus has been identified with electron microscopy, and forms huge intracytoplasmic inclusion bodies, which are diagnostic and easily recognizable on smears and biopsies. Serologic tests are not available and diagnosis is dependent on a high index of clinical suspicion and cytologic evaluation of the cheesy material removed from a lesion.

Consider: Molluscum lesions are usually multiple and separated from one another by a considerable distance. They may occur in close groups, however, and look much like a cluster of herpetic vesicles. Central umbilication helps to identify them as molluscum contagiosum, but this is a variable feature. At times, a giant molluscum will look like a pyogenic granuloma. Young molluscum lesions are papular; older lesions tend to collapse and assume a pedunculated appearance closely resembling a skin tag or an isolated condyloma acuminatum.

Treatment. VD alert.   When few in number, tiny, and isolated, the preferred treatment is evacuation and curettage. This can be accomplished without anesthesia simply by inserting a large hypodermic needle beneath the pseudocapsule and lifting upward. The base of the clean cavity is then touched with a silver nitrate stick, or lightly treated with electrodesiccation. Large lesions present a diagnostic problem, easily solved by a curative excisional biopsy. Cryosurgery with a point probe may be used without anesthesia and gives excellent results. Electrodesiccation is painful without prior local anesthesia and topical caustics are not recommended.

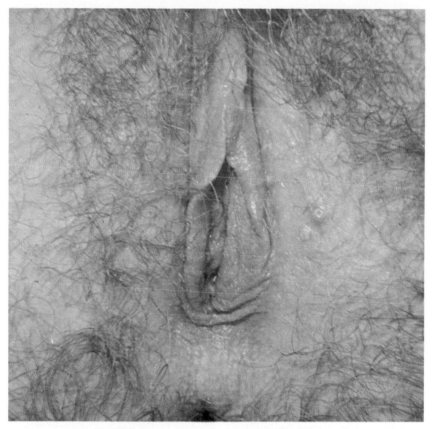

Molluscum contagiosum with umbilication.

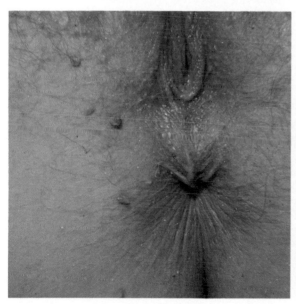

Molluscum contagiosum.

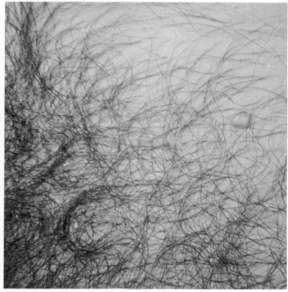

Molluscum contagiosum—single water wart.

199

Epidermal (Keratinous, Sebaceous, Inclusion) Cysts

These are the most common small cystic tumors of the vulva. They are lined by a smooth layer of keratinizing squamous epithelium. The cyst contents are largely keratinous and composed of cellular debris that has a sebaceous appearance and odor. But true sebaceous cells are rarely found in the lining epithelium. Theories of their origin include keratinization (squamous metaplasia) of the sebaceous gland and duct unit, traumatic infolding of surface epithelium, and hair shaft aberration. But none of these explain all cases. Often a communication with the surface is visible, or microscopically demonstrable, but this does not always imply an inclusion process in their pathogenesis. Regardless of the debate, these cysts are clearly of epidermal structure and origin.

Epidermal cysts are usually multiple and less than 1 cm in diameter, but single, isolated lesions and large lesions may occur. Although histologically cystic, they are solid and firm to palpation and feel much like "BB shot." Their distinctly yellow color becomes more obvious if the thin overlying epidermis is stretched over the cyst wall by pinching the cyst between the fingers as if to "pop" it. When a fine 20-gauge needle is inserted into a cyst under this tension, a thick, pale yellow material exudes that has the consistency of putty. Such cysts may become infected or undergo fibrosis or calcification, but most do nothing at all and some may very slowly enlarge. Unless secondarily infected, epidermal cysts cause no symptoms other than the "knobby" feeling they impart to the vulvar surface.

Consider: When multiple, they may be confused with syringomas, which are rather rare and more deeply situated and lack the discrete "dried bean" appearance characteristic of epidermal cysts. If the lesions are large and single, they may mimic hidradenomas, accessory breast tissue, fibromas, or lipomas. In such cases, histologic evaluation alone can provide a diagnosis.

Treatment. In most cases the diagnosis is obvious and treatment is not necessary. Acutely infected cysts should be treated with warm packs, drainage, and later excision to prevent recurrence. Larger isolated epidermal cysts cannot be recognized by inspection, and excision may be needed for both diagnosis and cure.

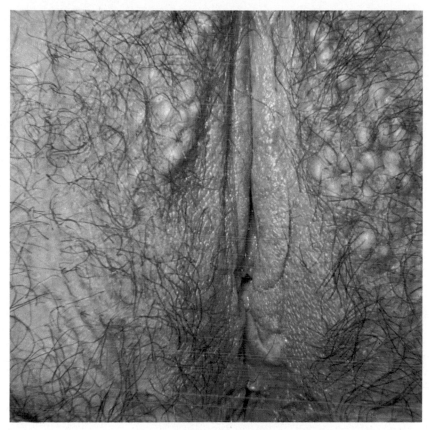

Epidermal cysts.

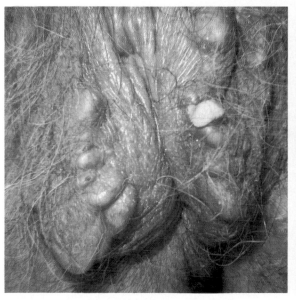

Epidermal cysts exuding contents.

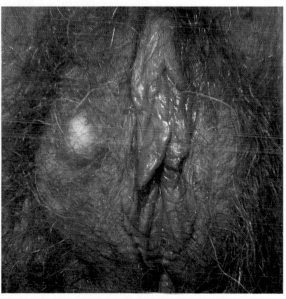

Epidermal cyst—single.

201

Vestibular Cyst

Cysts that are confined to the vestibular ring of the vulva are of two types: the fairly common mucous cyst of the adult vestibule and the rather uncommon simple cyst seen in the newborn.

Dysontogenetic mucous cysts of the adult vulvar vestibule occur with greater frequency than is generally supposed. Because of their asymptomatic nature, they are often ignored by the patient and the physician or dismissed as epidermal cysts. Two studies have now "mapped" their locations and they are classically found between the hymen and the pigmented epithelium of the minora. As Robboy has suggested, these cysts probably arise because of obstruction of the ducts of the minor vestibular glands. Such cysts have been called "urogenital sinus remnants" and "dysontogenetic mucous cysts," and both of these terms are fairly accurate. Other authors have called them "paramesonephric" or "müllerian," since their lining epithelium resembles that of the endocervix. Such an interpretation is embryologically unsound, however, as the müllerian ducts play no part in the development of the vulva.

In most patients, the cysts are single subepithelial tumors, averaging less than 1 cm in diameter. Their consistency or palpation is distincly cystic and they are nontender. They may be varying shades of blue or pale yellow in color, since they are usually overlaid by the nonpigmented surface epithelium of the vestibule. They are lined with a mucus-secreting columnar or cuboidal epithelium that stains with mucicarmine. Papillary folds and ciliated cells may be present and squamous metaplasia is not uncommon. Trichrome stains show no subepithelial layer of the smooth muscle characteristic of mesonephric duct anlage.

Mucous cysts of the vestibule may be found close to the urethral meatus, where their expansion could interfere with the urine stream. Larger cysts are often annoying because of their size, but most of these lesions are entirely asymptomatic.

In the newborn, small vestibular tumors that look exactly like mucous cysts may be seen. They are characteristically attached to the vestibule but are lined with a simple squamous epithelium and contain a sterile clear or milky white fluid. Undisturbed, they will rupture spontaneously and heal without complication within a few weeks of delivery.

Consider: When epidermal and mesonephric duct cysts and endometriosis are located within the confines of the vestibule, they mimic the appearance of mucous cysts and can be differentiated only on the basis of histology.

Treatment. Rarely are cystic tumors of the vulva malignant. Cysts in the newborn should be left alone to regress. Those causing a problem in the adult require excision.

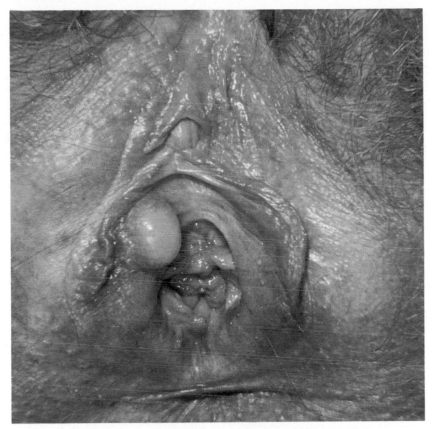

Vestibular mucous cyst.

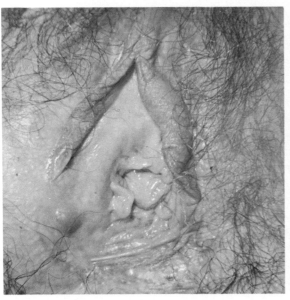

Vestibular mucous cyst.

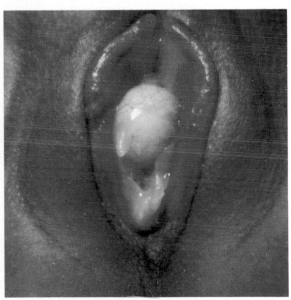

Vestibular cyst of the newborn.

203

Hemangioma

Three forms of hemangiomata affect the adult vulva with moderate frequency: the cherry angioma, the angiokeratoma, and the pyogenic granuloma.

Cherry angiomata are common, tiny (less than 2 to 3 mm) lesions, usually multiple, that arise on the labia majora and are associated with advancing age. They begin to appear in the fourth or fifth decade, so the term "senile" is not really appropriate. Numerous dilated capillaries in the superficial dermis account for their reddish dusky color. The gross appearance of these lesions is so characteristic that diagnostic biopsy is rarely needed. These tumors are generally asymptomatic, but bleeding can result from surface trauma.

Consider: Cherry angiomata should be considered in the differential diagnosis of postmenopausal bleeding.

Treatment. Lesions that cause external bleeding may be treated by cryotherapy, laser, or excision, but as a rule no treatment is required.

Angiokeratomas are not uncommon tumors found on the scrotum as well as the vulva. Although frequently multiple, they are not as abundant as are cherry angiomas, and the individual lesions are generally larger in size, averaging 5 mm in diameter. Telangiectasia, venous stasis, and pregnancy are all thought to play a role in their development, and the majority of patients are of reproductive age. The color of the lesion is generally darker than that of cherry angiomas, varying from deep to pale purple. This reflects a distinct tissue architecture that interposes layers of squamous epithelial cells around and between the vascular spaces. Hyperkeratosis and parakeratosis commonly cover the surface of the tumor and further mask the red color of the circulating blood.

Consider: When dark and sessile, the angiokeratoma resembles a nevus or melanoma. Exophytic lesions may look like condylomata acuminata.

Treatment. Uncertainty of diagnosis, rapid growth, and irritative bleeding prompt excisional biopsy, which is both diagnostic and curative.

Pyogenic granulomas are curious proliferations of capillary vessels that most often arise on the labia during pregnancy. As such, they are analogous to the pregnancy granulomas of the gingiva. While some degree of regression may occur postpartum, the lesions are prone to linger and recur. They are the largest (1 cm) and most symptomatic of adult vulvar hemangiomas. Bleeding is common and infection almost always presents, resulting in a chronic purulent exudate. Clinically, these growths show a beefy red "granulation tissue" surface, or they are enclosed by a thin sac of epidermis, which imparts a purple color. Often a raised "collarette" of surrounding skin encircles the base of the lesion. A fair amount of underlying induration may be appreciated on palpation, and the tumor is sometimes tender. Diagnosis depends on clinical appearance and histologic study showing granulation tissue with dense, acute, and chronic inflammatory infiltrate.

Consider: The pyogenic granuloma may closely resemble the basal cell carcinoma, melanoma, and hidradenoma.

Treatment. When the diagnosis is made during pregnancy, therapy may be delayed until after delivery. But a wide and deep wedge resection is the only treatment that does not result in early recurrence.

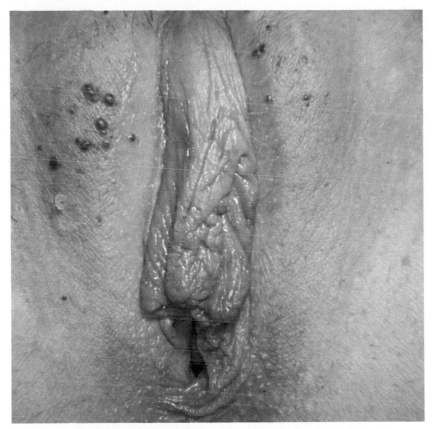

Cherry angiomas.

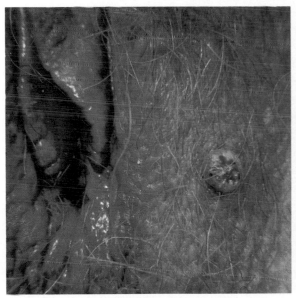

Angiokeratoma.

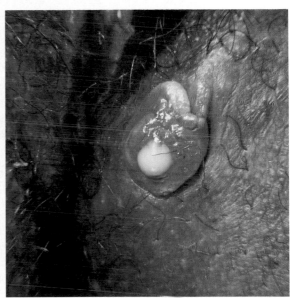

Pyogenic granuloma.

205

Hidradenoma

The hidradenoma papilliferum is a tumor peculiar to the vulva of sexually mature Caucasian women. The majority of these growths are single lesions arising from the labia or interlabial sulcus. In rare cases, more than one tumor is present. Their origin from sweat glands is clear, and they appear to arise from apocrine, rather than eccrine, anlage. The benign intraductal papilloma of the breast, also an apocrine structure, is an analogous tumor that may have similar histologic characteristics. The earlier literature erroneously reported the hidradenoma of the vulva as a form of andenocarcinoma, thus branding it with an undeserved reputation. At low power, the histologic pattern of random papillary formation resembles that of andenocarcinoma seen in other sites, but high-power scrutiny by an experienced eye identifies the benign appearance of the individual cells. The papillary projections are covered by typical apocrine duct and glandular epithelium. Often a double layer of cells is present in which the larger secretory cells are seen to be supported by a flatter and more compact myoepithelial layer.

The average lesion is "button-like" and approximates 1 cm in diameter, although slightly larger and slightly smaller tumors have been seen. Intradermal expansion can result in pressure necrosis of the covering epithelium, at which point an ulceration appears. The red adenomatous tissue then wells up through this defect, and lesions at such a stage closely resemble pyogenic granulomas. Bleeding and secondary infection may occur in these "open" tumors, but the nonulcerated varieties are asymptomatic.

Consider: Any round or ovoid tumor occurring in the interlabial sulcus or on the labia majora may represent a hidradenoma. The presence of central umbilication or ulceration should increase the index of suspicion. The diagnosis can only be confirmed histologically, and lesions reported as "adenocarcinoma" should be thoroughly restudied lest a needless vulvectomy be performed.

Treatment. These tumors are sufficiently rare to warrant excisional biopsy, which is both diagnostic and curative.

Accessory Breast Tissue

Lying along the "milk line," the vulva and axilla are both rich in apocrine glands. The normal breasts are modifications of these glands, so it is not surprising that breast tissue is sometimes found in these apocrine-rich areas. In fact, the vulva is the normal location for the breasts of some sea mammals (whale, porpoise). For this reason, vulvar breast tissue is not really "ectopic," but rather accessory. All degrees of development may be seen, from the small nonspecific button of subcutaneous tissue to bilateral labial masses capable of lactation. Many cases of accessory vulvar breast tissue are first manifested during pregnancy, when their enlargement is physiologically stimulated. All of these have been benign. Rarely do these growths result in mechanical dystocia, so their removal is best delayed until after the puerperium. Accessory breasts, especially those that arise in the nonpregnant state, have a somewhat higher incidence of neoplasia than do the normal breasts, and both fibroadenomas and adenocarcinomas have been reported in vulvar breast tissue.

Consider: A wide variety of tumors, therefore, need to be considered in the differential diagnosis, including hidradenoma, fibroma, lipoma, lymphedema, varicosities, and labial hernia.

Treatment. Because of uncomfortable enlargement with pregnancy and the danger of secondary neoplasia, such tumors should be removed.

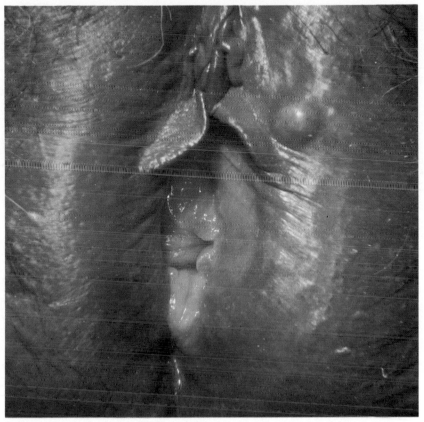

Hidradenoma.

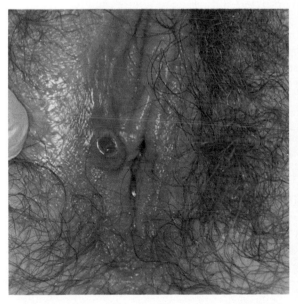

Hidradenoma—umbilicated. (Courtesy Dr. R. H. Kaufman.)

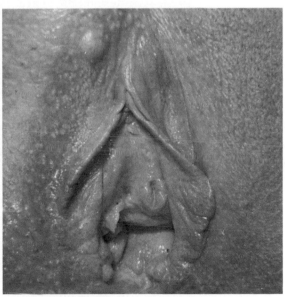

Accessory breast tissue nodule.

Endometriosis

External foci of ectopic endometrium may arise by metaplasia from the peritoneal mesothelium or from the accidental implantation of viable endometrium at the time of surgery or delivery. The latter mechanism explains most cases of vulvar involvement that often present at the site of a previous episiotomy. Superficial implants may give rise to a red or purple mass, while deeper involvement appears blue in color. Nodules without surface discoloration occur if the endometriosis is buried within the perineal body. Although none of these surface features are diagnostic, location on the posterior fourchette or within an episiotomy scar is suspicious. A history of cyclic enlargement with menses is highly suggestive.

Consider: Nevi, mucous cysts, mesonephric duct cysts, and melanomas can be differentiated only on the basis of histology.

Treatment. Excision is both diagnostic and curative.

Mesonephric Duct Cyst

During embryologic development of the female, the paired mesonephric ducts lie lateral and parallel to the müllerian ducts. Accordingly, remnants of the mesonephric duct may be found anywhere from the introital area of the vulva to the ovaries. While cystic dilatation of these ductal remnants can occur on the vulva, vaginal involvement is much more common. Characteristically, the mesonephric duct cysts occupy a lateral location, but only careful histologic evaluation of the cyst wall is absolutely diagnostic. Mucicarmine stains are negative, while Masson-trichrome preparations often reveal a layer of smooth muscle cells beneath a lining of transitional epithelium.

Consider: When present on the vulva, these dysontogenetic tumors lie close to the introitus and may have a slightly bluish tinge resembling the more frequent mucous cysts of the vestibule. External endometriosis may be similar in appearance, especially if the cysts occur within a mediolateral episiotomy scar, but often the endometriosis is betrayed by cyclic symptomatology.

Treatment. When located near the vaginal opening, their presence may interfere with coitus. Excision is both diagnostic and curative.

Pilonidal Sinus

A number of these tumors have now been reported and most have been in close approximation to the clitoris. When they occur over the coccyx, they are considered to be congenital malformations, but at other sites, this may not be the case. At least some lesions are acquired, with a definite adult onset, and probably arise as foreign body abscesses containing buried hair. Their location and inflammatory nature are sufficiently alarming that few cases are discovered incidentally.

Consider: The pyogenic granuloma and hidradenoma look very much like this lesion, as does any small abscess or infected epidermal cyst.

Treatment. Excision is the only known treatment but the depths of the lesion may be quite complex and what seems like an easy dissection becomes difficult. Unless the deep projections are completely removed, recurrence is frequent. Suture material may establish a new abscess, so cautery should be used when possible for hemostasis.

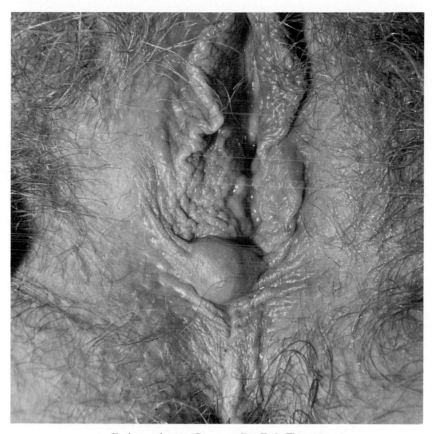

Endometrioma. (Courtesy Dr. F. J. Fleury.)

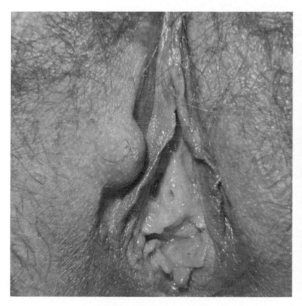

Mesonephric duct cyst.

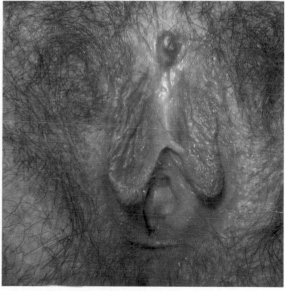

Pilonidal sinus.

Neurofibroma

Multiple neurofibromatosis (von Recklinghausen's disease) affects the vulva as well as the rest of the body. One study noted vulvar involvement in 18 per cent of women affected with this genetic disorder. Café au lait spots, dermal neurofibromata, and subcutaneous cordlike nodules may all occur. The latter are more common during the "pretumorous" childhood phase of the disease. Indiscriminate removal of the asymptomatic dermal tumors is not justified. As a rule there is little doubt about the diagnosis, in view of the multiple lesions elsewhere on the body and the presence of the café au lait macules. Excisions may be required, however, if the tumors interfere with the urine stream or have grown larger than 1 cm in diameter.

Consider: Isolated subcutaneous nodules on the vulva present a problem if the diagnosis has not yet been established. Rapid, asymmetric enlargement of the genitalia in young girls may cause psychologic difficulties. In such cases, a diagnostic excision of the mass can be combined with a plastic reduction of the affected labium.

Treatment. Rapid growth, symptomatology, and the need for diagnosis may all prompt excisional biopsy, but as a rule no therapy is required.

Acrochordon

Acrochordons are small, soft, fibroepithelial polyps that may be sessile or pedunculated. They are also known as skin tags. Their surface appears gently wrinkled or "mulberry"-like, and they are soft, in contrast to the gritty filiform surface of the condylomata acuminata, which they resemble. The color is generally that of the skin from which they arise, but the tip of the lesion may at times be slightly lighter in color. Frequently, the lesions look like small empty sacs of skin. When multiple, they are usually widely separated. The growths are not significant and are asymptomatic unless a twisted stalk causes an infarction. Their presence on the vulva, however, may bother the patient who palpates a "bump." Giant acrochordons have been seen, and diagnostic excisional biopsy may be needed for lesions larger than 1 cm.

Consider: Acrochordons of varying size mimic intradermal nevi, accessory breast tissue, hidradenomas, and neurofibromas.

Treatment. If the diagnosis is in doubt, excisional biopsy should be performed, or the pedicle may be tied at its base prior to excision of the tag. Typical lesions can also be destroyed with electrocautery, cryosurgery, or the laser.

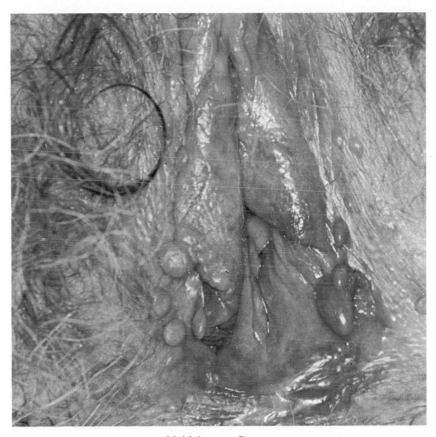

Multiple neurofibromas.

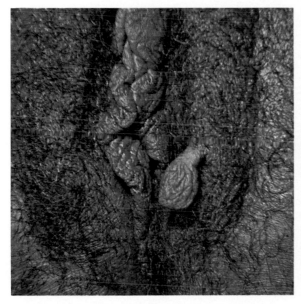

Acrochordon.

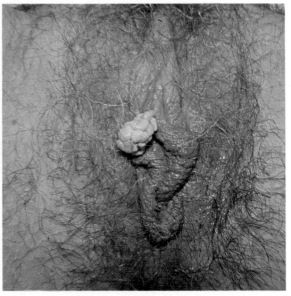

Acrochordon.

Fox-Fordyce Disease

Fox-Fordyce disease occurs almost exclusively in women who are postpubertal and premenopausal. It may affect the vulva or the axilla or both, and is basically a disorder of the apocrine sweat gland openings. The ducts become plugged with keratin, and subsequent dilatation of the duct and gland leads to the formation of retention vesicles. Apocrine secretion, leaking out into the dermis and epidermis, is thought to be responsible for the intense itching that is the hallmark of this disease. Most patients have undergone many unsuccessful attempts at relief of their pruritus before the diagnosis is finally made. The disease should be considered, along with pubic lice, in any woman who complains of intractable pubic itching without an obvious lesion.

The skin change is subtle and consists of multiple tiny flesh-colored papules, without the surrounding erythema or induration found in folliculitis. When scratch marks are present, they document the severity of the pruritus. The history of postpubertal onset and variations in the intensity of pruritus, which relate to the menstrual cycle, are characteristic. The endocrinologic relationships of this disease are not completely clear, but a definite inverse correlation of severity with estrogen levels seems certain. Remissions are frequently noted in pregnancy and have been experimentally produced with estrogen.

Consider: Axillary involvement helps to secure the diagnosis. Biopsy may not be helpful unless multiple sections are examined by an experienced dermatopathologist. Syringoma may look like Fox-Fordyce disease but it is not usually pruritic.

Treatment. Plugging of the ducts is an acnelike process. Antiacne measures are therefore helpful and include the new topical dermatologic agents. Oral contraceptives administered in the routine manner, especially those with a high estrogen content, reduce the apocrine activity and result in sustained remissions. Finally, this condition is probably the only indication in vulvar disease for a trial of topical estrogen. An ointment may be compounded using 1 mg of estrone in peanut oil (Theelin) per ounce of petrolatum. Applied three times daily, this therapy has been helpful in some cases.

Syringoma

Benign adenomatoid tumors of the eccrine sweat glands may affect any part of the body, especially the eyelids. When present on the vulva, they appear as multiple skin colored papules that are often confluent, forming short ridges. When deeply situated, they are almost invisible, especially if covered over by labial hair.

As a rule these tumors are not pruritic, but the presence of itching does not rule out the diagnosis. Some patients complain of a rough texture of the vulvar skin or have noted an isolated tumor, but most are asymptomatic.

Consider: The papules and cords may resemble epidermal cysts, Fox-Fordyce disease, herpes vesicles, and vulvar varices. Syringomas elsewhere on the body make the diagnosis more likely.

Treatment. Biopsy is the only sure method of diagnosis. No treatment is necessary, but the symptomatic patient may require surgical excision of the involved skin and deep dermis.

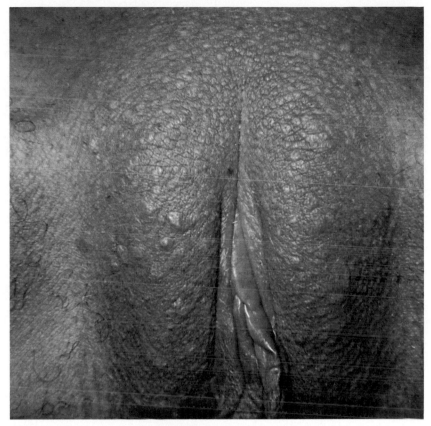

Fox-Fordyce disease.

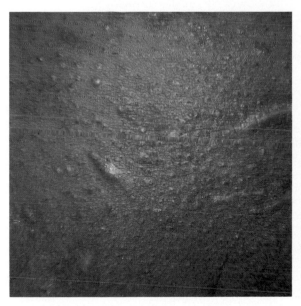

Fox-Fordyce disease—note excoriation scars.

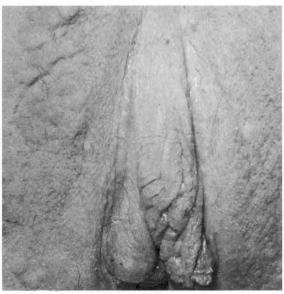

Syringoma. (Courtesy Dr. H. I. Borkowf.)

213

FURTHER READING

CONDYLOMATA

Dunn, J., Weinstein, L., Droegemueller, W., and Meinke, W.: Immunologic detection of condylomata acuminata specific antigens. Obstet. Gynecol. 57:351–356, 1981.
Beautiful color photos of immunofluorescent sections demonstrating condyloma antigen on location.

Gissmann, L., de Villiers, E.M., and zur Hausen, H.: Analysis of human genital warts (condylomata acuminata) and other genital tumors for human papillomavirus type 6 DNA. Int. J. Cancer 29:143–146, 1982.
A sophisticated study using a radio-labelled cloned DNA probe showed 93 per cent of all condylomata examined were positive for type 6 as were three verrucous carcinomas.

Graber, E.A., Barber, H.R.K., and O'Rourke, J.J.: Simple surgical treatment for condyloma acuminatum of the vulva. Obstet. Gynecol. 29:247–250, 1967.
This was the classic introduction of electrodesiccation and curettage as the treatment of choice.

Lynch, P.J.: Warts and cancer, the oncogenic potential of human papilloma virus. Am. J. Dermatopathol. 4:55–60, 1982.
A clear and cogent statement of the problem, present and future.

Oriel, J.D.: Natural history of genital warts. Brit. J. Vener. Dis. 47:1–13, 1971.
This is a landmark paper on the epidemiology of this infection and was the doctoral thesis of a world authority on the subject.

Quick, C.A., Watts, S.L., Krzyzek, R.A., and Faras, A.J.: Relationship between condylomata and laryngeal papillomata. Ann. Otol. 89:467–471, 1980.
Another landmark reference, which clinically and experimentally established the link between the two conditions.

Seski, J.C., Reinhalter, E.R., and Silva, J.: Abnormalities of lymphocyte transformations in women with condylomata acuminata. Obstet. Gynecol. 51:188–192, 1978.
Underlying immunosuppression characterizes cases of recalcitrant condylomata.

Tang, C.K., Shermeta, D.W., and Wood, C.: Congenital condylomata acuminata. Am. J. Obstet. Gynecol. 131:912–913, 1978.
A premature breech infant delivered 24 hours after membrane rupture had multiple condylomata around the anal orifice. The mother had a single labial lesion.

Woodruff, J.D., Braun, L., Cavalieri, R., et al.: Immunologic identification of papillomavirus antigen in condyloma tissues from the female genital tract. Obstet. Gynecol. 56:727–732, 1980.
One of the first breakthroughs utilizing the immunoperoxidase system to identify viral presence in a variety of lesions.

MOLLUSCUM CONTAGIOSUM

Wilkin, J.K.: Molluscum contagiosum venereum in a women's outpatient clinic: a venereally transmitted disease. Am. J. Obstet. Gynecol. 128:531–535, 1977.
An excellent article with a good bibliography and a unique "map" of lesions noted on the vulva.

CYSTS

Junaid, T.A., and Thomas, S.M.: Cysts of the vulva and vagina: a comparative study. Int. J. Gynaecol. Obstet. 19:239–242, 1981.
A high incidence of epidermal cysts in young Nigerian girls may relate to the trauma of circumcision in that country.

Kligman, A.M.: The myth of the sebaceous cyst. Arch. Derm. 89:141–144, 1964.
A landmark paper showing the true nature of the epidermal or keratinous cyst.

Merlob, P., Bahari, C., Liban, E., and Reisner, S.H.: Cysts of the female external genitalia in the newborn infant. Am. J. Obstet. Gynecol. 132:607–610, 1978.
An incidence of 6 per 1000 female births was noted, and the morphology and spontaneous course are nicely demonstrated.

Robboy, S.J., Ross, J.S., Prat, J., Keh, P., and Welch, W.R.: Urogenital sinus origin of mucinous and ciliated cysts of the vulva. Obstet. Gynecol. 51:347–351, 1978.
Extended and confirmed earlier work on the nature of these cysts and noted the presence of vestibular glands in 53 per cent of an autopsy series.

OTHER

Betson, J.R., Chiffelle, T.L., and George, R.P.: Pilonidal sinus involving the clitoris. Am. J. Obstet. Gynecol. 84;543–545, 1962.
An early paper that reviewed the literature, reported a case, and contributed new evidence for an acquired etiology.

Davies, M.G., Barton, S.P., Atai, F., and Marks, R.: The abnormal dermis in pyogenic granuloma. J. Am. Acad. Dermatol. 2:132–142, 1980.
Explains the abnormal proliferation of both endothelial and epidermal components as disordered growth of the papillary dermis.

Garcia, J.J., Verkauf, B.S., Hochberg, C.J., and Ingram, J.M.: Aberrant breast tissue of the vulva. Obstet. Gynecol. 52:225–228, 1978.
A complete review of the literature since 1900 with good case discussion and recommendations for management.

Imperial, R., and Helwig, E.B.: Angiokeratoma of the vulva. Obstet. Gynecol. 29;307–312, 1967.
A landmark paper from the AFIP detailing the aspects of 25 cases.

Lieb, S.M., Gallousis, S., and Freedman, H.: Granular cell myoblastoma of the vulva. Gynecol. Oncol. 8:12–20, 1979.
Discusses the benign and malignant variants, advocates wide excision for diagnosis, and summarizes the prior literature on this rare entity.

Messina, A.M., and Strauss, R.G.: Pelvic neurofibromatosis. Obstet. Gynecol. 47:63s–66s, 1976.
This report describes a case presenting as clitoral enlargement with café au lait spots and reviews the literature on this disease.

Woodworth, H., Dockerty, M.B., Wilson, R.B., and Pratt, J.H.: Papillary hidradenoma of the vulva: a clinicopathologic study of 69 cases. Am. J. Obstet. Gynecol. 110:501–508, 1971.
Combines a literature review with the largest known series of these tumors and remains a classic.

Young, A.W., Herman, E.W., and Tovell, H.M.M.: Syringoma of the vulva: incidence, diagnosis, and cause of pruritus. Obstet. Gynecol. 55:515–518, 1980.
An excellent paper on a rare disorder that is well illustrated and discussed.

11

LARGE TUMORS

BARTHOLIN CYST–ABSCESS

EDEMA

HEMATOMA

VERRUCOUS CARCINOMA

INVASIVE SQUAMOUS CARCINOMA

LYMPHOGRANULOMA VENEREUM

HERNIA–CYST OF THE CANAL OF NUCK

FIBROMA–LIPOMA

LARGE VARIANTS

216

LARGE TUMORS

The old books and articles on vulvar disease were criticized for their apparent preoccupation with gross tumors and relative lack of emphasis on the smaller, more common problems. Such criticism implies that the authors' intention was to produce amazement rather than education, but this was not their aim. Rather, their works accurately reflected the clinical experience of the time; a time when small, asymptomatic lesions were rarely seen. In previous generations, reticence and modesty on the part of both patient and physician made vulvar examination a rare event in the absence of gross abnormality. As a result, only symptomatic diseases were encountered with any regularity. In the case of most tumorous conditions of the vulva, symptoms arose only if the tumor became quite large, and the clinical authors faithfully reported this experience.

At present, women have been educated to accept the routine observation of both internal and external genitalia on a regular basis for the purposes of early cancer detection. This in turn has led to the greatly increased frequency with which small asymptomatic tumors have been discovered—and a corresponding decrease in the incidence of large dramatic growths.

Prompted by the psychologic denial that often accompanies the clinical signs of cancer, some patients still postpone examination. Such delay accounts for the fact that not many invasive squamous cell carcinomas are encountered under 1 cm in diameter. Some tumors like Bartholin gland duct cysts and fibromas-lipomas grow slowly, but because they arise in deep or hidden locations, they do not become clinically manifest until they have reached a large size. The initial ulcerative event in lymphogranuloma venereum is evanescent and easily ignored; only the scarring, edema, and bubo formation finally demand medical attention. For some lesions there exists an inherent size quality. Edema from whatever cause presents as a large tumor. Hematomata are instantly large and remain so until resolution. Hernias result from fascial defects that are themselves of generous proportion.

The lesions discussed in this chapter are presented in order to alert rather than astound. Some are common, others rather rare. But all are clinically important symptomatic entities that may be encountered from time to time in almost any practice.

Bartholin Duct Cyst–Abscess

Dilatation of the duct of Bartholin's gland is unquestionably the most common cause of large vulvar tumors. This intraluminal expansion results from blockage of the major duct or one of its larger branches. The cause of such obstruction cannot always be determined. Accidental or obstetric trauma, a relative congenital atresia, epithelial hyperplasia, and infection with secondary edema have all been implicated. It was once thought that the presence of a Bartholin duct cyst could be considered evidence of previous gonorrheal infection, but this is no longer the case. Most cysts of the duct occur because of purely mechanical factors that block the outflow of mucus. They contain sterile fluid and are not associated with infection or abscess formation. Many of these cysts will remain completely asymptomatic, and never enlarge beyond 1 or 2 cm in diameter. In those young women who are not inconvenienced by the presence of the introital mass, the cysts may be left untreated, with only periodic observation. Rapid enlargement, pain, hemorrhage, or secondary abscess formation would all constitute indications for therapy. On the other hand, primary abscesses of the duct (as opposed to cysts) may harbor a number of organisms, and anaerobic species are the most common. *Neisseria gonorrhoeae* is isolated from about 10 per cent of Bartholin duct abscesses and warrants the culture of all cases.

The Bartholin gland is composed of numerous mucus-secreting acini, which are situated near the vestibular bulb at the lower pole of the labium majus. The duct, lined with transitional epithelium, opens into the posterolateral vestibule just external to the hymenal ring. As the obstructed duct expands, due to continued mucus secretion from the gland cells, it forms a palpable enlargement in the deep lateral portion of the posterior fourchette. Further expansion causes a visible tumor to appear. Quite often, a prominent skin fold will overlie the cyst and appear to bisect it. This is the lower portion of the labium minus beneath which the normal duct courses. This sign is good evidence that the origin of the tumor is indeed the Bartholin gland duct.

Consider: Large epidermal cysts are more superficial in location and more ovoid in shape. Hernias, hydroceles, fibromas, lipomas, and masses of accessory breast tissue usually expand from above downwards along the course of the labium majus. Rarely do any of these involve the lateral corner of the posterior fourchette as does the Bartholin duct tumor. Carcinomas of the Bartholin gland mimic the asymptomatic benign duct cysts, and generally occur in women over the age of 40. In these patients, all new enlargements of the Bartholin area should be explored under general anesthesia with tissue specimens obtained for histologic examination.

Treatment. The treatment of choice for both cysts and abscesses is the creation of a fistulous tract from the dilated duct to the vestibule. This can be accomplished either by marsupialization or by use of the Word catheter technique. Both of these procedures are fully discussed in Chapter Four. An acute abscess, treated with hot compresses until it "points," usually results in spontaneous rupture through the labial skin and carries a high risk of recurrence. Incision, with insertion of a gauze wick to insure drainage, is not sufficient to prevent recurrence and should be avoided.

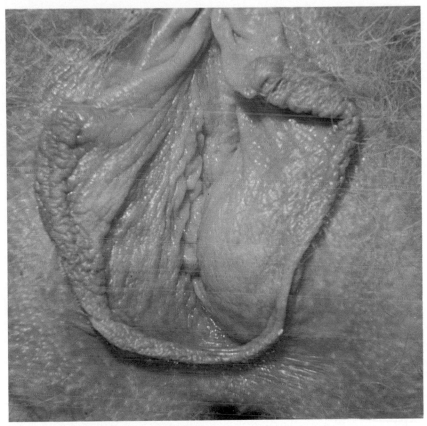

Bartholin gland duct cyst.

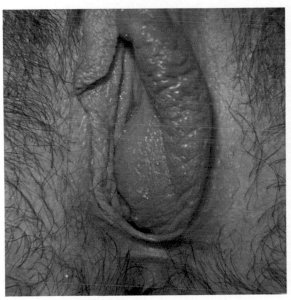

Bartholin gland duct abscess.

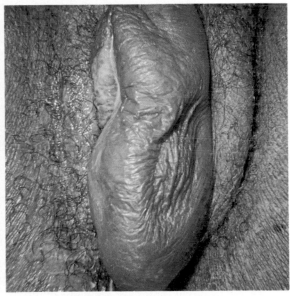

Acute abscess with edema.

Edema

Vulvar edema is a sign rather than a disease. But it may be the only presenting sign for a number of diseases, and it is sufficiently common to warrant inclusion as a separate entity. There is no specific etiology for vulvar edema. Vascular and lymphatic compromise may occur in a variety of conditions, but the major causes may be grouped into six categories: systemic, allergic, inflammatory, neoplastic, neurologic, and traumatic. Some forms of vulvar edema relate specifically to pregnancy and are discussed under that heading.

Like the eyelids, the labia minora are largely composed of loose connective tissue richly supplied with blood vessels and lymphatics. Systemic disorders such as hypoproteinemia, malignant ascites, congestive cardiac failure, and the nephrotic syndrome may result in vulvar swelling just as readily as they produce puffy eyelids. The same is true of allergic reactions. Ragweed allergy (hayfever) and heavy metal allergy (from gold injections) may be manifested in the vulva as well as in the tissues of the face. In addition, local contact reactions may be produced by topical deodorants, perfumes, detergents, fabrics, dyes, antibiotics, anesthetics and saliva.

Secondary edema is associated with herpes, Bartholin gland duct abscesses, lymphogranuloma venereum, and Crohn's disease as well as other inflammatory conditions. Local neoplasia may obstruct the cutaneous lymph vessels and result in an asymmetric induration, but if the deep regional lymph nodes are replaced by tumor, a softer and more generalized vulvar enlargement occurs.

Hypesthesia of the genital area can be produced by such neurologic disorders as multiple sclerosis or spinal cord injury, and chronic lymphedema may result. The accidental squeezing or entrapment of a single labium leads to a minor reactive edema, followed by progressive enlargement. Once begun, this process is self-perpetuating and ordinarily would cause pain. Voluntary abduction of the thighs would relieve the pressure, but when afferent sensation is lost, the process is inadvertently allowed to continue, resulting in marked distortion. The "peau d'orange" characteristic of the involved labial skin easily distinguishes this from the more common hyperplasia of the labia seen sometimes as a normal variant. Both conditions respond well to cosmetic labiectomy.

Consider: Vulvar edema has been described after paracentesis for ascites. In this latter procedure, ascitic fluid is thought to leak from the punctured peritoneum and dissect downward in the tissue planes of the abdominal wall.

Treatment. Just as there is no specific etiology for vulvar edema, there is no specific therapy. Systemic edema will usually resolve spontaneously if the causative disorder can be corrected. Allergic reactions respond well to identification and avoidance of the allergen, antihistamines, and local corticosteroids. Specific therapy should be directed at underlying inflammatory diseases and neoplastic processes. In cases of neurologic disorders, the therapy depends on the prognosis for the sensory involvement. If the nerves are irreversibly damaged, bilateral excision of the labia minora is at once curative and prophylactic. Traumatic edema is usually self-limited. Ice packs will retard the rate and extent of the edema formation in acute situations. Thereafter, warm compresses or baths will stimulate local circulation.

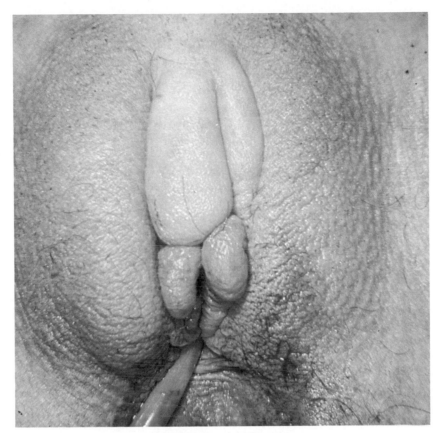

Diffuse edema—pre-eclampsia.

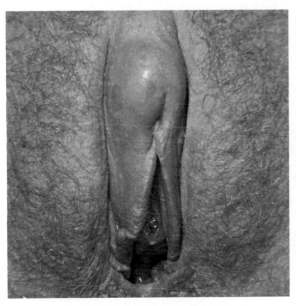

Clitoral edema—gold allergy.

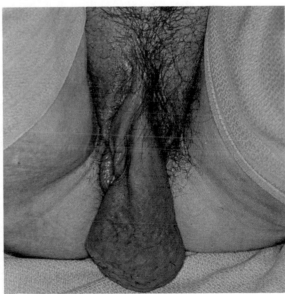

Chronic lymphedema—neurologic patient.

Hematoma

The vulva is supplied anteriorly by branches of the superficial and deep external pudendal arteries, which arise from the femoral artery near the fossa ovalis in the upper thigh. These external pudendal branches communicate in the labia with superficial and deep branches of the internal pudendal artery, which arises within the pelvis as one of the terminal branches of the hypogastric artery. This rich anastomosis offers little opportunity for the control of vulvar hemorrhage via compression or by ligation of a single major vessel. The venous system draining the area follows the arteries. In addition, a venous plexus surrounds the bulb of fat and erectile tissue present beneath each labium majus.

When sharp or blunt injury is sustained by the vulva and these vessels are damaged, a hematoma results. Most hematomas result from falls against a sharp object or from straddle injuries. Coital trauma and deliberate kicks account for others. A wet suit with a thick protective crotch is worn by all professional water skiers. Amateurs without this equipment run the risk of vulvar hematoma and perineal laceration if they fall at speed. Amusement rides, like the "mechanical bull," have also been reported as causal. In children, the circumstances of the injury are sometimes out of proportion to the findings. An innocent fall from tripping over the furniture may be accompanied by bleeding vulvar laceration and hematoma. Children should therefore be carefully examined after any history of trauma.

Whatever the injury, the likelihood of hematoma formation is increased in the presence of an underlying coagulopathy such as von Willebrand's disease or thrombocytopenia. These would be especially suspect in spontaneous hematoma formation. Finally, the vulvar wound may signal deeper damage, and the possibilities of urethral compromise and pelvic fracture may need to be explored.

Consider: Repetitive vulvar trauma in children may not be accidental, and the battered child syndrome must be kept in mind. In adults, look-alike lesions are generally ruled out by the history.

Treatment. If intact, these tumors are usually self-limiting, and their own expansion frequently provides enough compression to stop the hemorrhage. Aspiration is therefore a mistake. An icepack and pressure dressing will often help to stop the progression of the lesion. After 24 hours, in the absence of clotting abnormalities, warm wet packs or baths are used to promote circulation and encourage resolution of the extravasated blood. Patency of the urethra must be maintained, and some cases will require a catheter until bladder and urethral control is re-established. If enlargement continues despite these measures, a major vessel is probably involved. Incision and drainage of the mass with careful placement of hemostatic sutures is indicated. Rarely can an individual vessel be identified and ligated. Pressure packing may be necessary as a last resort, but the rate of infection after such a procedure is high and the pack should be removed as soon as possible. Hematomas may be secondarily infected from surface abrasion occurring at the time of original insult or from skin necrosis resulting from the subcutaneous pressure. Such lesions should be treated with incision and drainage, and systemic antibiotics are frequently necessary.

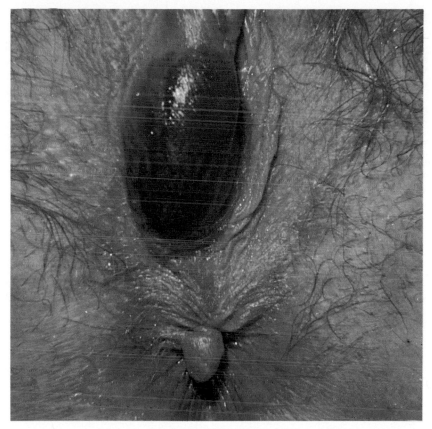

Hematoma—spontaneous.

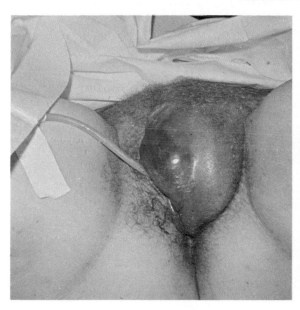

Hematoma—traumatic.

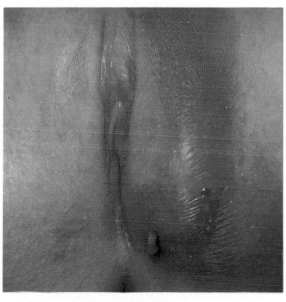

Infected hematoma in a child.

223

Verrucous Carcinoma

A spectrum of malignant potential exists among tumors, from the benign squamous papilloma and the condyloma acuminatum to the invasive squamous cell carcinoma. Verrucous carcinoma falls somewhere between these extremes, but the borders of differentiation are uncertain.

In some populations, condylomata acuminata are recognized as premalignant conditions. They are also included among the granulomatous diseases that may precede the development of invasive carcinoma. Giant forms of condylomata sometimes occur. These were first described on the penis by Buschke and Lowenstein, who noted their locally invasive tendency. Such tumors are clinically indistinguishable from invasive carcinomas. Histologically, however, they resemble benign condylomas except for their inversion, the downward growth that is observed in the dermis. In the absence of prior podophyllin application, few mitoses are noted, but intraepithelial pearl formation may occur.

The "pushing" growth of broad fronts of normal-appearing condyloma cells characterizes this tumor. When found in a lesion clinically resembling a giant condyloma, the term verrucous carcinoma is applied. The median age of patients with this disease is much older than that which characterizes the common sexually transmitted condyloma. Podophyllin has no effect on such lesions, and only makes histologic differentiation a more difficult task. Radiation therapy is contraindicated, and many reports attest to the sudden transformation of verrucous carcinoma into anaplastic squamous carcinoma following such attempts.

These lesions are prone to recur locally, even after radical excision. While they may have spread into the connective tissue of regional node–bearing areas, nodal and distant metastases do not occur. The occurrence of gigantic condylomatous growths in the absence of pregnancy or immunosuppression should alert the examiner to the possibility of verrucous carcinoma. Similarly, lesions resembling condylomata grossly and histologically, in women beyond the reproductive years, are highly suspect. Such tumors are more likely to fall in the middle portion of the malignant spectrum and should not be assumed to be totally benign.

Consider: On visual inspection, these lesions resemble invasive carcinomas, exuberant condylomas, and the exophytic forms of granuloma inguinale. Only large biopsies can differentiate these lesions.

Treatment. Podophyllin and radiation therapy are contraindicated. Optimum treatment consists in wide local resection. Recurrences are not uncommon and are best managed with additional surgery.

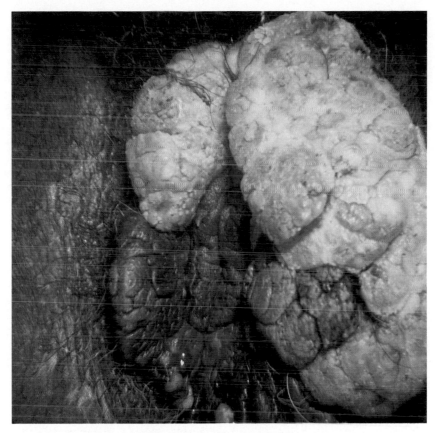

Verrucous carcinoma—massive.

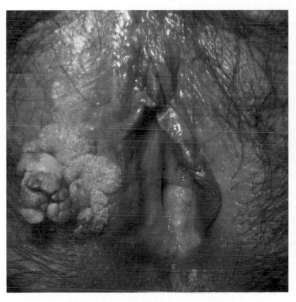

Verrucous carcinoma—polypoid.

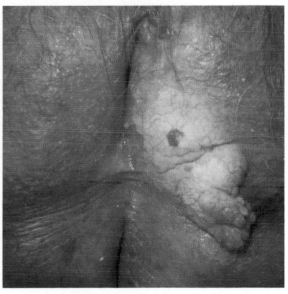

Verrucous carcinoma—sessile.

225

Invasive Squamous Cell Carcinoma

Invasive squamous cell carcinoma is the most common form of malignant neoplasia encountered on the vulva. Ninety per cent of most series of vulvar cancers are assigned to this category. Usually patients present because of their awareness of a mass that may have been preceded by long-standing pruritus and mild discomfort. Both ulceration and erythema are common, but the most striking feature is the presence of three-dimensional enlargement. These are not subtle lesions. The exophytic tumor surface may be friable and bleed easily on contact. In long-neglected tumors secondary infection is common. Rarely are patients truly surprised by the diagnosis, but a positive statement regarding the presence of carcinoma should never be made without histologic confirmation. Biopsy is mandatory and should be taken from a mature, but not necrotic, portion of the lesion. Multiple biopsy samples are usually more helpful and more representative than single specimens alone.

Squamous carcinomas may develop into huge tumors prior to diagnosis. To some extent, prognosis can be directly correlated with lesion size, but this relationship does not always hold for such giant growths. Massive tumors are predominantly exophytic and their growth rate is relatively slow. If a significant tendency to lymphatic invasion were present, distant metastases would have been evident long before the tumor reached such extraordinary proportions. Another unusual feature of large carcinomas is their occasional production of an unidentified substance with parathormone-like activity. The resultant hypercalcemia may cause severe mental aberration such that the patient initially appears to be psychotic. Attempts to correct the hypercalcemia by metabolic means have been universally unsuccessful. Once the tumor mass is excised, however, serum calcium levels return to normal, accompanied by dramatic improvement in the patient's mental status.

Consider: Other diseases such as granuloma inguinale, lymphogranuloma venereum, and verrucous carcinoma may result in a similar clinical appearance. These same diseases may also precede or be associated with the development of invasive squamous cell carcinoma.

Treatment. The management of invasive squamous cell carcinoma of the vulva is discussed in detail in Chapter Five. The prognosis for most cases is dependent on node involvement. If the nodes are free of tumor even though the primary growth is quite large, the prospects for survival are very good.

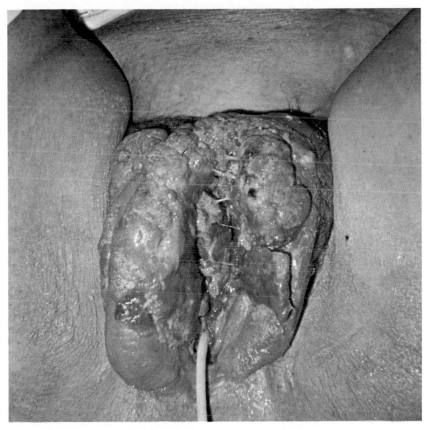

Invasive squamous carcinoma—massive exophytic.

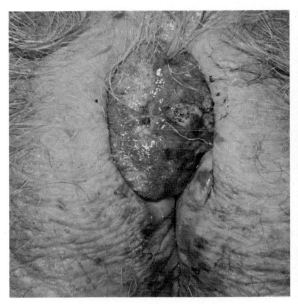

Invasive squamous carcinoma—clitoral.

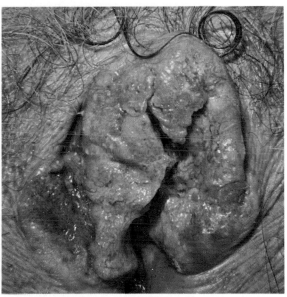

Invasive squamous carcinoma.

227

Lymphogranuloma Venereum
(*LGV*)

One of the classic venereal diseases, LGV is now recognized to be caused by *Chlamydia trachomatis,* serotype L. Other chlamydia cause nongonococcal urethritis and conjunctivitis. The clinical manifestations of LGV vary with the sex of the host and the country of origin. Worldwide in its distribution, LGV is declining in some areas. It is more common in blacks and in tropical and subtropical climates. Except for isolated pockets in some urban areas, the disease is relatively rare in the United States.

A nonspecific syndrome of fever and malaise often accompanies the development of a papule, which becomes a painless vulvovaginal ulcer after an incubation period of one to four weeks from the time of infection. This stage frequently goes unrecognized. About one month later, adenitis develops in either the groin or perirectal/pelvic nodes. Inguinal lymphadenitis, especially if unilateral, is highly suspicious for LGV. At first, the nodes are enveloped by a soft edema of the surrounding tissue. Later, they become matted and form bubos that enlarge and may rupture unless aspirated. The "groove" sign, a double genitocrural fold, is highly suggestive. When the adenitis is largely perirectal and pelvic, few clinical signs are evident until late in the course of the illness, when fibrosis, rectal stricture, sinus tract formation, and rectovaginal fistulas occur. These cases, with delayed diagnosis, may exhibit a tattered vulva with multiple buttonhole fenestrations and elephantiasis-like edema (esthiomene). In such patients, there is an increased incidence of squamous cell carcinoma of the vulva developing at a relatively young age.

All cases of acute, tender, inguinal adenitis are suspect and should be considered to be LGV unless another cause can be assigned. The differential diagnosis must include syphilis, which may also result in bubo formation. Biologic false-positive VDRL tests occur in about 20 per cent of patients with LGV. The FTA–ABS test must then be used to distinguish these conditions. The intradermal Frei test is no longer used because of its lack of accuracy. Instead, a complement fixation test (LGV–CFT) is employed, although it is group specific against all chlamydial infections. Even so, titres of 1:64 or higher are suggestive of LGV.

Consider: Besides syphilis, other diseases occasionally confused with LGV include chancroid, infectious mononucleosis, cat scratch fever, and tularemia. Old lesions resemble granuloma inguinale, hidradenitis suppurativa, and Crohn's disease.

Treatment. VD alert. Supportive therapy includes bed rest and ice packs applied to the enlarging inguinal glands. Fluctuant bubos should be aspirated through healthy skin via an 18-gauge needle. Avoid rupture, incision, or excision of bubos, since extension and aggravation of the infection may result. Tetracycline, 500 mg every six hours, is the drug of first choice. Sulfamethoxazole, 1 gm twice daily after a 2-gm loading dose, is also effective. Either drug should be continued for a minimum of three weeks, and repeat courses may be necessary. In the chronic destructive phase, the same antibiotics are used along with surgical excision and reconstruction after careful search for concomitant squamous cell carcinoma.

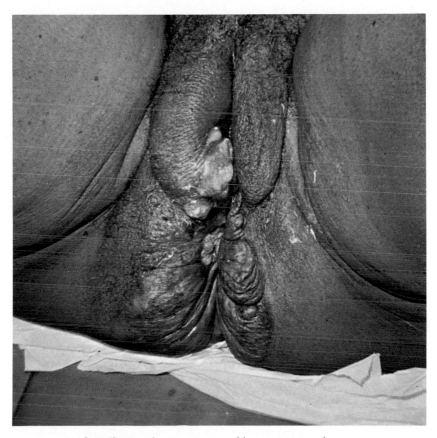

Lymphogranuloma venereum with squamous carcinoma.

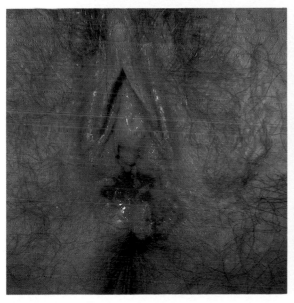

Evanescent LGV ulcer.

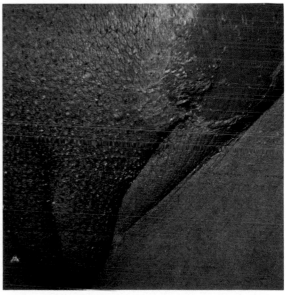

Lymphogranuloma venereum—bubo with "groove" sign.

229

Hernia

Pudendal hernias can present as vulvar masses and often masquerade as large cysts or soft-tissue tumors. These lesions may be asymptomatic, but some impart a subjective sensation of localized heaviness. Hernias are generally reducible and can be quickly differentiated from other tumors by careful palpation. This distinction is most important, since direct incision of such a mass could result in injury to the prolapsed abdominal viscera contained within the hernial sac. Fascial defects resulting from congenital deficiency or previous trauma, as well as respiratory illnesses accompanied by a chronic cough, may play a role in their etiology.

Inguinal hernias may also present on the vulva after downward progression along the course of the round ligament. At an earlier stage, such tumors appear as nonspecific inguinal masses, and pose problems in differential diagnosis. Enlarged inguinal nodes from a variety of causes, and ectopic testes (in the androgen insensitivity syndrome) may be confused with developing inguinal hernias and should be considered in the list of possibilities. Reducibility is again the most important diagnostic feature. Hernias may transilluminate, depending on the contents of the sac. Inguinal testes and lymph nodes do not.

Cysts of the canal of Nuck, while not true hernias per se, are analagous to hydroceles in the male. Anton J. Nuck was a professor in anatomy and surgery at Leyden. His interest in the pathogenesis of inguinal hernia in women prompted his discovery of the peritoneal diverticulum that in cystic form bears his name. Cysts of the canal of Nuck are of varying size and are somewhat mobile beneath the skin. They transilluminate well and are painless.

Consider: Hernias are generally above and lateral to the common location for Bartholin duct masses, but any large soft-tissue tumor can mimic a hernia. To prevent injury, reduction, palpation, and transillumination should always be attempted.

Treatment. Surgical repair is usually indicated, and the route of the approach is determined by the anatomical structures involved.

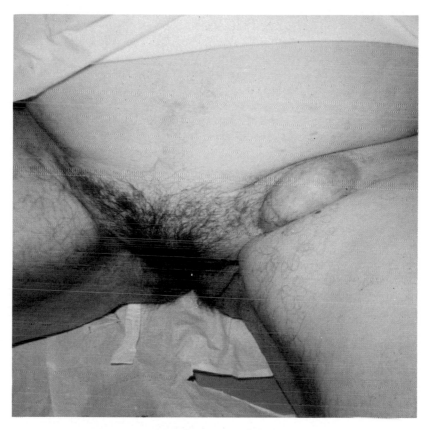

Cyst of the Canal of Nuck.

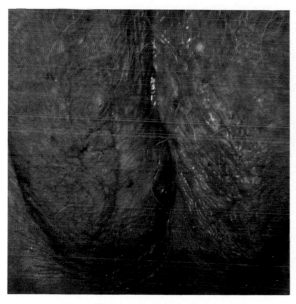

Right pudendal hernia.

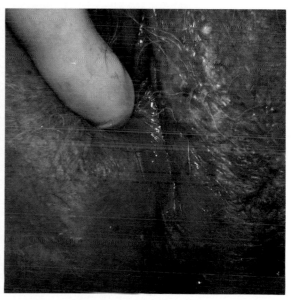

Pudendal hernia—reduced.

231

Fibroma-Lipoma

The fibrofatty and muscular tissues of the labia, rectovaginal septum, and ischiorectal fossa may occasionally give rise to benign fibromas, lipomas, and leiomyomas. Despite their prominence in the older literature, these solid, soft-tissue tumors are relatively infrequent. Such growths may be of any size and may occur at any age. Some have been noted at birth. Rarely do they cause symptoms other than the presence of a mass. Pain emanating from such a tumor is unusual and suggests rapid growth or degeneration.

These lesions arise from the connective tissue deep within the pudendal structures. Since their normal growth rate is slow, their appearance on the surface of the vulva generally suggests that they have actually been present for some time. Rapid enlargement under observation is an ominous sign that may signal malignant transformation. Leiomyosarcomas, epithelioid sarcomas, and fibrosarcomas are the most common varieties of soft-tissue vulvar malignancy, excluding melanomas, but development from a pre-existing benign tumor is not their usual mode of onset.

Depending on the relative amounts of fibrous and lipomatous content, the benign tumors vary in their consistency from very firm to soft. Lipomas tend to be more bulky than fibromas, but histologically most tumors contain a mixture of the two elements. These lesions have a smooth surface contour, since the overlying epithelium is not primarily involved. Origin from the deeper, posterior and lateral aspects of the vulva is common and may be a helpful feature in the differential diagnosis of these lesions. Some fibromas develop a broad pedicle that lengthens as the weight of the mass increases, but many of these pedunculated "fibromas" actually represent large variants of the common acrochordon.

A nonspecific vulvar mass of uncertain origin should always be investigated. The initial observer cannot be certain of the true duration of the lesion, and the patient's own estimate of onset and growth rate is often little more than a guess. The minimal hazards of anesthesia must therefore be weighed against the rare, but devastating, occurrence of sarcoma.

Consider: When still relatively small, they may resemble epidermal, mesonephric duct, or mucous cysts, or foci of endometriosis. The larger varieties are easily confused with Bartholin gland duct cysts and inguinal or pudendal hernias.

Treatment. Whenever possible, these growths should be excised. Pedunculated lesions may be amenable to office management under local anesthesia. Broad-based pedicles, however, may contain large vessels that require accurate ligation. Large tumors involving the ischiorectal fossa may pose formidable problems in dissection, and should only be approached under general anesthesia.

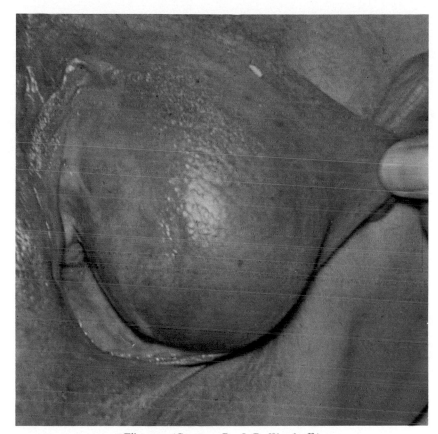

Fibroma. (Courtesy Dr. J. D. Woodruff.)

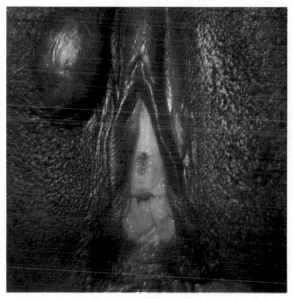

Leiomyoma.

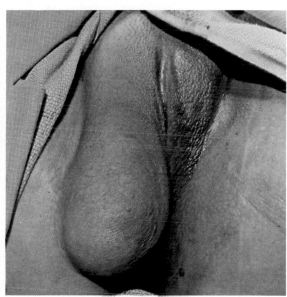

Lipoma. (Courtesy Dr. W. C. Fetherston.)

Large Variants

Some tumors, while frequently observed in their "smaller editions," sometimes present as large growths. As such, they may be confused with other pathologic entities and their true nature not suspected until histologically verified.

The acrochordon, or skin tag, is generally a small tumor with little likelihood of enlargement. The rate of growth is slow, but some may attain considerable size if they are conscientiously ignored for many years. The tumor tends to maintain the general architectural features seen in smaller acrochordons: a pedicle is present, and the apical portion is frequently folded or dimpled. The synonym "fibroepithelial polyp" has been applied to this growth, and since only benign fibrous connective tissue is present in the matrix, the lesion is sometimes simply called a "fibroma." While malignant degeneration has not been reported, these tumors should be excised, since twisting of the pedicle may cause infarction and necrosis.

Epidermal cysts occasionally reach diameters exceeding 1 cm. When single, such cysts may mimic fibromas, lipomas, leiomyomas, accessory breast tissue, or cysts of the canal of Nuck. The diagnosis is generally a retrospective one after the cyst lining has been microscopically evaluated.

Von Recklinghausen's multiple neurofibromatosis is associated with both epidermal and subcutaneous tumors. The latter are less common, but may achieve a much larger size. Synonyms for these gigantic nodules include "plexiform neuromas" and "elephantiasis nervorum." In children, even small subcutaneous nodules seem large in comparison with other body features. A cordlike consistency is often noted on palpation, and the presence of other manifestations of von Recklinghausen's disease greatly supports the diagnosis. Malignant transformation into sarcoma is reported to occur in 5 to 15 per cent of these tumors. Those exhibiting rapid enlargement are particularly suspect.

Consider: These masses may be confused with enlarged accessory breast tissue, fibroma-lipomas, or thrombosed varicosities.

Treatment. Accurate diagnosis of large variant tumors is usually made postoperatively. Whenever possible, these tumors should be completely excised. Surgical removal is increasingly more important, as well as increasingly more difficult, when a rapid growth rate is observed in one of these lesions.

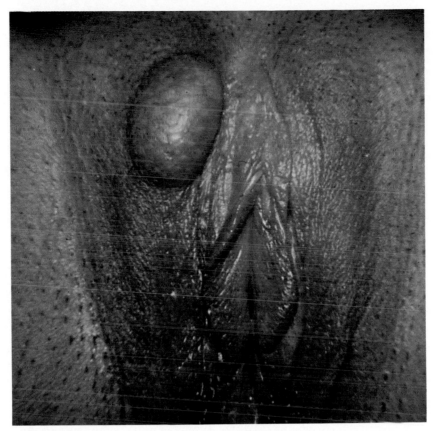

Giant epidermal cyst.

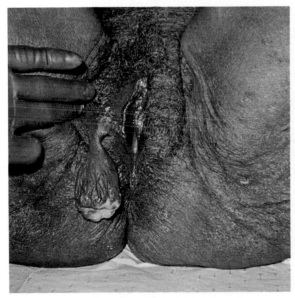

Giant acrochordon.

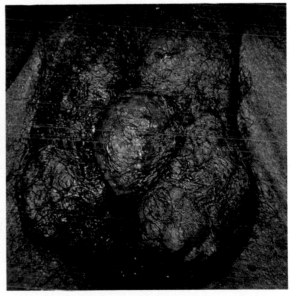

Giant neurofibromas. (Courtesy Dr. K. Zelle.)

FURTHER READING

BARTHOLIN CYST–ABSCESS

Lee, Y.H., Rankin, J.S., Alpert, S., et al.: Microbiological investigation of Bartholin's gland abscesses and cysts. Am. J. Obstet. Gynecol. 129:150–153, 1977.
Percutaneous aspirates from 12 cysts and 34 abscesses were analyzed with qualitative microbiology.

HEMATOMA

Ezell, W.W., Smith, E.I., McCarthy, R.P., et al.: Mechanical traumatic injury to the genitalia in children. J. Urol. 102:788–792, 1969.
Injuries in the pediatric age group often result in profuse bleeding and require surgical hemostasis.

Hudock, J.J., Dupayne, N., and McGeary, J.A.: Traumatic vulvar hematomas. Am. J. Obstet. Gynecol. 70:1064–1073, 1955.
The most informative and comprehensive article yet written on an ageless subject.

VERRUCOUS CARCINOMA

Partridge, E.E., Murad, T., Shingleton, H.M., et al.: Verrucous lesions of the female genitalia—verrucous carcinoma. Am. J. Obstet. Gynecol. 137:419–424, 1980.
A good review of the literature with excellent illustrations of the key pathologic features and a discussion of the clinical and therapeutic problems involved.

INVASIVE SQUAMOUS CARCINOMA

Neibyl, J.R., Genadry, R., Friedrich, E.G., et al.: Vulvar carcinoma with hypercalcemia. Obstet. Gynecol. 45:343–348, 1975.
Literature review and a report of two cases with this association—both were excessively large tumors.

LYMPHOGRANULOMA VENEREUM

Felman, Y.M., and Nikitas, J.A.: Lymphogranuloma venereum. Cutis 25:264, 1980.
This excellent overview of the disease includes epidemiology, diagnosis, and treatment.

HERNIA

Anderson, W.R.: Pudendal hernia. Obstet. Gynecol. 32:802–804, 1968.
Contains a good diagram and photographs that illustrate this timeless problem of anatomy.

FIBROMA–LIPOMA

Fukamizu, H., Matsumoto, K., Inove, K., and Moribucki, T.: Large vulvar lipoma. Arch. Dermatol. 118:447, 1982.
A report of a case in a newborn that reviews the few other cases documented in the last 20 years.

Tavassoli, F.A., and Norris, H.J.: Smooth muscle tumors of the vulva. Obstet. Gynecol. 53:213–217, 1979.
An excellent collation of the clinical and pathologic features of 32 such tumors seen at the AFIP.

LARGE VARIANTS

Venter, P.F., Rohm, G.F., and Slabber, C.F.: Giant neurofibromas of the labia. Obstet. Gynecol. 57:128–130, 1981.
Two cases of these large variants are illustrated and discussed.

12

SPECIAL PROBLEMS

VULVAR PAIN

PREGNANCY

VARICOSITIES

ANATOMIC VARIANTS

CIRCUMCISION

SPECIAL PROBLEMS

There are significant disorders of the vulva that present no visible features for recognition. The syndrome of idiopathic pain and burning is one of these. Every physician who has dealt with a patient with vulvar pain knows the difficulty and frustration involved in trying to find a treatable cause. Unfortunately, the condition is not rare.

Pregnancy is a physiologic state that affects the entire woman. The vulva shares in the gestational adaptation and also presents problems particular to the pregnant state. Other common disorders (trichomoniasis, condylomata, herpes) assume special significance in pregnancy, where they pose a particular therapeutic challenge.

Variation is present throughout all of biology. The human body is not mass-produced nor computer-designed, so anatomic variations are frequently encountered. Most are so subtle that they cause no concern, but others result in symptoms or may be confused with pathologic conditions. When not recognized as such, a variation may be mistakenly treated, resulting in real pathology. By the same token, physicians are reluctant to treat what they recognize as variation because of its "normalcy" and may refuse to perform a corrective procedure fully justified by the symptoms.

International travel is now commonplace. Diseases and conditions once confined to a specific geographic area are now global. Customs and rituals have also been shared. Among some of the peoples of Africa, especially in the Sudan and Nigeria, the circumcision or infibulation of young girls is still widely practiced. For some it retains a religious significance, but for most it is simply a matter of custom much like male circumcision in the United States. Increasing numbers of circumcised women now present for care, and it is important to know how they may be helped.

Vulvar Pain

In a philosophic sense, the problem of pain has occupied many centuries of thought. But on a practical level, the patient and physician seek only to have the pain stop.

In a neurophysiologic sense, pain represents a point on the perceptive spectrum. A stimulus is applied and a specialized nerve ending is activated and transmits an electrochemical signal to the brain via a network of conductors. The signal is received and then enhanced or dampened by the library of past experience and current events instantaneously available to the cortex. The result may be anything from no response, through tingling, itching, and burning, to excruciating pain. Most vulvar skin disorders produce itching; only a few acute inflammatory conditions like herpes and abscesses cause frank pain.

It is all the more curious then that some women complain bitterly of pain in the vulva when there is no visible disorder to account for it. In 1886, *The Practical Home Physician* listed only five diseases of the vulva: inflammation, abscess, eczema, pruritus, and excessive sensitiveness. Under the last heading the authors noted that even light touch stimulus could bring on convulsions, that it interfered with sexual function, that it was found in "hysterics and those at the change of life." The authors recommended unspecified surgery and improvement in general health as possibly beneficial. One century later, we are not much further ahead.

However, *pudendal neuralgia* is described in neurologic texts as a distinct entity, usually found in the male, characterized by an increased sensitivity to touch such that even light pressure on the genitalia may be intolerable. Cyclists, horsemen, and those with old straddle injuries are among the affected, but most are thought to be "neurotic". That the condition occurs in both men and women, with about equal frequency, is important knowledge. Now it is possible to dismiss those exclusively female factors of hormonal aberration, menopause, and vaginitis from the list of probable causes. In all likelihood, the basic problem lies above the level of the external genitalia and involves neural pathophysiology. The term *pudendal neuralgia* can be applied to vulvar pain, and this may give the patient the security of a label for her disorder. Both the patient and her physician should understand that pudendal neuralgia can result from a variety of possible causes located at one of many levels in the nervous system.

In following the course of the afferent nervous system from the genital skin to the cerebral cortex, a nerve impulse travels from specialized receptors and unmyelinated nerve endings via fine branches to the pudendal nerve, which hooks around the ischial spine and runs along the pelvic wall, passes between the leaves of the coccygeal and piriform muscles, and joins the lumbosacral plexus. The sacral nerves carry the message to their dorsal roots, which enter the spinal cord between the bony processes of the vertebrae. There the fibers join one of the sensory bundles in the cord and ascend to the cortex via the thalamus.

Possible causes of vulvar pain may now be considered from the cortex downwards. Among the "cortical" factors, anxiety and depression can reinforce many kinds of pain responses. When these form part of the picture, certain psychoactive drugs have been helpful. Trigeminal neuralgia is a well-recognized entity of facial pain brought on by mild stimuli like a cold breeze and is treated successfully with anticonvulsant drugs like carbamazepine (Tegretol) and phenytoin (Dilantin). Some cases of pudendal neuralgia have been similarly responsive to Dilantin in daily doses of 300 mg.

Spinal cord injury is generally secondary to a skeletal event in the vertebral column. Herniated discs and bony spurs in the cervical or lumbar regions are the most common examples. Many patients have suffered silent disc herniation or vertebral collapse from osteoporosis and this should always be considered in the patient with pudendal pain. One woman who complained of vulvar pain "like brimstone" noted that she suffered most when in church. A functional etiology seemed obvious until it was learned that the church had only backless stone benches for seats. Radiologic studies showed a herniated lumbar disc. The presence of leg weakness, foot drop, bladder dysfunction, or back pain mandates investigation of the lower spine. X-ray studies, urodynamic studies, nerve conduction tests, and the noninvasive scanning techniques now available may all be quite helpful.

Patients who have had genital herpes infections may develop a latent viral infection in the pelvic nerves and ganglia. It is not known for certain that the presence of latent virus can be responsible for pain. But the condition of post-herpetic neuralgia is recognized and at least provides an explanation for some cases with known exposure. Serologic tests for herpes antibody would identify those patients at risk.

All nerve tissue depends on a delicate biochemical balance to maintain its normal function. There are some medical diseases that are notorious for their ability to interfere with this balance and cause neuropathy. Classically, such metabolic causes result in paresthesia rather than pain, but diabetes, pernicious anemia, and vitamin and mineral deficiencies should all be considered in the evaluation of pudendal pain. Diabetics whose disease is controlled by diet and oral agents and who note burning vulvar pain are often dramatically relieved when small amounts of insulin are added to their regimen.

The nerve impulse is carried to the high CNS centers by more than a simple wave of electrical energy. It depends on a complex neurotransmission mechanism. Locally produced prostaglandins may sensitize neuroreceptors to a variety of chemical mediators involved in the itch/pain response. Perhaps for these reasons, many women with pudendal neuralgia are relieved by taking one of the nonsteroidal anti-inflammatory agents that are also prostaglandin antagonists. Ibuprofen (Motrin) 300 mg q.i.d. has given excellent results for some patients after the first week or two of administration.

As the pudendal nerve traverses the pelvis, it passes between the leaves of the levator ani muscle and can become trapped and irritated by a spasm of those fibers. Muscle spasms occur in varying degrees. When brought on by pressure at the introitus, the spasms result in vaginismus, and a definite firm edge of levator ani muscle can be palpated through the lateral vaginal wall in patients who suffer with this condition. Vaginismus may then be either a cause of pudendal neuralgia or one result of "oversensitivity" in the introital area. In either case, it is amenable to conscious adjustment, and muscle-relaxing exercises, along with counseling, can be of great benefit.

Some patients with pain have been operated in the past for Bartholin duct masses or have persuaded well-meaning surgeons to excise areas producing pain. Neuromas may form and nerves may become trapped in the scar tissue. If the pain preceded the surgery, there is little to be gained by re-excision, but patients will seize on the surgical episode as "the cause" like drowning victims seize upon the rescuer. In cases of postsurgical onset, while the temptation is great to "revise" the scar, relief of pain should never be guaranteed. If pudendal block relieves the pain, it is more likely, but not necessarily, due to a peripheral cause. If a single small area is noted that alone seems responsible for the pain and if the pain disappears when this area is infiltrated with a small amount of a local anesthetic, only then might additional dissection be warranted. As an alternative to surgery, corticosteroid injection, described in Chapter Four, has been found to be quite effective.

One common entity that is easily overlooked, but that usually presents as pain or dyspareunia, is vestibular adenitis: an inflammation of the minor vestibular glands, especially those near the posterior fourchette. This entity is illustrated and discussed as a red lesion in Chapter Six, but should always be considered in the differential diagnosis of pudendal neuralgia and dyspareunia. Laser ablation or vestibular excision with vaginal advancement is indicated for permanent relief.

Patients with vulvar pain are often difficult and demanding. They want a name for their problem, and pudendal neuralgia is one that seems to fit. Of course, what they want most is relief. The previous discussion covers a lot of territory and a complete evaluation is time-consuming. In the end, genuine concern and a sympathetic willingness to explore all possibilities may be the most that can be offered. There will remain that group of patients whose symptoms are in fact functional and who may benefit from professional psychiatric exploration and intervention.

Pregnancy

The vulva takes part in the total body changes that occur with pregnancy. The skin turgor is increased and pigmentation is more pronounced. Alterations in vascular dynamics result in congestion and some "puffiness" of the labia that can be appreciated from time to time. These same factors also lead to the edematous conditions of the pregnant vulva and to vulvar varices.

Eastman noted that vulvar edema in pregnancy was usually associated with an hypertensive disorder or with multiple gestation. Certainly, the vulva responds like the eyelid to hypertensive and hypoproteinemic states. Vulvar edema is not at all unusual in nonpregnant women with nephrotic syndrome and so may almost be expected in patients with toxemia of pregnancy.

But vulvar edema that begins postpartum has a completely different significance. Swelling is frequent at the episiotomy site, and a mild generalized edema is present after delivery over an intact perineum. But a series of maternal deaths have been recorded in which unilateral vulvar edema began on the second postpartum day and heralded development of a generalized perineal induration that eventuated in rapid sepsis and vascular collapse. No common pathogen could be identified nor did a necrotizing fasciitis ever develop.

Among the more curious pregnancy-induced changes is that of gingival hyperplasia and the so-called "epulis" tumor of the gum. On histologic section numerous endothelial-lined spaces are evident within a granulation tissue matrix. The same histology marks the pyogenic granuloma that occurs on the vulva and frequently arises during pregnancy. Both may be analogous processes—manifestations of the same stimulus in different locations. As a rule, no treatment other than local cleanliness is recommended for the gingival tumor and the same is true for the vulva. Postpartum regression is usual at the oral site. The vulvar tumor may remain, however, and require wide and deep wedge resection to reduce the chances of recurrence.

Marine mammals have their breasts located on the vulva. Accessory breast tissue may also occur on the human vulva, which is in the "milk line." Often these adenomatous rests are dormant until stimulated by pregnancy. The diagnosis of accessory breast should therefore be considered in those vulvar enlargements that begin during pregnancy, especially in the primi-gravida.

Three sexually transmitted diseases pose special problems during pregnancy. Trichomoniasis is a common vaginitis that can be particularly severe in pregnancy and lead to the rarely seen colpitis emphysematosa. In this condition little blebs of carbon dioxide gas form beneath the vaginal epithelium and produce clusters of small cysts. The gas presumably comes from the organism. Ordinarily, trichomonal infection is easily managed with metronidazole. But the drug is contraindicated during the first trimester. During this time, then, alternatives are necessary. Hypertonic saline (20 per cent) douches are very effective when given once a day for a week and then weekly until the discharge has cleared or until metronidazole can be used. The fungicide clotrimazole as a vaginal cream has been reported effective for trichomonas in half the cases studied and may also be tried.

Condylomata acuminata thrive during pregnancy for reasons that may be related to the relative immunosuppression that occurs in gestation. But because they pose a hazard to the newborn, giving rise to later laryngeal papillomata, it is important to eradicate growths within the birth canal. Electrocoagulation and curettage has been used with success for this purpose, as has the carbon dioxide laser.

Herpes simplex infection also needs special attention in pregnancy. Viral infection of the newborn carries a high mortality and neurologic morbidity rate. For this reason, cesarean section has been advocated for mothers who have had documented herpes infections during gestation. As viral cultures have become widely available, it is now possible to monitor viral shedding. For women with active lesions in labor, examination should be avoided and cesarean section performed. But the infant of the patient with no active lesion, who has had a herpes episode during the pregnancy, is not at increased risk if the latest herpes cultures (especially from the cervix) are negative. Known herpes patients should ideally have weekly cultures during the last four to eight weeks of gestation. Intrapartum management may then be based on these results.

241

Varicosities

In a way, these large tumors of the vulva are another of the problems associated with pregnancy, since rarely are they encountered apart from gestation. While about 2 per cent of pregnant women have vulvar varices, not all of these are symptomatic and most regress markedly postpartum. Rarely, thrombosis may occur and require surgical intervention.

Clinically, these tumors have a bluish-purple cast, but in dark women there may be little or no color change evident. Numerous "wormlike" irregularities are noted beneath the surface skin, and the involvement is almost always unilateral. They may be mistaken for multiple epidermal cysts, but on palpation, varices are soft and reducible with minimal pressure. As a rule, varicosities of the leg veins will be noted along with those of the vulva. Rarely do these venous dilatations cause significant symptoms. Yet some may enlarge to such size that patients complain of heaviness and pressure. Reports of spontaneous rupture, hematoma formation, massive hemorrhage, and thrombosis can be found, but such occurrences are most unusual.

Consider: Vulvar breast tissue may first become evident in pregnancy. Varicoceles resemble giant neurofibromas or syringomas, but the history and association with pregnancy direct the diagnosis.

Treatment. For relatively small localized varices, no treatment is necessary and many of these tumors subside spontaneously after delivery. Those that enlarge or cause sensations of increased vulvar weight can be adequately managed by the use of support garments. Cases of massive involvement causing severe symptoms or threatening hemorrhage may require excision of the distended segments through a longitudinal labial incision after the branches have been doubly ligated both above and below the dilated vessels. In rare instances, ligation of the external pudendal and internal saphenous veins is necessary. Sclerosing therapy may also be used and works well for residual disease. Definitive therapy of any kind, however, is best delayed until four to six months postpartum.

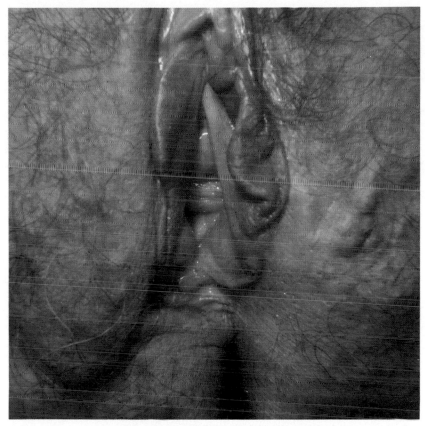

Bilateral varices with single varicocele.

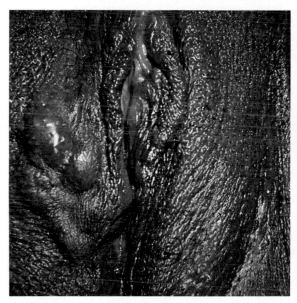

Varicosities.

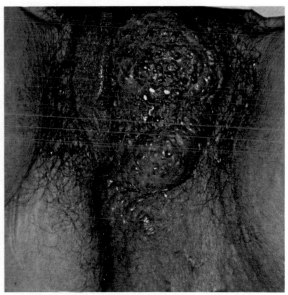

Varicosities—massive. (Courtesy Dr. E. Delfs.)

Anatomic Variants

Severe congenital anomalies of the vulva are rare, but complete absence of the genitalia has been reported along with isolated failure of clitoral development. There are nine recorded cases of total vulvar reduplication, usually associated with a double vagina and failure of müllerian fusion. But such occurrences are extremely rare. Common, however, are the subtle variations.

Minor accessory labia are frequently seen presenting as "extra folds." These ridges of skin run upwards, from the point where the minora turn mediad to form the periclitoral structures, and parallel the normal majora. These structures may at times be so well developed that they resemble supplementary labia minora. Additional sulci are thus created. If these are deep, they require special hygienic attention to keep them clear of smegma and squamous debris. Plain mineral oil on a cotton ball works extremely well for this purpose. Otherwise, they require no special regard.

Labial elongation is another common problem. The labia minora develop asymmetrically in about 12 per cent of women. Their dimensions are also highly variable. When spread like wings on minimal tension, the horizontal distance from the vaginal midline to the outer curve is usually 3 to 5 cm in the adult. Some women have minora that exceed these measurements and they cause no difficulty. But others are troubled when they wear tight clothing or engage in sports, even with labia of more modest size.

It was truly once the practice of some African tribes to attach weights to the labia of youngsters in order to produce what they considered to be an attractive degree of lengthening. But it is a myth that labial elongation is a result of masturbation. The young girl or woman who complains that her labia are too long and interfere with her normal dress and activity should be considered for a reduction labioplasty. Carefully done, such simple trimming should not reduce sexual function but can restore symmetry and allow the minora to remain protectively enclosed by the lateral major labia.

Vestibular papillae have not been well described. Yet this is perhaps the most common and—since it is so often confused with condylomata acuminata—the most mistreated variant. Tiny papillae, not unlike those found on the lateral surfaces of the tongue, are seen on the lateral vestibular surfaces. Under the colposcope, these are simple papillary projections similar to the grapelike structures of the endocervix, having a single central capillary loop and covered with a thin layer of squamous epithelium. Most arise independently from the surface and are soft and pliable when probed. True condylomata, on the other hand, show multiple papillae more heavily coated with keratin, with multiple spikes arising from a common stalk, and their vessels are less prominent.

Histologic examination shows a core of fibromyxomatous connective tissue in the vestibular papillae and a covering of squamous epithelium without the koilocytotic or other viral changes expected in true condylomata. Nor do the papillary cells contain HPV antigen.

Consider: When this condition is noted, it is often mistaken for a condylomatous infection and usually treated with a topical caustic solution. Burning results, but the "lesion" does not respond. Because a diagnosis of condylomata carries the onus of a sexually contracted disease and has far-reaching implica-

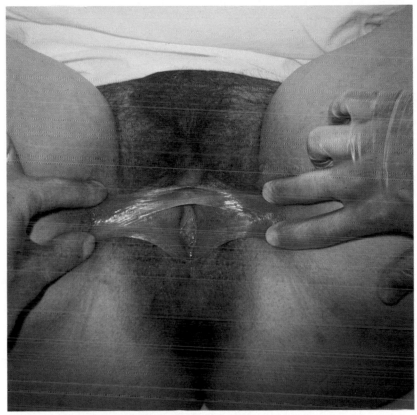

Labial elongation.

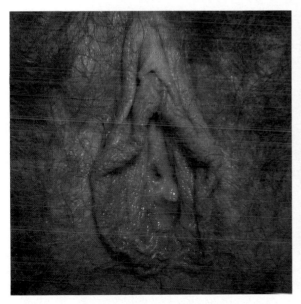

Reduplication—upper minora.

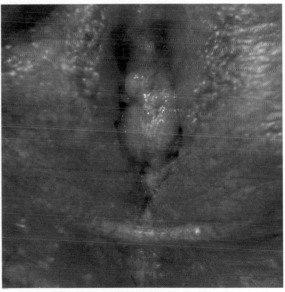

Vestibular papillae.

245

tions, it is important to confirm the diagnosis with biopsy. When the change is confined to the vestibule and manifest only by a "rough" or "pebble-grain" epithelium, perhaps it represents simply a papillary vestibule that requires no treatment. Colposcopy can be used for confirmation. Histologically, a report of "squamous papilloma" is usually found and would be consistent with a diagnosis of vestibular papillae.

Circumcision

The custom of routine circumcision of the male penis began as a Jewish religious tradition centuries ago and has been practiced widely by others in this country during most of the twentieth century. The lack of hygienic necessity for the procedure is now recognized, and it has fallen from fashion as a routine hospital service provided with delivery.

In a similar way, other civilizations of the Great Crescent developed female circumcision as a ritual of religion that grew to become a custom. It too was widely practiced until declared illegal in 1945 in most localities. Both Nigeria and the Sudan continue to circumcise young females on an illegal basis, and the work is now performed mainly by midwives.

This is an age of international travel conducted on an unprecedented scale. Not only tourism but also periods of prolonged academic work by foreign students and the permanent immigration of many people from other lands has extended the scope of American medicine. It is therefore worthwhile for today's practitioner to be familiar with the major types of female circumcision-infibulation. For indeed, a patient from the Sudan, Nigeria, Kenya, or Sierra Leone, or from an Indian tribe in Peru, Eastern Mexico, or Western Brazil, or from the Malay Archipelago may have been circumcised as a young girl.

If done, it is likely to have been performed in one of three ways: (1) The Sunna circumcision consists mainly of removal of the prepuce and most closely parallels the male circumcision in a qualitative and quantitative sense. (2) The Modified Pharaonic or reduction circumcision, now becoming more common, removes prepuce and glans with the adjacent minora. (3) The Pharaonic procedure is the most drastic, excising the whole of the clitoris, minora, and majora, with midline approximation by means of a clip (infibula) or suture leaving little but a midline scar penetrated by small openings for urine and menses.

The cosmetic appearance of the vulva after circumcision is distinctly abnormal but seems to cause little distress to the patient. Restoration is not usually desired. One couple who sought correction of a ritual female circumcision, which produced a bridge-like band of tissue across the introitus and had removed the minoral structures, were offered an extensive plastic repair with "like new" results all but guaranteed. They had to convince the surgeon that all they wanted was removal of the tissue band, which required only one ml of xylocaine, two ties and cuts, and three minutes of office time! How important it is for all of us, always, to *listen to the patient!*

The special problems in vulvar disease are a fascinating area. And so also are the other categories. Vulvar diseases are generally visible, an accurate diagnosis can be made, and effective therapy is available for most conditions. But the greatest reward of the work is the relieved patient, grateful for the skill and the study applied by a caring physician.

FURTHER READING

PAIN

Greaves, M.W., and McDonald-Gibson, W.: Itch: role of prostaglandins. Brit. Med. J. iii:608–609, 1973.
Suggests the action of prostaglandins as sensitizers of the nerve endings to other agents occurring in the skin as part of an inflammatory response.
Krantz, K.E.: Innervation of the human vulva and vagina. Obstet. Gynecol. 12:382–396, 1958.
A landmark paper in anatomy and the only study to investigate the nerve endings in the vulva.
Lamont, J.A.: Vaginismus. Am. J. Obstet. Gynecol. 131:632–636, 1978.
This study of 80 patients presents the evidence for muscular spasm and the success of counseling techniques.

PREGNANCY

Ewing, T.L., Smale, L.E., and Elliott, F.A.: Maternal deaths associated with postpartum vulvar edema. Am. J. Obstet. Gynecol. 134:173–179, 1979.
A careful account of four cases of this entity.
Grossman, J.H., Wallen, W.C., and Sever, J.L.: Management of genital herpes simplex virus infection during pregnancy. Obstet. Gynecol. 58:1–4, 1981.
Proposes weekly cultures of the cervix and affected sites allowing vaginal delivery with negative cultures and advising precautions for lactation.
Malfetano, J.H., Marin, A.C., and Malfetano, J.H., Jr.: Laser treatment of condylomata acuminata in pregnancy. J. Reprod. Med. 26:574 576, 1981
Describes a typical case which details the technique, postoperative care, and results to be expected.
Morgan, I.: Metronidazole treatment in pregnancy. Int. J. Gynaecol. Obstet. 15:501–502, 1978.
Standard courses of the drug were given to 597 pregnant women (62 in the first trimester) with trichomonas. Their obstetric outcome was the same as a control group.
Vontver, L.A., Hickok, D.E., Brown, Z., et al.: Recurrent genital herpes simplex virus infection in pregnancy: infant outcome and frequency of asymptomatic recurrences. Obstet. Gynecol. 143:75–84, 1982.
Well written and well discussed, this study found that silent shedding does occur. Recurrences during pregnancy were documented in 84 per cent of the study group.
Young, R.L., Acosta, A.A., and Kaufman, R.H.: The treatment of large condylomata acuminata complicating pregnancy. Obstet. Gynecol. 41:65–73, 1973.
A classic paper describing in detail the technique of electrosurgery applied to large lesions.

VARICOSITIES

Veltsman, L.L., and Ostergard, D.R.: Thrombosis of vulvar varicosities during pregnancy. Obstet. Gynecol. 39:55–56, 1972.
The successful surgical management of this unusual complication is described.
Zelikovski, A., Sternberg, A., Haddad, M., and Urca, I.: Varicosities of uncommon sites: therapeutic aspects. Int. Surg. 66:73–77, 1981.
A rare case report of vulvar varices successfully treated postpartum with sclerotherapy

ANATOMIC VARIANTS

Breen, J.L., and Weinberg, C R · Genitourinary and intestinal duplication. Obstet. Gynecol. 26:804–810, 1965.
The classic paper on vulvar duplication and anomalies.
Dickinson, R.L.: Human Sex Anatomy. Robert E. Krieger Publishing Co., Huntington, N.Y., 1971.
A case and sketch book in which are logged the labial measurements of a large series along with the incidence of asymmetric development.
Radman, H.M.: Hypertrophy of the labia minora. Obstet. Gynecol. 48:78s–80s, 1976.
Two cases are described that well illustrate the problem and its surgical therapy.

CIRCUMCISION

Aziz, F.A.: Gynecologic and obstetric complications of female circumcision. Int. J. Gynaecol. Obstet. 17:560–563, 1980.
A short summary of this problem giving an overview of the major techniques employed in the Sudan.
Shandall, A.A.: Circumcision and infibulation of females. Sudan Med. J. 5:178–212, 1967.
A scholarly and complete treatise on the subject, well worth the effort required to obtain the article. The history of the procedure throughout the world is documented and the various techniques and complications are illustrated and discussed.

Index

Note: Page numbers in italics refer to illustrations; page numbers followed by (t) indicate tables.

Abscess
  I & D of, 68
  of Bartholin gland duct, 218, *219*
  vaginal, 23
  Word catheterization of, 70–71, *72*
Accessory breast tissue, *207*
  common site of, *191*
  differential diagnosis of, 206
  in pregnancy, 241
Acetic acid
  for douching, 14
  halogenated, for condylomata acuminata, 54–55, 194
Acid-base balance, of vagina, 12
Acidophilus milk, as douche solution, 14, 30
Acrochordon, 210, *211*
  giant, 234, 235
Acyclovir
  as topical agent, 56
  in HSV-2 infections, 170
Adenitis, vestibular, vulvar pain due to, 240
Adenocarcinomas, and vulva, 104
Adriamycin (doxorubicin), 103
Adson mousetooth forceps, 65
Albinism, partial, 144, *145*
Alcohol injections
  technique of, 72–74, *73*
  vs. Mering procedure, 71
  vs. total vulvectomy, 71
"Alert," for VD. See *VD alert*.
Ampicillin, for vaginitis, 22
Anectomy, 85
Anemia, and candidal overgrowth, 16
Anesthesia
  "fieldblock" technique in, 63, *63*
  for marsupialization technique, 70
  for vulvar biopsy, 62–63
  regional techniques in, 65
Angiokeratoma, 204, *205*
  common site of, *191*
Angiomatous tumor, *205*
  common site of, *191*
  differential diagnosis of, 204
Antibiotics
  for candidal overgrowth, 12, 16
  for gardnerella vaginitis, 22
  for syphilis, 127

Anus, and vulvar carcinoma, 93, *93*
Aqueous solutions, in wet dressings, 50
Aristocort (triamcinolone acetonide), 51
Atrophic leukoplakia. See *Lichen sclerosus*.
Atrophic vulvitis. See *Lichen sclerosus*.
Atrophy, definition of, 25
Auspitz's sign, 109
  in psoriasis, 116
Autoimmune disorders
  and VDRL reactions, 47–48
  Behçet's disease as, 167, 174, *175*
  in lichen sclerosis, 134
  pemphigoid as, 178
  pemphigus as, 176

Bacteria
  adherence of, in vagina, 11
  anaerobic, in vaginitis, 21–22
  in pyoderma infection, 182
  pH range of, *13*
Balanitis xerotica obliterans, 134
Bartholin gland duct
  abscess of, 218, *219*
  adenocarcinomas of, 104
  cyst of, 218, *219*
    I & D of, 68
    marsupialization of, 68, *69*, 70
Basal cell, 10
  in post-menopausal vagina, 27
Basal cell carcinoma, 98, *181*
  dark lesions due to, 150(t)
  differential diagnosis of, 180
  vulvar ulcer due to, 167
Behçet's disease
  etiology of, 167
  genital lesions of, 174, *175*
  oral lesions of, 174, *175*
  treatment of, 174
Benzathine penicillin, for syphilis, 172
Betamethasone valerate (Valisone), 51
Biopsy
  anesthesia for, 62–63
  diagnostic punch for, 63, *64*, 65
  equipment for, *66*
  excisional, 67

249

Biopsy (*continued*)
  management of bleeding in, 65
  punch, technique for, 65, *66*
  specimen, handling of, 67–68, *68*
  toluidine blue test as guide for, 40–41, *42–43*
Bipolar instruments, 74, 75
Bleeding
  due to atrophic vaginitis, 27
  in electrosurgery, 75, 76
  in vaginitis, 9
  management of, in surgery, 65
Bleomycin, 103
Blood, effect of, on vaginal pH, 12
Blood cells, finding of, in vaginal smear, 9
Boric acid, 20
Borofax (boric acid in lanolin), 20
Bovie loop, *193*
Bowen's disease, 90
Bowenoid papulosis, 90, 196, *197*
Breast, carcinoma of, and vulva, 104, 105
Breast tissue, in vulva. See *Accessory breast tissue.*
Burow's solution, 50
  for HSV-2 infections, 170
  for podophyllin "burns," 54
Burrow ink test, 46
Buttermilk, as douche solution, 14

Calymmatobacterium granulomatis, 44, 182
Canal of Nuck, cysts of, 230, *231*
Candida. See also specific species.
  as yeast infection, 15
  culture for, 47
  gentian violet therapy for, 19
  infection
    differential diagnosis for, 16
    pruritus due to, 16
    recurrent, 20
  pH range of, *13*
  suppression of, in vagina, 12
  vaginitis due to, 9, *17*
  vulval infection due to, 109–110, *111*
Candida albicans, 122
  gentian violet therapy for, 19
  imidazole drugs for, 20
  in vaginitis, 16, *17*
Candida glabrata, 16–17, *18*
  gentian violet therapy for, 19
Carcinoma
  basal cell. See *Basal cell carcinoma.*
  in situ. See *Carcinoma in situ.*
  invasive, 180. See also *Invasive carcinomas.*
    vulvar ulcer due to, 167
  invasive squamous cell. See *Invasive carcinomas.*
  microinvasive. See *Microinvasive carcinoma.*
  of cervix, HSV-2 and, 168
  of vulva
    chemotherapy for, 103
    node involvement with, 102–103
    partial vulvectomy for, 82, *83*
    radiotherapy in, 103
    staging of, *102*

Carcinoma (*continued*)
  of vulva, total vulvectomy for, 82, *84, 85*
    wide excision for, 80, *81*
  Pap smears for, 167
  verrucous. See *Verrucous carcinoma.*
Carcinoma in situ, *197*
  and Paget's disease, 97
  of cervix
    and condylomata acuminata, 93
    Pap smear for, 41
  of vulva, *43,* 90–95, *121, 155*
    5-FU therapy for, 55–56
    and condylomata acuminata, 93
    and contiguous structures, *93*
    and sexually transmitted disease, 92
    clinical hallmarks of, *93*
    dark lesions due to, 150(t)
    description of, 91, *91*
    differential diagnosis of, 196
    DNCB therapy for, 57–58
    laser vaporization for, 77–78
    red lesions due to, 120
    treatment of, 94–95
    white lesions due to, 142, *143*
Carcinoma simplex, 90
Cephalosporin, for vaginitis, 22
Cephradine, for vaginitis, 22
Cervix, carcinoma of
  and condylomata acuminata, 93
  and HSV-2, 168
  Pap smear for, 41
CF (complement fixation) test, 48
Chancroid, vulvar, 167
Chemotherapy
  for carcinoma of vulva, 103
  herpes infection and, 168
Cherry angiomata, *191,* 204
  common site of, 191
Chlamydia trachomatis, 228
Chlorambucil, in Behçet's disease, 174
Circumcision, 246
Clitoris
  carcinoma in situ of, *143*
  invasive carcinoma of, *227*
Clotrimazole
  for *Candida albicans,* 20
  for *Trichomonas vaginalis,* 20, 24
  in pregnancy, 241
"Clue cell"
  description of, 21
  finding of, in vaginal smear, 9
  in *Gardnerella vaginalis,* 21–22
  in *Hemophilus vaginalis,* 22
Coagulation, in electrosurgery, 75
Collins, Conrad G., 39
Colpitis emphysematosa, 241
Colposcopy, 37
  and toluidine blue test, 40
  in identification of pubic louse, 46
Complement fixation test, 48
Compound nevus, *157*
  dark lesion as, 150(t), 156
Condom
  and vaginal pH, 13
  in vaginitis therapy, 14

Condylomata acuminata, 29, *195*
  and carcinomas, 93
  common site of, *191*
  cryosurgery for, 78
  differential diagnosis of, 192–193
  douching and, 14
  electrosurgery for, 74–77, 193, *193*
  5-FU therapy for, 55
  immunosuppression and, 192
  in pregnancy, 241
  laser vaporization for, 77–78
  malignant transformation of, 191
  partial vulvectomy for, 82, *83*
  podophyllin and, 29
  transmission of, 13
  treatment of, 53, 193–194
  vs. vestibular papillae, 244, 246
Condylomata lata, *173*
Connective tissue, sarcomas of, and vulva, 104
Corps ronds, 91, *91*
Cortdome (hydrocortisone), 51
Corticosteroids
  as topical agents, 51
  injection of, 74, 240
Corynebacteria
  effect of antibiotics on, 12
  in vagina, 12
Corynebacterium minutissimum, 38, 126
Corynebacterium vaginale, 21
Cosmetics, for vagina, 6
Creams, in vulvar disease, 49
Crohn's disease, 176
  and total vulvectomy, 82, *84,* 85
  treatment of, 176
  ulcers due to, *177*
  vs. Behçet's disease, 174
Crotamiton (Eurax), 51, 138
Cryosurgery, 78, 79
Cultures, laboratory
  for fungus, 46–47
  for virus, 47
Cysts
  epidermal. See *Epidermal cysts.*
  mesonephric. See *Mesonephric duct cysts.*
  mucous. See *Mucous cysts.*
  of Bartholin gland duct, 218, *219*
    I & D of, 68
    marsupialization of, 68, 69, 70
  vestibular. See *Vestibular cysts.*
  Word catheterization for, 70–71, 72
Cytotoxic agents, 53–56
  and candidal overgrowth, 16
  in HSV-2 infections, 170

Dark lesions of vulva
  description of, 150–151
  due to carcinoma in situ, 154, *155*
  due to pubic lice, 162, *163,* 164
  due to reactive hyperpigmentation, 158, *159*
  histiocytoma as, 162, *163*
  histologic diagnosis of, 150(t)
  lentigo as, 152, *153*
  melanoma as, 150(t), 156, 160, *161*

Dark lesions of vulva (*continued*)
  nevi as, 156, *157*
  seborrheic keratoses as, 158, *159*
Denervation, surgical, vs. alcohol injections, 71
Deodorants, vaginal, 6
Deoxyribonucleic acid in carcinoma cells, 94, *94*
Depigmentation disorders, 144, *145*
Dermatitis, seborrheic, *115*
  red lesions due to, 114
Dermatofibromas, 162, *163*
Dermatophyte test medium, 47, 110
Desiccation, in electrosurgery, 75
Desquamative vaginitis, 176
Diabetes mellitus
  and candidal overgrowth, 16
  red lesions and, 110, *111*
  vaginal glycogen in, 11
  vulvar pain with, 239
Dilantin (phenytoin), 110
  for vulvar pain, 239
2,4-Dinitrochlorobenzene (DNCB) sensitization,
    57–58
DiPaola, G. R., 3
Discharge, vaginal
  due to candidal overgrowth, 16
  iatrogenic, 29
  in atrophic vaginitis, 25, 27
  in gardnerella vaginitis, 21
  in purulent vaginitis, 30
  in trichomonas vaginitis, 23
  in vaginitis, 9
  physiologic, 28–29
DNA
  histogram of, *94*
  in carcinoma cells, 90, 94
DNCB (2,4-dinitrochlorobenzene) sensitization,
    57–58
Domeboro tablets, 50
Donovan bodies, in granuloma inguinale diagno-
    sis, 182
Douching
  equipment for, 15
  for purulent vaginitis, 30
  indications for, 14
  post-coital, and vaginal pH, 13
  saline, for trichomonas vaginitis, 24
  solutions for, 14
  technique for, 15
  with povidone-iodine solutions, 30
Douglas, Charles P., 2
Doxorubicin (Adriamycin), 103
Drugs, topical, 49
  cytotoxic agents as, 53–56
  steroids as, 51–53
  vehicles for, 50–51
DTM (dermatophyte test medium), 47, 110
Dyspareunia, 240
Dystrophy, vulvar, *42*
  alcohol injection for, 71–74, *73*
  as premalignant condition, 120–132
  classification of, 131(t)
  hyperplastic, laser vaporization for, 77–78,
    79
  lichen sclerosus. See *Lichen sclerosus.*
  mixed, 133, 140, *141*

Ecosystem, vagina as, 10, *11*
Edema, of vulva, 220, *221*
Efudex (5-fluorouracil), 55
   for condylomata acuminata, 194
Ejaculate, and vaginal pH, 12
Electrosurgery
   and recurrent lesions, 77
   anesthesia for, 75
   bipolar technique of, *76*
   monopolar technique of, *76*
   types of apparatus for, 74–75
Elephantiasis nervorum, 234, *235*
Endometrioma, *209*
   common site of, *191*
   differential diagnosis of, 208
Endometriosis, 208
Enovid E, in Behçet's disease, 174
Enterobius vermicularis, 26
Epidermal cysts, *201*
   common site of, *191*
   differential diagnosis of, 200
   giant, 234, *235*
Erythrasma, 38, *127*
   red lesions due to, 126
Erythroplasia of Queyrat, 90, 120, *121*
Escherichia coli, 25
Estrogen
   atrophy of vagina and, 11
   effect of, on vaginal epithelium, 10
   glycogen formation and, 11
   topical
     in atrophic vaginitis, 28
     in Fox-Fordyce disease, 212
Eurax (crotamiton), 51, 138
Examination
   laboratory, in vaginitis, 9
   medical, of vulva, 36–37
     equipment for, 37, *37*
     photography and, 38–39
Excision
   wide, 80, *81*
   wide local, for basal cell carcinoma, 98

FADF (fluorescent antibody dark field) test, 44
Fibroepithelial polyp, 234
Fibromas, *233*
   common site of, *191*
   differential diagnosis of, 232
   giant, 234
Fibrosarcomas, 232
Fluocinolone acetonide (Synalar), 51
Fluocinonide (Lidex), 51
Fluorescent antibody dark field test, 44
Fluorescent treponemal antibody absorption test, 48
5-Fluorouracil (Efudex)
   as topical agent, 55–56
   for condylomata acuminata, 194
Folliculitis, 127
   red lesions due to, 126, 128
Fox-Fordyce disease, *213*
   common site of, *191*
   differential diagnosis of, 212
   retinoid therapy for, 56

"Freckles," vulvar, 152, *153*
Frei test, 48, 228
FTA-ABS (fluorescent treponemal antibody absorption) test, 48, 172
   in LGV, 228
5-FU (fluorouracil)
   as topical agent, 55–56
   for condylomata acuminata, 194
Fulguration, in electrosurgery, 75
Fungus
   infection due to, douching for, 14
   smears for identification of, 45

Gardner, Herman L., 2, 21
Gardnerella vaginalis
   "clue cells" in, 21
   infection due to, douching for, 14
   pH range of, 13
   therapy for, 22
   transmission of, 13
Genetic aspects, of lichen sclerosus, 134
   of depigmentation, 144
Genital warts. See *Condylomata acuminata.*
Gentian violet
   contact reactions with, 19
   for candidal vaginitis, 19
Giant condyloma of Buschke-Lowenstein, 98–99
Glycogen, in vagina, 11
Gonorrhea
   herpes infection and, 170
   transmission of, 13
Granuloma inguinale, 44, *183*
   differential diagnosis of, 182

Halcinonide (Halog), 51
Halogenated acetic acid, for condylomata acuminata, 54–55
Hemangiomas, 204, *205*
   common site of, *191*
   sclerosing. See *Histiocytoma.*
Hematomas, of vulva, 222, *223*
Hemophilus, pH range of, *13*
Hemophilus ducreyi, 167
Hemophilus vaginalis. See *Gardnerella vaginalis.*
Hemosiderin deposit, dark lesion due to, 150(t)
Hernia
   inguinal, 230
   pudendal, 230, *231*
Herpes simplex virus, 90
   acyclovir therapy for, 56, 170
   common site of, *191*
   culture for, 47
   identification of, 41, 44, 45
   infection due to
     and sexually transmitted diseases, 170
     and vulvar pain, 239
     in pregnancy, 241
     treatment of, 170
   Pap smears for, 167
   transmission of, 13

Herpes simplex virus (*continued*)
  type 2, 29
    Burow's solution for, 50
    cytotoxic agents for, 170
    recurrence of, 168, *171*
    vulvar ulcers due to, 168, *169*, *171*
Hewitt, Jean, 3
Hidradenitis suppurativa, 178
  electrosurgery for, 74–77
  partial vulvectomy for, 82, *83*
  treatment of, 178
  ulcers due to, *179*
Hidradenoma, *207*
  common site of, *191*
  differential diagnosis of, 206
  vulvar ulcer as, 167
Histiocytoma, *163*
  dark lesion as, 162
Histogenesis, theory of, 96
Histogram, of DNA, *94*
History, medical, obtaining of, 35–36
Hormones, impact of, on vaginal epithelium, 10
HPV (human papilloma virus), 29, 90
HPV (human papovavirus), 191
HSV (herpes simplex virus). See *Herpes simplex virus.*
Human papilloma virus, 29, 90
Human papovavirus, 191
Hunt, Elizabeth, 2
Hydrocortisone (Cortdome), 51
Hydrogen peroxide
  for douching, 14
  for Gardnerella vaginitis, 22
Hygiene, vaginal deodorants and, 6
Hypercalcemia, due to invasive carcinomas, 226
Hyperkeratosis, *40*, *41*
Hyperplastic dystrophy, 130, *133*
  as premalignant condition, 130–132
  classification of, 131(t)
  white lesions due to, 138, *139*
Hyphae, finding of, in vaginal smear, 9

I & D (incision and drainage) technique, 68
Ibuprofen (Motrin) in vulvar pain, 239
Immunotherapy, 56–58
Incision and drainage technique, 68
Inclusion cysts. See *Epidermal cysts.*
Intermediate cell, 10
International Federation of Obstetrics and Gynecology, 3, 101
International Society for the Study of Vulvar Disease, founding of, 3
  terminology proposed by, 131
Intertrigo, 146, *147*
Intradermal nevus, *157*
  dark lesion as, 150(t), 156
Invasive carcinomas, *121*, *181*, *227*
  differential diagnosis of, 180, 226
  granuloma inguinale and, 182
  incidence of, 99
  metastatic tumors of, 102–103
  red lesions due to, 120
  staging of, 102(t)

Invasive carcinoma (*continued*)
  treatment for, 99–100, 102–103
  vulvar ulcer due to, 167
  with LGV, *229*

Jeffcoate, T.N.A., 132
Junctional nevus, 157
  dark lesion as, 150(t), 156

Kaufman, Raymond H., *2*
Kenalog (triamcinolone acetonide), 51
  injection of, for vulvar pruritus, 74
Keratinous cysts. See *Epidermal cysts.*
Keratosis, seborrheic, 159
  dark lesion as, 150(t), 158
Ketoconazole, 20
Keyes cutaneous punch, *64*, *65*
Koebner phenomenon, 116
Koilocytotic atypia, 29
Kraurosis vulvae. See *Lichen sclerosus.*
Kwell (lindane, benzene hexachloride), 164

Labia minora
  anatomic variants of, 244
  elongation of, 244, *245*
Laboratory examinations, in vaginitis, 9
Lactation, and glycogen storage, 11
Lactobacillus(i)
  effect of antibiotics on, 12
  in vagina, 12
  solution of, for douche, 14, 30
Laryngeal papillomata, of newborn, prevention of, 241
Larynx, tumors of, 192
Laser vaporization, 77–78, *79*, 126, 170, 193
Leiomyoma, *233*
Leiomyosarcoma, 232
Lentigo, *153*
  dark lesion as, 150(t), 152
Lesions, vulvar
  dark. See *Dark lesions.*
  red. See *Red lesions.*
  white. See *White lesions.*
Leukemia, herpes infection and, 168
Leukoderma, 144
  postherpetic, *145*
Leukoplakia, terminology for, 3–4
LGV. See *Lymphogranuloma venereum.*
LGV-CFT (lymphogranuloma venereum-complement fixation test), 228
Lichen sclerosus, *132*
  childhood, *137*
  classification of, 131(t)
  description of, 132–133
  treatment of, 53, 136
  white lesions due to, 134, *135*, *137*
Lidex (fluocinonide), 51
Lidocaine, in local anesthesia, 62
Light amplification by stimulated emission of radiation, vaporization by, 77–78, *79*

Lipoma, *233*
    common site of, *191*
    differential diagnosis of, 232
Louse
    crab, smears for identification of, 45–46, *45*
    pubic, *163*
        dark lesion due to, 162
        life cycle of, 164
LS & A (lichen sclerosus et atrophicus). See *Lichen sclerosus*.
Lupus erythematosus, discoid, vulvar ulcer as, 167
Lymphogranuloma venereum, 48–49
    differential diagnosis of, 228
    with invasive carcinoma, *229*
Lymphogranuloma venereum-complement fixation test, 228
Lynch, Peter J., 5

Marsupialization technique
    description of, *69, 70*
    vs. I & D, 68
Mebendazole, 26
Medical history, obtaining of, 35–36
McKelvey, John L., 99
Melanin, 150
Melanocyte, 150
Melanoma, *161*
    dark lesion due to, 150(t), 160
    nevus transformation to, 156
    staging in, 104–105, 104(t)
Melanosome, 150
Menstruation
    and candidal overgrowth, 16
    and vaginal pH, 12
    history of, obtaining of, 36
Mering procedure, 71
Mesonephric duct cysts, *209*
    common site of, *191*
    differential diagnosis of, 208
Metronidazole
    for Gardnerella vaginitis, 22
    for Trichomonas vaginitis, 24
    in pregnancy, 241
Miconazole, for candidal infection, 20
Microinvasive carcinoma, 100–103
    measurement in, *101*
Mineral oil, as vulvar cleanser, 6, 49
Minor accessory labia, 244
Mixed dystrophy, 133, *141*
    white lesions due to, 140
Mole, *157*
    dark lesion as, 150(t), 155
Molluscum contagiosum, *199*
    common site of, *191*
    cryosurgery for, 80
    differential diagnosis of, 198
    electrosurgery for, 74–77
    retinoid therapy for, 56
Monopolar instruments, 74, 75
Monsel's solution, in bleeding, 65
Motrin (ibuprofen), in vulvar pain, 239

Mucous cysts, *203*
    common site of, *191*
    differential diagnosis of, 202
Myoblastoma, granular cell, vulvar ulcer as, 167

Neisseria gonorrhoeae, 218
Neoplasm(ia). See also *Carcinoma* and *Carcinoma in situ*.
    detection of, 89–90
    development of, 90
    intraepithelial vulvar
        definition of, 90
        5-FU therapy for, 56
        terminology for, 3
    vulvar ulcer as, 167
Neovascularization, 109
Nerve block
    for vulvar biopsy, 62
    pudendal, 65, 70
Neurofibroma, 210, *211*
    giant, 234, *235*
Nevitol, for condylomata acuminata, 194
Nevus(i), *157*
    dark lesion as, 150(t), 155
Nickerson's media, 110
Nits, louse, *163*
    dark lesions and, 162, 164
Nystatin, in candidal vaginitis, 20

Odors
    "fishy," in Gardnerella vaginitis, 21
    in vaginitis, 9
Ointments, in vulvar disease, 49
Oral contraceptives
    and candidal overgrowth, 16
    and glycogen storage, 11
    and vaginitis, 12
    in treatment of Behçet's disease, 174

Paget's disease, of vulva, *119*
    and concomitant carcinomas, 97
    description of, 95–96, *96*
    differential diagnosis of, 118
    5-FU therapy for, 55–56
    recurrence in, 97–98
    study of, 4
    total vulvectomy for, 82, *84*, 85
    treatment for, 97–98
Pain, vulvar, differential diagnosis of, 238–240
    vestibular adenitis as cause of, 240
Pap smear. See *Papanicolaou smear*.
Papanicolaou smear
    and vulvar diagnosis, 41
    in differential diagnosis of ulcers, 167
Papule, formation of, *93*
Parabasal cell
    finding of, in vaginal smear, 9
    in atrophic vaginitis, 27

Parakeratosis, *91, 93*
  definition of, 39–40, *40*
  vs. cancer, 41, *42–43*
Parasite, smears for identification of, 45–46
Partial albinism, 144, *145*
Paste, 49
"Pearl," of squamous cells, 91, *92*
Pemphigoid, 178
  autoimmune response and, 167
  bullous, *179*
  treatment of, 178
Pemphigus, 176
  autoimmune response and, 167
  treatment of, 176
  ulcers due to, *177*
Penicillin
  benzathine, for syphilis, 172
  beta-lactamase-resistant, 32
pH
  in atrophic vaginitis, 27
  in bacterial overgrowth, 12
  in Trichomonas vaginitis, 23
  in vaginitis, 9
  of organisms, *13*
  vaginal, in Gardnerella vaginitis, 21
  with purulent vaginitis, 30
Phenytoin (Dilantin), 110
  for vulvar pain, 239
Photography
  equipment for, 38–39
  in diagnosis, 38
Phthirus pubis, 45–46, *45*
  dark lesions and, 162, 163
  life cycle of, 164
Piebaldism, 144, *145*
Pigment, cellular
  disorders of, 144, *145*
  incontinence of, *93*
Pilonidal sinus, *209*
  differential diagnosis of, 208
Pinworms, *26*
  diagnosis of, 26
Pityriasis versicolor, *123*
  red lesions due to, 122
Pityrosporum orbiculare, 122
Plexiform neuromas, 234, *235*
Podophyllin, 29
  "burns" due to, 54
  composition of, 53
  for condylomata acuminata, 194
  proper usage of, 54
Podophyllotoxin, 53
Porphyrin, 38
Potassium sorbate
  for candidal vaginitis, 20
  for douching, 14
Povidone-iodine solution, 30
Poxvirus, 198
Pregnancy
  accessory breast tissue in, 241
  candidal overgrowth and, 16
  glycogen storage and, 11
  HSV-2 infection in, 168
  "strawberry" vaginal epithelium in, 23
  treatment of *Candida albicans* in, 20

Pregnancy (*continued*)
  treatment of condylomata in, 77
  vaginal pH and, 12
  vulva in, 240–241
Progesterone
  and glycogen storage, 11
  as topical agent, 53
  effect of, on vaginal epithelium, 10
Prostaglandins
  herpes infection and, 168
  vulvar pain and, 239
Protozoa, finding of, in vaginal smear, 9
Pruritus
  due to lice, 45–46, 162–164
  due to pinworms, 26
  in candidal vaginitis, 16
  in trichomonas vaginitis, 23
  in vaginitis, 9
  vulvar
    alcohol injection for, 71–74, *73*
    corticosteroid injection for, 74
Psoriasis, *117*
  red lesions due to, 116
  retinoid therapy for, 56
Pudendal neuralgia, 238–239
Pyoderma, *183*
  differential diagnosis of, 182
Pyogenic granuloma, 204, *205*
  common site of, *191*
  in pregnancy, 241
Pyrantel pamoate, 26

Radiation therapy
  in vulvar carcinoma, 103
  reaction to, 146, *147*
Rapid plasma reagin, 48
Reactive hyperpigmentation, *159*
  dark lesions due to, 150(t), 158
Reactive vulvitis, *113*
  red lesions due to, 112
Red lesions of vulva
  description of, 109
  due to candidal infection, 110, *111*
  due to carcinoma in situ, 120, *121*
  due to contact irritants, 112, *113*
  due to erythrasma, 126, *127*
  due to folliculitis, 126, *127*, 128
  due to Paget's disease, 118, *119*
  due to pityriasis versicolor, 122, *123*
  due to psoriasis, 116, *117*
  due to seborrheic dermatitis, 114, *115*
  due to squamous cell carcinoma, 90, 120, *121*
  due to tinea cruris, 122, *123*
  due to vestibular adenitis, 124, *125*, 126
Rete peg, 91, *96*
Retinoids, as topical agents, 56
RID, 164
RPR (rapid plasma reagin), 48, 172

Sabouraud's slants, 47
Saline solution, for douching, 14, 15

Sarcomas, 105, 232
Sarcoptes scabiei, 45–46, *45*
  Burrow ink test for, 46
Scabies
  Burrow ink test for, 46
  identification of, 45–46
Sclerosing hemangioma, 162, *163*
Sea water, for vulvar soaks, 50
  use after laser, 78
Sebaceous cyst. See *Epidermal cysts.*
Seborrheic dermatitis, *115*
  red lesions due to, 114
Seborrheic keratosis(es), *159*
  dark lesions as, 150(t), 158
Senile atrophy. See *Lichen sclerosus.*
Serologic tests
  and autoimmune disease, 47–48
  for herpes simplex virus, 48
  for LGV, 48–49
  for syphilis, 47–48, 172
  in differential diagnosis of ulcers, 167
Sexual intercourse
  and candidal overgrowth, 16
  and vaginal pH, 12
  odor upon, in Gardnerella vaginitis, 21
Silver nitrate, in bleeding, 65
Silver nitrate solution, for wet pack therapy, 50
Sinus, endodermal tumors of, and vulva, 104
Skin, hydration of, 4
Skin tag, 210, *211*
  giant, 234, *235*
Smears, diagnostic
    for fungi, 45
    for granuloma inguinale, 44
    for herpes, 41, 44, 45
    for parasites, 45–46
    for syphilis, 44–45
    Pap. See *Papanicolaou smear.*
Squamous cell carcinoma. See *Invasive carcinoma.*
Staphylococcus, 25
Staphylococcus aureus, in toxic shock syndrome, 31, 32
Steroids, 51–53
  and candidal overgrowth, 16
  as topical agents, 51
Streptococcus, 25
Superficial cells, 10
  and glycogen storage, 11
Sweat glands
  adenocarcinomas of, and vulva, 104
  adenoma of, vulvar ulcer as, 167
Synalar (fluocinolone acetonide), 51
Syphilis, 44–45
  detection of, 47–48
  differential diagnosis of, 172
  herpes infection and, 170
  Pap smears for, 167
  treatment of, 172
  ulcers due to, 167, *173*
Syringoma, *213*
  common site of, *191*
  differential diagnosis of, 212

Tampon
  and toxic shock syndrome, 31
  in vaginal disease, 31–32
Taussig, Frederick J., 1–2
Testosterone, as topical agent, 51–53
Tetracycline, and vaginitis, 12
Tetracycline-induced fluorescence test, 38
Thrush, in vaginal mucosa, 16
Thymol solution, 30
TIFT (tetracycline-induced fluorescence test), 38
Tinea cruris, 45, *45*, *123*
  red lesions due to, 122
TNM (tumor-node-metastasis) classification, 101
Toluidine blue test
  and colposcopies, 40
  as guide for biopsies, 40–41, *42–43*
  description of, 39
Topical drugs, 49
  cytotoxic agents as, 53–56
  steroids as, 51–53
  vehicles for, 50–51
Torulopsis glabrata, 16
Toxic shock syndrome, 31–32
Treponema pallidum, 45, 48
Triamcinolone acteonide (Aristocort, Kenalog), 51
  injection of, for vulvar pruritus, 74
Trichloracetic acid, 194
Trichomonas vaginalis, 22–25, *23*
  infection, douching for, 14
  in pregnancy, 241
  in vaginitis, 9
  pH range of, *13*
  transmission of, 13
Trichophyta, culture for, 47
Trichophyton rubrum, 45, 122
Tuberculosis, of vulva, 185
  differential diagnosis of, 184
  ulcer as, 167
Tumors
  large vulvar
    Bartholin duct cyst as, 218, *219*
    development of, 217
    due to invasive carcinoma, 226, *227*
    due to LGV, 228, *229*
    due to verrucous carcinoma, 224, *225*
    edema as, 220, *221*
    fibroma as, 232, *233*
    hematoma as, 222, *223*
    hernia as, 230, *231*
    in pregnancy, 241
    lipoma as, 232, *233*
    variants of, 234, *235*
  small vulvar
    accessory breast tissue as, 206, *207*
    acrochordon as, 210, *211*
    carcinoma in situ as, 196, *197*
    condyloma acuminatum as, 191–194, *195*
    definition of, 190
    due to endometriosis, 208, *209*
    due to Fox-Fordyce disease, 212, *213*
    epidermal cysts as, 200, *201*
    hemangiomas as, 204, *205*
    hidradenomas as, 206, *207*

Tumors (*continued*)
  small vulvar, mesonephric duct cysts as, 208, *209*
  molluscum contagiosum as, 198, *199*
  neurofibromas as, 210, *211*
  pilonidal sinus as, 208, *209*
  sites for, *191*
  syringoma as, 212, *213*
  ulcer as, 167
  vestibular cysts as, 202, *203*
Tumor-node-metastasis classification, 101
Tyrosine, 150

Ulcers of vulva
  and sexually transmitted diseases, 170
  description of, 167–168
  due to basal cell carcinoma, 180, *181*
  due to Behçet's disease, 174, *175*
  due to Crohn's disease, 176, *177*
  due to granuloma inguinale, 182, *183*
  due to hidradenitis suppurativa, 178, *179*
  due to HSV, 168, *169*, *171*
  due to invasive carcinoma, 180, *181*
  due to pemphigoid, 178, *179*
  due to pemphigus, 176, *177*
  due to pyoderma, 182, *183*
  due to syphilis, 172, *173*
  due to tuberculosis, 184, *185*
Urethra
  caruncles of, electrosurgery for, 74–77
  in total vulvectomy, 85
  prolapse of, cryosurgery for, 80

Vaccine, autogenous, 56
  for condylomata acuminata, 56
  preparation of, 57
Vaccinia, 184, *185*
Vaccinotherapy, 56–58
Vagina
  abscess of, 23
  acid-base balance of, 12
  and vulvar carcinoma, *93*
  as ecosystem, 10, *11*
  atrophy of, 9
  Candida albicans overgrowth in, 12
  candidal infection of, 110, *111*
  corynebacteria in, 12
  epithelium of
    glycogen in, 11
    "pavement" cells of, 11
    response of, to hormones, 10
    "strawberry" appearance of, 23
  lactobacilli in, 12
  ulcer of, and tampons, 31, *31*
  walls of, erythema of, 16
Vaginismus, 239
Vaginitis
  atrophic, 25–28
  candidal, 15–21
    recurrent, 20
    gentian violet for, 19

Vaginitis (*continued*)
  "clue cells" in, 21–22
  condom usage with, 14
  condylomata acuminata and, 193
  desquamative, 176
  diagnosis of
    differential, 9
    equipment for, 9, 10
    "fresh look" approach for, 10
  due to antibiotic usage, 12
  due to bacteria, 21–22
  due to pinworms, 26
  due to protozoa, 22–25
  due to viral infections, 29–30
  due to yeast, 15
  Gardnerella vaginalis, 21–22
  iatrogenic, 32
  in pregnancy, 241
  in virgins, 13
  male infection and, 13
  psychosomatic, 30–31
  purulent, 30
  reinfection with, 13–14
  sexually transmitted, 21, 23
  tampon related problems and, 31–32
  transmission of, 13
  treatment of, during menstruation, 12
  Trichomonas vaginalis, 22–25, *23*
  vs. vulvar disease, 9
Vaginitis emphysematosa, 23
Vaginocervicitis, due to herpes, 29–30
Valisone (betamethasone valerate), 51
Varicosities, vulvar, *243*
  differential diagnosis of, 242
VD alert, 167
  carcinoma in situ and, 154
  dark lesions and, 154, 164
  for condylomata acuminata, 193
  for granuloma inguinale, 182
  for HSV infection, 170
  for LGV, 228
  for molluscum contagiosum, 198
  for syphilis, 172
  pubic lice and, 164
VDRL (venereal disease research laboratories), 172
  in LGV, 228
  reactions, and autoimmune disease, 47–48
Venereal disease research laboratories testing. See *VDRL*.
Venereal disease, alert for. See *VD alert*.
Venereal warts. See *Condylomata acuminata*.
Verrucous carcinoma, *225*
  description of, 98
  differential diagnosis of, 224
  partial vulvectomy for, 82, *83*
  treatment for, 99
Vestibular adenitis, 124, *125*, 126
  vulvar pain due to, 240
Vestibular cyst, *203*
  differential diagnosis of, ·202
  mucous, common site of, *191*
Vestibular glands, minor
  inflammation of, 124, *125*, 126

Vestibular melanosis, *153*
Vestibular papillae, *245*
  differential diagnosis of, 244, 246
Vinegar, white, as douche solution, 14, 15
Vitiligo, 144, 145
von Recklinghausen's disease, 210, *211*
  giant neurofibromas in, 234, *235*
Vulva
  anatomic variants of, 244, *245*
  atypia of
    DNCB therapy for, 57–58
    laser vaporization for, 77–78
    wide excision for, 80, *81*
  breast carcinoma and, 104, 105
  bumps on, 29
  circumcision and, 246
  dark lesions of. See *Dark lesions*.
  diseases of, vs. vaginitis, 9
  early study of, 1–2
  endodermal sinus tumors and, 104
  hydration of, 4
  hygiene of, 6
  in history, 1
  inspection of, 36–37
    equipment for, 37, *37*
    photography and, 38–39
  pain in, 238–240
  pioneers in study of, 1–2, 4
  pregnancy and, 240, 241
  red lesions of. See *Red lesions*.
  skin of, functions of, 4
  tumors of. See *Tumors*.
  ulcers of. See *Ulcers*.
  varicosities of, 242, *243*
  white lesions of. See *White lesions*.
Vulvectomy
  partial, 82, *83*
  radical, 85, *86*, 87
    and bilateral groin dissection, 102
  total, *84*, 85

Vulvectomy (*continued*)
  total, anectomy in, 85
    vs. alcohol injections, 71

Water wart, 198, *199*
Way drainage system, *86*
Way, Stanley, 100
Wet dressing, 49
Wet smear
  for trichomonas diagnosis, 25
  in vaginitis, 9
White blood cells, finding of, in vaginal smear, 9
White lesions, of vulva
  description of, 130
  due to carcinoma in situ, 142, *143*
  due to depigmentation disorders, 144, *145*
  due to radiation reaction, 146, *147*
  hyperplastic dystrophy as, 138, *139*
  intertrigo as, 146, *147*
  lichen sclerosus as, 134–138
  mixed dystrophy as, 140, *141*
  terminology for, 3
Wood's light, 37
  for erythrasma diagnosis, 38
Woodruff, theory of histogenesis by, 96
Woodruff, J. Donald, 4–5
Word catheter, 70, *71*
Word catheterization
  anesthesia for, 70
  technique of, 70–71, *72*

Yeast, vaginitis due to, 15
Yogurt, as douche solution, 14, 30

Zelle, Kane, 3